Pharmaceuticals: Drug Development, Design and Manufacturing

Pharmaceuticals: Drug Development, Design and Manufacturing

Edited by Rodrik Ledger

hayle
medical

New York

Hayle Medical,
750 Third Avenue, 9th Floor,
New York, NY 10017, USA

Visit us on the World Wide Web at:
www.haylemedical.com

ISBN: 978-1-63241-900-2

Cataloging-in-Publication Data

Pharmaceuticals : drug development, design and manufacturing / edited by Rodrik Ledger.
    p. cm.
Includes bibliographical references and index.
ISBN 978-1-63241-900-2
1. Drugs. 2. Drug development. 3. Drugs--Design. 4. Pharmaceutical industry.
5. Pharmaceutical chemistry. I. Ledger, Rodrik.
RM301 .P43 2020
615.1--dc23

Table of Contents

Preface

Over the recent decade, advancements and applications have progressed exponentially. This has led to the increased interest in this field and projects are being conducted to enhance knowledge. The main objective of this book is to present some of the critical challenges and provide insights into possible solutions. This book will answer the varied questions that arise in the field and also provide an increased scope for furthering studies.

A pharmaceutical drug is a compound which is used for the diagnosis, treatment and prevention of a disease. It can be classified depending on the level of control, mode of action, route of administration and therapeutic effects, among others. Some classes of medicine are antibiotics, antipyretics, analgesics, antiseptics, oral contraceptives, tranquilizers, stimulants, etc. The development of pharmaceutical products traverses a number of stages from drug discovery to commercialization. There exists a clear distinction between small molecule drugs and biologic medical products. While small molecule drugs are developed through chemical synthesis; biologic medical products include vaccines, recombinant proteins, gene therapy and cell therapy. This book brings forth some of the most innovative concepts and elucidates the unexplored aspects of pharmaceuticals. It presents researches and studies performed by experts across the globe on potential pharmaceutical agents. With state-of-the-art inputs by acclaimed experts of this field, this book targets students and professionals.

I hope that this book, with its visionary approach, will be a valuable addition and will promote interest among readers. Each of the authors has provided their extraordinary competence in their specific fields by providing different perspectives as they come from diverse nations and regions. I thank them for their contributions.

Editor

Roles of Heat Shock Proteins in Apoptosis, Oxidative Stress, Human Inflammatory Diseases, and Cancer

Paul Chukwudi Ikwegbue [1], Priscilla Masamba [1], Babatunji Emmanuel Oyinloye [1,2] (iD) and Abidemi Paul Kappo [1,*] (iD)

[1] Biotechnology and Structural Biochemistry (BSB) Group, Department of Biochemistry and Microbiology, University of Zululand, KwaDlangezwa 3886, South Africa; pikwegbue@yahoo.com (P.C.I.); presh4u@rocketmail.com (P.M.); tunji4reele@yahoo.com (B.E.O.)

[2] Department of Biochemistry, Afe Babalola University, PMB 5454, Ado-Ekiti 360001, Nigeria

* Correspondence: KappoA@unizulu.ac.za

Abstract: Heat shock proteins (HSPs) play cytoprotective activities under pathological conditions through the initiation of protein folding, repair, refolding of misfolded peptides, and possible degradation of irreparable proteins. Excessive apoptosis, resulting from increased reactive oxygen species (ROS) cellular levels and subsequent amplified inflammatory reactions, is well known in the pathogenesis and progression of several human inflammatory diseases (HIDs) and cancer. Under normal physiological conditions, ROS levels and inflammatory reactions are kept in check for the cellular benefits of fighting off infectious agents through antioxidant mechanisms; however, this balance can be disrupted under pathological conditions, thus leading to oxidative stress and massive cellular destruction. Therefore, it becomes apparent that the interplay between oxidant-apoptosis-inflammation is critical in the dysfunction of the antioxidant system and, most importantly, in the progression of HIDs. Hence, there is a need to maintain careful balance between the oxidant-antioxidant inflammatory status in the human body. HSPs are known to modulate the effects of inflammation cascades leading to the endogenous generation of ROS and intrinsic apoptosis through inhibition of pro-inflammatory factors, thereby playing crucial roles in the pathogenesis of HIDs and cancer. We propose that careful induction of HSPs in HIDs and cancer, especially prior to inflammation, will provide good therapeutics in the management and treatment of HIDs and cancer.

Keywords: apoptosis; cancer; heat shock proteins; inflammation; reactive oxygen species; tumour necrosis factor-α

1. Introduction

Although some heat shock proteins (HSPs) are constitutively produced, most are molecular chaperones that are normally over-expressed by cells in response to inducible signals that may lead to protein denaturation [1]. These stressors include heat, nutrient deficiency, oxidative stress, acute or chronic inflammatory diseases, viral infections, ischemia, heavy metals, exercise, gravity, and bacterial infections [2–5]. These responses enable cellular protection against protein denaturation and possible degradation of misfolded proteins, which may, in turn, result in protein aggregation and cancer [6]. Some of these constitutively-expressed heat shock polypeptides are involved in protein folding and translocation of organelles across cellular membranes, prompting many authors to label them "molecular chaperones" [5–8].

Since the discovery of heat shock proteins in 1962 by Ritossa in the salivary glands of the *Drosophila* larvae, the important functions of heat shock proteins in response to various stressful signals including human cancer and cystic fibrosis, has been well elucidated [9–11]. Upon discovering these proteins, it is not surprising that HSPs have made a very large impact in various areas of research, including medical and biological fields, because of their diverse functions in both pathological and normal conditions [12,13].

Molecular chaperones, which are found in all living cells and form part of the defence system against both internal and external stressors, are primarily grouped into two major groups according to their amino acid composition, molecular weight, as well as their specific cellular function as the high molecular weight and the small molecular weight HSPs [14,15]. The high molecular weight HSPs which range from 60 to 110 kDa are ATP-dependent and their primary cellular function is binding and folding of nascent proteins through ATP-dependent allosteric organization, even though assembling, transportation, vaccination against cancer metastasis, and degradation of improperly-folded peptides have also been reported [16,17]. Small molecular weight HSPs or heat shock protein β (HspBs), which range from 15 to 43 kDa, are ATP-independent molecular chaperones, of which their functions have been documented in embryo developmental processes, formation of respiratory organs, like cardiac muscles, as biomarkers for tumour formation, in exercise-induced stress, as well as in protein folding [5,15,18]. The classification, localization, and roles of HSPs are highlighted as shown (see Table 1).

Table 1. Classification of heat shock protein families.

Classification	Location	Cellular Function	Reference
Hsp10	Mitochondria	Serves as biomarker in endometrial cancer and helps protein folding	[19,20]
Hsp27	Cytosol, endoplasmic reticulum & nucleus	Facilitates refolding of denatured proteins (chaperoning activity) and serves as a biomarker in many cellular diseases such as cancer	[21]
Hsp40	cytosol	Assists HSP70 in protein folding (co-chaperoning with HSP70)	[22]
HSP60	Cytoplasm & mitochondria	Assists in protein folding, prevents protein aggregation and assembling of unfolding proteins via the formation of the hetero-oligomeric complex	[23]
Hsp70	Cytoplasm & nucleus	Aids protein assembling, protein folding, degradation of improperly folded peptides and translocation of organelles	[5]
Hsp90	Cytoplasm	Assists in protein folding, refolding and degradation. It also facilitates signal transduction and important roles in cancer and sarcomere formation as well as in myosin folding	[5,24]
Hsp100	Cytoplasm	Complexes with other HSPs to refold aggregated or misfolded proteins	[25]
Hsp110	Cytosol & nucleus	Helps immune response and complexes with HSP70 to promote protein refolding and cell survival under stress	[26]

The roles of HSPs in the pathology of many diseases including human inflammatory diseases (HIDs), has been well documented. Hsp70 and Hsp60 in particular have been reported to form part of the auto-antigen complex capable of eliciting immunoregulatory cascades, thus suppressing the immune response which is commonly observed in various HIDs, such as Type 1 diabetes, atherosclerosis, rheumatoid arthritis, asthma, and allergies [27]. Hsp functions in the immunology of HIDs could be attributed to their diverse properties: (1) their ability to assemble immune system apparatus to infectious sites; (2) they are capable of interacting with antigen-presenting cells and initiating CD8+ immune responses and are, therefore, seen as potential cancer vaccines; (3) their ability to refold denatured proteins, including most immune cells, thus promoting their survival under stressful conditions [28,29]. In this review, we discuss in detail the interplay between HSPs, apoptosis, reactive oxygen species (ROS) and inflammatory diseases, as well as possible roles and potential target HSPs hold in HIDs and cancer.

2. Role of HSPs in Apoptosis

Apoptosis, which is alternatively called programmed cell death or "cellular suicidal", is a process by which cells are selectively killed without deteriorating neighbouring tissues [30]. This process is normally induced during embryo development, cell division, aging, as well as maintenance of cellular homeostasis, although it has also been reported to form part of the immune defence mechanism in response to cellular damage including the onset of cancer, and neurodegenerative and human inflammatory diseases (HIDs) [31–33]. Inappropriate stimulation of apoptosis has been associated with a variety of human diseases, such as ischemic damage, neurodegenerative disorders, autoimmune diseases, as well as cancer, making it a good therapeutic candidate against human diseases [32].

Studies have shown that apoptosis is mediated following the activation of caspases (a group of aspartate-specific cysteine proteases) that catalyses the addition or removal of specific cysteine or aspartic acid residues from target substrates, thereby activating or inhibiting the action of the targeted substrate [34,35]. These endoproteases are produced in an inactive state as zymogenes but upon activation, they play a central role in controlling apoptosis-mediated cell death, pyroptosis, necroptosis, as well as inflammatory reactions [36]. Caspases are broadly classified according to their roles in biological processes: apoptotic caspases (-7,-8, and -9) and inflammatory caspases (-1, -4, -5, and -12) in human and (-1, -11, and -12) in mice, respectively. The pro-inflammatory cytokines (such as interleukin 17, IL1β, TNF-α, IL-8, among others) and other inflammatory mediators are up-regulated as a result of the activation of caspases that are involved in inflammatory responses resulting in the innervation of innate immunity responses to cellular insults [36,37].

Caspase mediation of apoptosis falls into two broad categories: intrinsic and extrinsic mechanisms. Intrinsic or mitochondrial apoptotic pathway is a highly regulated and active pathway that cells use to antagonize mitochondrial stimulations as a result of stressors such as DNA damage, hypoxia, growth factor deprivation, as well as the accumulation of misfolded proteins. In response to cell death signals which activate the diverse functions of Bcl-2 families, intrinsic apoptosis is known to induce mitochondrial-membrane permeability through the opening of the permeability transition pore (PTP), thus allowing the release of cytochrome c (a pro-apoptotic factor that plays an important role in intrinsic apoptosis) into the cytosol. Inside the cytosol, cytochrome c complexes with apoptotic protease activating factor-1 (Apaf-)—an adaptor peptide—to recruit and activate pro-caspase-9, thereby forming a complex called apoptosome. The active caspase-9, on the other hand, triggers the activation and release of downstream 'executioner' caspase-3, which facilitates the degradation of the targeted substrate [34,36,38].

The extrinsic apoptosis pathway is characterised by interactions between Fas receptors (TNFR1, DR3 or death receptor 3, TRAIL-R1 or DR4, and Fas or CD95) and Fas ligands (TNF, Apo2-L, and FasL) on the surface of lymphocytes in response to suicidal signals. The binding of Fas ligand to FADD adaptor protein causes the dimerization of Fas associated death domains (FADDs) found in both Fas receptor and FADD adaptor proteins. This interaction allows the death effector domain (DED) to relate with pro-caspase-8 resulting in the formation of a complex called the death inducing signalling complex (DISC). The subsequent innervation of pro-caspase-8, which then triggers the activation of other pro-caspases, which then leads to the suicidal execution of cells [31–34,36,39,40].

Cells respond to numerous stressors, ranging from external to internal stressors, by expressing highly-regulated proteins upon thermal induction, called heat shock proteins (HSPs). These highly-conserved proteins are known for their diverse functions including protein folding, translocation of organelles across membranes, assembling and disassembling of proteins, signalling transduction, degradation of misfolded proteins, as well as ROS generation in the mitochondria capable of inducing apoptosis [41]. Overwhelming evidence has shown that HSPs have a wide array of functions in apoptosis, which in most cases, leads to the suppression of apoptotic pathways. Interestingly, the same stress signals that trigger apoptosis also stimulate the expression and release of HSPs. However, induction of HSPs represses apoptosis through inhibition of pro-apoptosis factors, such as p53, Bax, Bid, Akt, Apaf-1, and other Bcl-2 families. So far, numerous mechanisms of how HSPs incite cytoprotective effects against apoptosis has been proposed; one of them being the ability of Hsp27 to interact with cytochrome c and block its dimerization with Apaf-1, hence preventing the formation of apoptosome complex, which is the hallmark of mitochondrial cell suicide [36,42].

Work by Rane and colleagues have shown that Hsp27 relates directly with the serine/threonine (Akt) signalling pathway and this association inhibits neutrophil-mediated apoptosis in a phosphorylation-dependent manner [43]. Although the exact mechanism is still obscure, subsequent studies have shown that another molecular chaperone, Hsp70, directly associates with Apaf-1, blocking the production of apoptosome in an ATPase-dependent manner rather than its chaperoning activity [34,38,44]. Goto and co-workers and Beere reported that Hsp70 together with its co-chaperone Hsp40 homologs, inhibits nitric oxide mediated apoptosis by blocking the mitochondrial translocation of Bax, a pro-apoptotic member of Bcl-2 family in both ATPase and chaperoning dependent-fashion [34,45]. In spite of all the negative functions of HSPs in attenuating apoptosis, members of Hsp60 located in the mitochondria, in complexes with Hsp10, are involved in the signalling complex that results in pro-caspase-3 activation in cytochrome c-dependent apoptosis. In addition, several studies have shown that cytosolic Hsp60 associates with Bcl-2 proapoptic protein, Bax, leading to its activation, as well as its mediated apoptosis [46,47]. This observation suggests HSPs' roles in apoptosis to be complex, complicated, and controversial [34,38].

3. HSPs and Oxidative Stress

Due to continuous mitochondrial oxidative respiratory reactions and other cellular and non-cellular processes, including phagocytosis, inflammatory reactions, ionizing radiation, air pollutants, exercise, cigarette smoking, and ozone [48–50], cells frequently generate reactive oxygen species (ROS) and reactive nitrogen species (RNS), which disturb normal oxidant and antioxidant cellular homeostasis, leading to oxidative stress [51,52]. These oxygen-containing compounds can be broadly categorized according to their oxygen-containing capacity: superoxide anion (O_2^-), hydroxyl radical (OH), alkoxyl radical (RO), peroxyl radical (HOO), nitric oxide radical (NO), nitrogen oxide (NO_2), as well as potent non-radicals, such as hydrogen perioxide (H_2O_2), ozone (O_3), and oxygen singlet ($^1O_2$) [53,54]. Both ROS and RNS in accumulated levels are very reactive and more potent than normal oxygen and nitrogen, thus causing deleterious effects to the living system.

In spite of all negativities associated with accumulated cellular ROS, several studies have shown that, at low or moderate levels of unknown concentration, ROS perform important cellular beneficial roles, including acting as secondary messengers in signal transduction, in immune defence, in antibacterial infections in the phagosome and vascular tone, as well as in ROS-induced programmed cell death in cancer cells [52,54–58]. The hydroxyl radical (OH^-) which is the most reactive and most dangerous radical, is regenerated when H_2O_2 (a product of enzymatic reactions) decomposes slowly in the presence of Fe^{2+} in a process called the Fenton reaction and through other cellular reactions, including one between NO and O_2^- to form a perioxynitrite intermediate which immediately decomposes to OH^- [59]. Upon OH^- formation, OH^- is capable of abducting electrons from biomolecules, especially lipids (polyunsaturated fatty acids), thereby inflicting DNA, carbohydrate, protein, and lipid oxidation and, most importantly, resulting in oxidative stress when the antioxidant system is supressed [58]. The body uses the antioxidant system to neutralise free radical cellular damage by converting them to less harmful substances under physiological conditions; however, this balance can be disrupted upon cellular stress leading to the accumulation of cellular levels of free radicals, especially ROS, thus activating many inflammatory cascades which have been implicated in various human inflammatory diseases (HIDs), such as arthritis, asthma, stroke, atherosclerosis, trauma, hepatitis, and in cancer [52,60–62].

The deteriorating cellular effects of free radicals in accumulated levels has been well documented; however, it is not surprising that biological systems protect themselves by increasing the expression level of highly-regulated proteins termed "heat shock proteins" in response to these reactive species (ROS) that may otherwise lead to oxidative stress. HSPs are known for their cytoprotective activities in response to a variety of cellular insults through their chaperoning activities ranging from polypeptide folding, assembling, and translocation of organelles across membranes, to conducting repairs, and the degradation of irreparable peptides [8,63]. Nevertheless, DNA fragmentation has been observed in cells undergoing ROS-mediated genotoxicity, but this effect has been rescued with the addition of the Hsp70 family, thereby suggesting that the cytoprotective effects of HSPs could be by protecting

DNA breaks in response to ROS-induced insults [64]. Interestingly, HSPs have been reported to work hand-in-hand with the antioxidant system to inhibit or neutralise the cellular effects of ROS [65,66]. Accumulated ROS levels are said to induce apoptosis and are associated with a variety of inflammatory reactions, which is the hallmark of human inflammatory disease (HID) pathogenesis [53]. Hence, it is tempting to suggest that HSPs could play cytoprotective roles in the pathogenesis of HIDs and could be targeted as drug candidates for immunotherapy against HIDs.

4. HSPs in Human Inflammatory Diseases (HIDs) and Cancer

Inflammation, which forms part of the human first line of defence in response to stressful insults (such as pathogen invasion, oxidants, and cell damage), is characterized by swelling, pain, heat, and redness in the infected area [67]. This response enables cellular injury repair as well as elimination of any sign of necrotic cells, thereby activating innate immunity [68]. The inflammatory reaction is considered beneficial to humans in response to cellular insults because of the fact that it helps to clear and repair damaged cells and tissues. However, long-term unregulated inflammation may result in chronic inflammatory reactions marked with massive tissue and cell destruction, and this has been reported to play central role in the pathogenesis of many human inflammatory diseases (HIDs) [53]. HSPs have been reported to prevent inflammation through the inhibition of pro-inflammatory cytokines including tumour necrosis factor-α (TNF-α). The following sections in this review will hereby focus on the roles of HSPs in adult respiratory distress syndrome, rheumatoid arthritis, asthma, and cancer.

4.1. Acute Respiratory Distress Syndrome

Adult Respiratory Distress Syndrome (ARDS), which is alternatively called acute respiratory distress syndrome, is a lung inflammatory disorder characterized by Diffuse Alveolar Damage (DAD) as a result of the influx of liquid into the alveoli sacs (the site of blood-oxygenation), as well as the imbalance between pro-and-anti-inflammatory cytokines (interferon, TNF-α, interleukins, platelets derived growth factor) which, in most cases, leads to severe hypoxemia, stiffness of the lungs, pulmonary infiltration and organ failure, without causing cardiogenic pulmonary oedema [69,70]. Although ARDS mortality depends on several factors such as age, critical illness and other medical complications, ARDS has been estimated according statistical reports, to affect approximately 50 in every 100,000 people, resulting in almost 40% of deaths in infected patients worldwide [71,72]. So far, the actual causes of ARDS are obscured but, in most cases, ARDS has been reported in trauma or critically ill patients. Age and other unhealthy lifestyles, like smoking and chronic alcoholism, have also been documented as predisposing factors associated with ARDS cases [73].

In response to severe DAD cases, alveoli sac permeability of lung membranes is increased; this allows for the influx of neutrophils, tumour necrosis, macrophage inhibitory factor, together with platelet activation and sequestration, which are believed to be the centre stage for the development, progression, and pathogenesis of ARDS. However, elimination of activated inflammatory cytokines that cause tissue and cellular destructions in inflamed area have been reported to decrease morbidity and deaths in HIDs [74]. Nevertheless, heat shock proteins are known for their cytoprotective effects in response to cellular insults including inflammatory diseases; these proteins are said to be up-regulated during this stage of infection. Wesis and colleagues demonstrated that Hsp70 has the ability to suppress inflammatory responses by initiating the refolding of protein aggregates, thereby preventing the cellular damage and destruction observed in the pathology of ARDS and sepsis [75]. In support of this finding, other studies have shown that decreased mortality rates immediately after heat shock protein administration to endotoxin may mark the events of ARDS after several hours of development, as previously observed in rats [72,76]. Overwhelming evidence has shown that loss of pulmonary cells promote cell division which contribute massively to the pathogenesis of ARDS and heat shock proteins, Hsp70 in particular, has been previously shown to limit inflammation in HIDs, by inhibiting the pathway that leads to nuclear factor (NF)-kB activation as observed in pneumocytes [75]. Although the mechanism of Hsp-cytoprotective action in ARDS is largely unknown, it has been reported to follow the same mechanism as previously observed in other lung inflammatory diseases, like sepsis and pneumocystis [77].

4.2. Rheumatoid Arthritis

Rheumatoid arthritis (RA) is a long-term autoimmune-inflammatory disease where, instead of the immune system defending the body, it attacks synovial fluid-membranes normally found in the wrist, hand, or joints of the feet. RA, like other inflammatory diseases, is characterised by stiffness, swelling, and warmness and pain of the joints which, if left untreated long-term, may result in severe inflammation, deformity, and several functional disabilities [78,79]. Severe inflammation is said to attract numerous immune cytokines, chemokine, lymphocytes, and other immune components to the area of the infection (normally in the joints), causing redness, warmness, and painful discomfort, which are the symptoms, observed in rheumatoid arthritis infection. To date, the exact cause of RA is poorly understood and there is no pronounced cure. However, RA has been reported to arise as a result of family history or genetics (people that are genetically predisposed to RA) and other predisposing factors, such as environmental effects, educational background, and low socio-economic status, as well as unhealthy lifestyles, such as smoking and lack of exercise [78,80–82].

In spite of all the efforts in treatment, different medications and improvement in lifestyle with added exercise and healthier nutrition, RA remains one of the leading inflammatory autoimmune diseases worldwide. According to statistical reports, 24.5 million people were effected by RA in 2015, with a rate of 100,000 people every year [78]. RA, which occurs more in middle-aged females than in males, and has shown 10% mortality increase between 1990 and 2013, making it one of the prevalent health concerns according to the National Institute of Health (NIH).

In response to RA infection which is characterized by severe inflammation, biological systems always increase the synthesis of heat shock proteins especially Hsp70, the most inducible protein upon stress. Hsp70 exerts its anti-apoptotic activities by inhibiting pro/inflammatory signals or factors that lead to apoptosis, inflammatory pathways, such as activation of caspases, JNK (Jun N-terminal) signalling pathway, the release of cytochrome c, and the formation of apoptosome, which is the hallmark of apoptosis and inflammation progression [34]. More so, it is not surprising that Hsp70 is, therefore, up-regulated in the synovial membrane during rheumatoid arthritis fibroblast-like synoviocyte (RA-FLSs) infection to modulate the effects of T-cells, as well as to control inflammation via inhibition of pro-inflammation signals [83]. Surprisingly, Kang and colleagues reported that repression of Hsp70 by siRNA in an in vitro experiment decreased inflammation by protecting RA-FLSs from nitric oxide mediated-programmed cell death, although the actual function of Hsp70 in the RA in vivo experiment is still not yet clear [84]. This observation suggests the pro-apoptotic and negative roles of Hsp70 in the pathogenesis of RA FLSs infection; thus, inhibition of Hsp70 expression in RA could be one of the mechanisms of controlling severe inflammation observed in rheumatoid arthritis. In addition, van Room and co-workers showed that T-cells taken from RA patients were able to react with human or self-Hsp60 and inhibit the activation of TNF-α (a pro-inflammatory factor) through the activation of Th2 cytokine regulator, whereas there were no regulatory effects observed in Hsp65 isolated from *Mycobacterium tuberculosis* [85,86]. Consistent with this finding, several studies have shown that T-cell response to self-Hsp70 and Hsp60 through production of interleukin-4 and interleukin-10 regulatory cytokines suppresses arthritis diseases in many animal models. These observations suggest that cross-reactivity of HSPs with T-cells could be one of the ways of controlling human inflammatory diseases, like RA, under stressed physiological states [86,87]. Taken together, the self-Hsp60 reactivity observed in Lewis rats and adjuvant arthritis [88] makes it easy to speculate that human Hsp60 and mycobacterial Hsp60 could be used as potential vaccines against autoimmune inflammatory diseases since they are capable of eliciting immune responses.

4.3. Asthma

Asthma is a multigenic and multifactorial bronchial chronic inflammatory disorder characterised by airway obstruction, bronchospasm and remodelling of the bronchial wall, thus resulting in thickness of airflow walls and difficulties in breathing [89]. The symptoms of asthma, which can be caused by genetic or environmental factors (allergens and air pollutions), or both, range from chest tightness and wheezing sounds when breathing, down to shortness of breath; all these symptoms may vary in individuals. The various associations of different cellular networks, such as smooth muscle, macrophages, fibroblasts, eosinophil and epithelial cells may result in airway remodelling and inflammation [90]. This process of remodelling promotes further thickening of bronchial walls and narrowing the airflow, leading to the breathing difficulties commonly observed in the pathogenesis of asthmatic patients [91].

Statistics have shown that asthma affects 358 million people worldwide which has, so far, resulted in 397,100 deaths in 2015 alone, as compared to the 183 million people who were affected in 1990 [92,93]. According to the Global Initiative for Asthma (GINA), South Africa remains the fourth leading country, globally, and the first on the African continent with the highest mortality resulting from asthma attacks [94]. Furthermore, an estimated 3.9 million South Africans were affected by asthma in 2012, accounting for 1.5% of deaths in this country every year [95]. Taking into account the cytoprotective roles of HSPs in response to cellular insults, several authors have reported the over-expression of Hsp70 in asthmatic patients [96,97]. Surprisingly, recent studies have suggested that intracellular synthesis of Hsp70 chaperones in airways and alveolar sacs of asthma patients correlate with the deleterious effects and severity of the disease, probably by forming part of the inflammatory complex, where it may up-regulate THP-1 synthesis by inducing CD23 expression in the Th2 environment [98–100]. Nevertheless, initial studies have proposed its autoprotective activities in response to asthma and lung complications by inhibiting TNF-α mediated-inflammation [96,101]. In support of this finding, many studies have conclusively stated with evidence that the interaction between anti-Hsp70 and anti-Hsp60 correlates with progression, poor prognosis, and severity observed in asthmatic patients, as previously suggested by Shingai and colleagues in a patient with autoimmune liver disease [102] and *Mycobacterium* Hsp65 in chronic human atherosclerosis [103]. Interestingly, serum Hsp70 circulation is said to increase in pregnant asthmatic patients and this elevated Hsp70 level correlates with foetal and maternal complications such as low birth weight in infants, pre-eclampsia and preterm delivery, and these result in an almost 35% increased death rate in asthmatic pregnant women [104]. Other factors such as smoking and maternal obesity, on the other hand, have also been reported to promote perinatal death [105].

The exact mechanism of Hsp70 activity during asthma development remains to be seen, although evidence has it that Hsp70 mostly targets T-cells and humoral immunity in response to infectious agents, and this may provide a link between T-lymphocyte cross-reactivity-induced autoimmunity and immune responses to infectious diseases [106]. Another possible explanation is the ability of Hsp70 to interact with antigen presenting cells (APCs) and amplify its activities, which plays a crucial role in the modulation and initiation of asthmatic attacks in chronic asthma patients [96,104]. Additional studies have shown the up-regulation of Hsp90 and Hsp72 in response to ROS-induced asthma attacks in young children. Even though the exact functions of Hsp90 and Hsp72 remain unknown, it has been suggested that the elevated levels of these heat shock proteins could be to refold denatured proteins that may result from ROS induced-oxidative stress [107], thereby preventing protein aggregates, cellular deteriorations, and further complications. Tong and Luo showed that elevated Hsp70 levels in peripheral blood mononuclear cells (PBMCs) suggest Hsp involvement in the pathogenesis of asthma infection [108]. Through these observations we, therefore, propose that enhancing Hsp inhibitors in asthmatic patients could reduce the severity in this disease and will become another interesting aspect in the management of asthma and other lung inflammatory diseases, nonetheless more research is needed in this area of study.

4.4. Cancer

Cancer is a term given to the group of diseases characterized by the abnormal invasion and proliferation of cells as a result of uncontrolled cell divisions or mutated tumour suppressor genes [109]. Cancer remains one of the major sources of global morbidity and mortality and persists as the leading cause of death in individuals below 85 years old in the United States despite recent improvements in treatment modalities [53,110]. This exponential increase in cancer cases could be due to increasing prevalence in related factors, such as obesity, unhealthy life styles (smoking, lack of physical activity and imbalance diet), as well as genetic predisposition [31].

Hanahan and Weiberg proposed that the mechanisms by which cancerous cells survive in the human body are by increased resistance to anti-proliferative signals and apoptosis induced-suicidal or abnormal cell death [111]. Interestingly, several studies have reported that this resistance to apoptosis and antiproliferative signals observed in cancerous cells are actually induced in the presence of HSPs, which favour the refolding of denatured peptides through Hop (Hsp70/Hsp90 organizing protein) chaperoning related activities instead of peptide degradation [112,113]. Previous studies have shown that HSPs inhibit both pro-inflammatory and pro-apoptotic caspases, by binding and blocking their activation, thus increasing cancer cell survival [114]. Overexpression of Hsp27 in prostrate, ovarian and bladder cancers have been shown to correlate with down-regulation of p53 induced-stimulation of the p21 gene and up-regulation of matrix metalloproteins (MMPs), proteins that are known to pave the way for cancer cell migration, invasion, proliferation, and metastasis, thereby inhibiting p53 mediated senescence, apoptosis and cell cycle arrest [115]. These observations are simple indications of the roles of Hsp27 in prognosis, angiogenesis, proliferation, as well as metastasis of cancer cells.

In line with this, Hsp27 has been reported to promote epithelial-to-mesenchymal transition (EMT) in prostate cancer patients. EMT is an important event that occurs during organ morphogenesis and embryogenesis, characterized by the actin cytoskeleton remodelling, loss of apico-basolateral polarity and cell-cell junction dissolving, thus resulting in proliferation and mobility of cancer cells [116]. Down-regulation of Hsp27 using OGX-427 (an antisense therapy) decreases cancer cell invasion, migration, phosphorylation of LL-6-dependent STAT3 (a major mediator of EMP in many cancer types) and nuclear translocation, as well as matrix metalloproteinase, thereby reversing EMT activity. This observation suggests that Hsp27 is needed for interleukin LL-6 to induce EMP possibly through the modulation of the STAT3 signalling pathway [117].

Similarly, overexpression of Hsp70 corresponds with an increased proliferation of malignant cells and knockdown of Hsp70 experiments in various malignant tumours have been shown to increase the susceptibility of cancer cells to certain chemotherapy agents, suggesting the negative roles of Hsp70 in the invasiveness and proliferation of cancerous cells [118]. In addition, Hsp70 also acts as a cancerous cell-surviving factor by inhibiting TNF-α mediated-apoptotic cell death, thus promoting carcinogenesis and cancer cell oncogenic potential through the mechanism of escape immunology [115]. Furthermore, studies have reported that either Hsp90 or Hsp70 can bind and block the activation of apoptotic protease activating factor 1 (Apaf-1) and indirectly inhibit pro-caspase activation, apoptosis, as well as enhance abnormal cell survival [119]. Nevertheless, Hsp60 has been reported to show pro-carcinogenic activity through the inhibition of dusterin in neuroblastoma cells, cyclophilin D mediated-mitochondrial cell death, and promotion of cell survival via nuclear factor-kB activation [120,121].

Conversely, previous in vivo experiments by Chalmin and colleagues showed that the down-regulation of Hsp70 correlates with cancer cell survival due to the reduced immune killing of cancer cells [122]. Consistent with this finding is that Hsp40 homolog-DNAJA3 has been shown to inhibit squamous cell carcinoma invasion, migration, growth, recurrence and proliferation in both in vivo and in vitro experiments [115], possibly through induction of mitochondrial apoptosis, as previously observed in MCF-7 breast cancer cells [123]. These findings suggest that Hsp70 could suppress tumour cells when co-expressed with DNAJA3 in the absence of other molecular chaperones, like Hsp90, via CHIP (C-terminal HSP70 interacting protein)-mediated protein degradation.

5. Association between Heat Shock Proteins, Oxidative Stress, Apoptosis, Human Inflammatory Diseases (HIDs), and Cancer

Although accumulated levels of ROS have been proposed to cause deleterious effects to biomolecules, such as lipids, carbohydrates, proteins, and nucleic acids, ROS at moderate levels of unknown concentrations have been documented to play significant roles, such as acting as secondary messengers in signal transduction, immune defence, antibacterial infections in the phagosome, as well as ROS-induced programmed cell death in cancer cells [52,54]. Biological systems employ antioxidants (reduced glutathione, catalase, superoxide dismutase) to nullify the negative effects of free radicals, as well as to prevent ROS-mediated cellular damages and functional impairments. However, this antioxidant system can be supressed under severe cellular stress conditions as a result of elevated ROS levels, resulting in oxidative stress and amplification of inflammatory reactions, as well as activation of immune system cascades, a proposed central stage in progression and pathogenesis of several HIDs [53,124,125].

Inflammation is said to be part of the first line of the innate immunity complex that responds to cellular damage caused by infectious agents or xenobiotics [53]. Onset of stress has been established to attract several inflammatory cells, such as cytokines, macrophages, and chemokines, at the site of damaged cells, which is a process mediated upon toll-like receptor (TLRs) activation. The aim of this TLR mediated-inflammatory response is to eliminate detrimental cells and promote cellular repair via the mechanism of apoptosis. However, long-term un-regulated inflammatory reaction may lead to excessive and amplified apoptosis, resulting in chronic inflammation characterized by massive tissue and cellular destruction, commonly seen in many chronic and neurodegenerative diseases [62,126].

The roles of ROS induced-apoptosis in inflammatory reactions can be viewed as a double-edged sword. ROS-induced apoptosis under normal cellular conditions performs beneficial roles in suicidal killing of cells via mitochondrial apoptosis, but the abnormal stimulation of this mechanism under stressful conditions could result in excessively amplified intrinsic apoptosis, leading to the massive cellular destructions observed in the aetiology of several HIDs [127,128]. In line with this, elevated levels of ROS in the airways of asthmatic and ARDS patients suggests their roles in the pathogenesis and progression of HIDs by inducing severe inflammation [129,130]. HSPs, on the other hand, are mostly induced upon heat stress and, therefore, it is not surprising that HSPs are highly expressed in the inflamed area, possibly to refold denatured peptides caused by ROS-induced reperfusion injury on the inflammation sites identified in rheumatoid arthritis [131]. Heat is also one of the major characteristics of inflammation, and excessive inflammation leads to HIDs. Although some HSPs perform pro-inflammatory/apoptotic functions, most HSPs are known for their anti-apoptotic/inflammatory potential, including the inhibition of pro-inflammatory/apoptotic factors or pathway capabilities such as through the nuclear factor (NF-kB), activation of caspases and c-Jun NH2-terminal kinase pathway [132]. Suppression of HSP expression levels, therefore, leads to worse inflammation cases, which can be linked to the severe inflammation seen in several HIDs.

6. Future Direction in the Use of HSPs as Therapeutic Candidates

From this point, it can be proposed that carefully regulation of inflammatory responses, induction of apoptosis and endogenous generation of ROS would definitely help in the management or treatment of HIDs. In many studies, HSPs have been reported to play crucial roles in the pathogenesis of HIDs and cancer due to their modulating effects in inflammation cascades that lead to the endogenous generation of ROS and apoptosis [27,34,133], possibly via their chaperoning activities of refolding misfolded proteins, or via inhibition of pro-inflammatory cytokines under pathological conditions. Under stressful conditions, HSPs has been suggested to play a prominent role by binding to the lipid rafts inside lipid membranes, thus maintaining lipid membrane stability, physical orderliness, as well as preventing lipid membrane functional impairments. Altered membrane functionality has been associated with cancer, neurodegenerative diseases, and diabetes, suggesting the possible role of HSPs as therapeutic targets in the management of these diseases [134].

Up–regulation of HSPs in cancerous cells has been well documented and has been associated with poor prognosis, proliferation, cell differentiation, invasion, progression, and metastasis [135,136]. Among others, Hsp90, Hsp70, and Hsp27 in particular, have been reported by many studies to increase tumour cell survival via inhibition of pro-inflammatory cytokines and ROS-mediated apoptosis [119,136,137]. Chauhan and co-workers demonstrated that Hsp27 can promote the survival of malignant tumours by conferring resistance to the inflammatory drug dexamethasone (a drug for treating HIDs such as rheumatoid arthritis, skin inflammation, and cancer) in myeloma cell lines via the inhibition of SMAC (mitochondrial release of second mitochondrial-derived activator of caspases) and cytochrome c, both of which are masters of intrinsic apoptosis mediators [138].

Hsp27 can also act as an anti-apoptotic factor by promoting the activities of nuclear factor-kB (NF-kB) while blocking apoptosis pathways mediated by NF-kB inhibitor (IkBα), thereby promoting cancer cell proliferation and survival [135]. Hsp27 involvement in cancer could be through phosphorylation at three-serine residues mediated by MAPKAPK2 (mitogen-activated protein kinase activated protein kinase). This phosphorylation enables the Hsp27 to form oligomers up to 100 kDa, making it ideal in preventing protein aggregation by refolding denatured peptides in an ATP-independent manner [119]. Similarly, Hsp70 and Hsp90 function in cancer cell survival has been previously elucidated. Work by Nylandsted and colleagues showed that selective inhibition of Hsp70 in breast cancer lines increased the susceptibility of cancer to chemotherapy and sensitized them to caspase-mediated apoptotic death [139]. Hsp90 is known to play a crucial role in cancer cell survival and has been reported as a drug target in many cancer types. Inhibition of Hsp90 in leukaemia, colorectal, breast, lung, melanoma, and bladder cancer correlates with decreased invasion, motility, and prognosis of cancer, as well as an increase in the susceptibility of cancer cells to therapy [115]. This may be possible via the inhibition of signalling pathways that confer resistance to chemotherapy. In view of this, Zuninga and Shonhai previously postulated that Hsp70 and Hsp90 are the most druggable HSPs due to the fact that most Hsp inhibitors either mimic or target their ATPase activity [140]. This could be via the inhibition of Hsp70/Hsp90 organizing protein (Hop), which favours the refolding of aberrant peptides while blocking CHIP-mediated peptide degradation. Interestingly, subset studies have shown that physical exercise induces Hsp expression [141–143], and is one of the ways of managing HIDs and cancer. Furthermore, one can then speculate that one of the health benefits of exercise is to induce Hsp expression, which is known for its cellular cytoprotective activities, probably by forming part of the immune protective system against infection.

The onset of stress increases ROS generation, as well as inflammatory reactions. The generated ROS and inflammation activates the immune response and induces apoptosis, which aims at fighting off the infectious agent. However, if this mechanism is not well stimulated, it could degenerate to chronic inflammation. Interestingly, heat shock factor-1 (HSF-1) is also upregulated during this stage of infection. HSF-1 increases the synthesis of protective HSPs, which stops inflammatory reactions and massive cellular destruction through apoptosis, as well as further ROS generation, possibly via inhibition of pro-inflammatory factors and activation of the immune system, thus preventing chronic inflammation, HIDs, and cancer progression, as proposed in Figure 1.

HSPs have been reported to perform beneficial cytoprotective effects when induced prior to inflammation and deleterious effects after propagation of pro-inflammation reactions [132]. We, therefore, proposed that induction of HSPs prior to inflammation and carefully regulation of ROS, inflammation and apoptosis through the induction of HSPs as well as the inhibition of HSPs in cancer and certain HIDs (asthma and ARDS) and enhancement of HSP activities in RA may, and will, serve as future study references as proposed in the model (Figure 1), which highlights the possible roles of HSPs in HIDs and cancer.

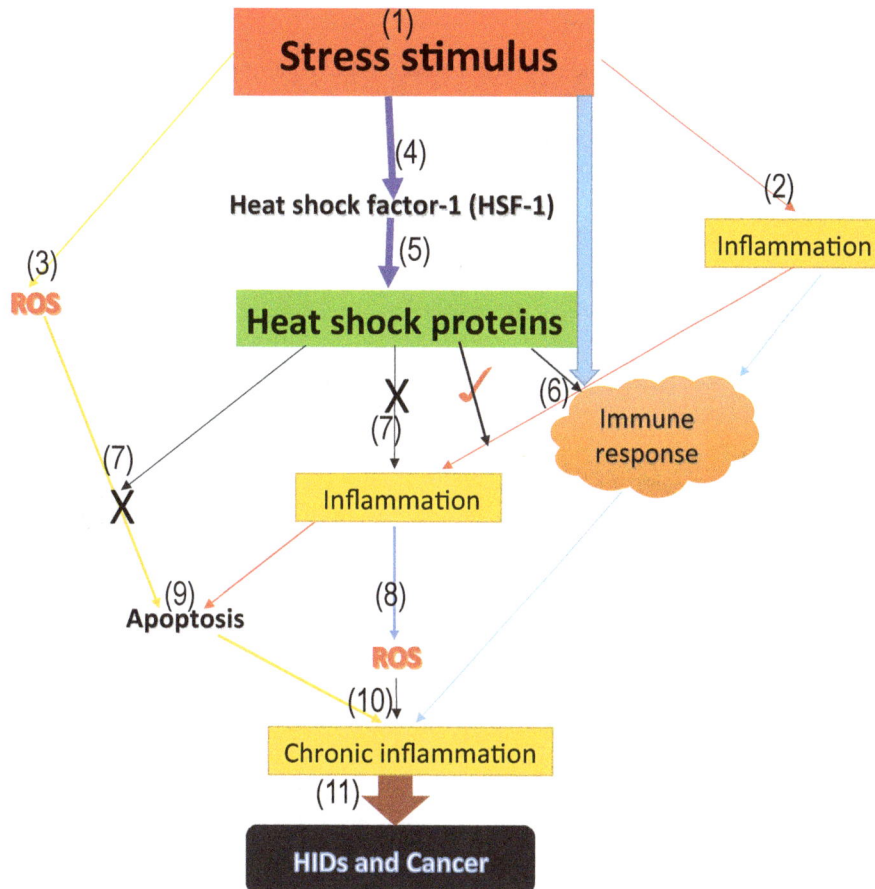

Figure 1. Model proposing the roles of heat shock proteins in HIDs and cancer. The above model represents the proposed roles that heat shock proteins play in human inflammatory diseases and cancer. (1) the onset of the stress signal; (2) stress activates inflammatory reactions which aims at repairing the damage caused by the stress; (3) generation of ROS from the infected area; (4) activation of the heat shock factor-1 (HSF-1), which increases the synthesis of the cytoprotective heat shock proteins; (5) activation of heat shock proteins; (6) stress, as well as inflammation and heat shock proteins, activate the immune response and form part of the innate immune response (7); cytoprotective heat shock proteins inhibit further generation of ROS, as well as inflammation, thus blocking excessive ROS and inflammation mediated-apoptosis via the inhibition of pro-inflammatory and pro-apoptotic factors; (9) excessive apoptosis mediated by ROS; (8) accumulated level of ROS leading to oxidative stress; (10) immune response, inflammatory reaction, accumulated ROS level and excessive apoptosis mediated by ROS as a result of antioxidant suppression, leading to oxidative stress and chronic inflammation marked with massive cellular and tissue destruction; and (11) long-term uncontrolled chronic inflammation degenerates to HIDs and cancer.

7. Conclusions

The search for new drugs for the treatment of HIDs and cancer continues, and new studies are now focused on discovering drugs that will have minimal side effects. Recently, HSPs have attracted a great deal of research interest because of their ever-present occurrence in a variety of human diseases, including HID-tested patients, even though their action in some HIDs is still unclear. From our perspective as proposed in the model (Figure 1). We, therefore, suggest that targeting HSPs in HIDs will serve as good potential candidates towards the treatment and management of many HIDs, as well as early detection of these diseases.

References

1. Srivastava, P. Roles of heat-shock proteins in innate and adaptive immunity. *Nat. Rev. Immunol.* **2002**, *2*, 185. [CrossRef] [PubMed]

2. Asea, A. Chaperokine-induced signal transduction pathways. *Exerc. Immunol. Rev.* **2003**, *9*, 25–33. [PubMed]

3. Searle, S.; McCrossan, M.V.; Smith, D.F. Expression of a mitochondrial stress protein in the protozoan parasite Leishmania major. *J. Cell Sci.* **1993**, *104*, 1091–1100. [PubMed]

4. Zügel, U.; Kaufmann, E. Role of Heat Shock Proteins in Protection from and Pathogenesis of Infectious Diseases. *Clin. Microbiol. Rev.* **1999**, *12*, 19–39. [PubMed]

5. Jee, H. Size dependent classification of heat shock proteins: A mini-review. *J. Exerc. Rehabil.* **2016**, *12*, 255–259. [CrossRef] [PubMed]

6. Sharma, G.; Nath, A.; Prasad, S.; Singh, N.; Dubey, P.; Saikumar, G. Expression and Characterization of Constitutive Heat Shock Proteins 70.1 (HSPA-1A) Gene in In Vitro produced and In Vivo-Derived Buffalo (Bubalis) Embryos. *Reprod. Domest. Anim.* **2012**, *47*, 975–983. [CrossRef] [PubMed]

7. De Maio, A. Heat shock proteins: Facts, thoughts, and dreams. *Shock* **1999**, *11*, 1–12. [CrossRef] [PubMed]

8. Shiber, A.; Ravid, T. Chaperoning proteins for destruction: Diverse roles of HSP70 chaperones and their co-chaperones in targeting misfolded proteins to the proteasome. *Biomolecules* **2014**, *4*, 704–724. [CrossRef] [PubMed]

9. Daugaard, M.; Kirkegaard-Sørensen, T.; Ostenfeld, M.S.; Aaboe, M.; Høyer-Hansen, M.; Ørntoft, T.F.; Rohde, M.; Jäättelä, M. Lens epithelium-derived growth factor is an HSP70-2 regulated guardian of lysosomal stability in human cancer. *Cancer Res.* **2007**, *67*, 2559–2567. [CrossRef] [PubMed]

10. Singh, O.V.; Pollard, H.B.; Zeitlin, P.L. Chemical rescue of ΔF508-CFTR mimics genetic repair in cystic fibrosis bronchial epithelial cells. *Mol. Cell. Proteom.* **2008**, *7*, 1099–1110. [CrossRef] [PubMed]

11. Zhang, H.; Liu, R.; Huang, W.A. 14-mer peptide from HSP70 protein is the critical epitope which enhances NK activity against tumor cells in vivo. *Immunol. Investig.* **2007**, *36*, 233–246. [CrossRef] [PubMed]

12. De Maio, A. Extracellular heat shock proteins, cellular export vesicles, and the Stress Observation System: A form of communication during injury, infection, and cell damage. *Cell Stress Chaperones* **2011**, *16*, 235–249. [CrossRef] [PubMed]

13. De Maio, A.; Santoro, M.G.; Tanguay, R.M.; Hightower, L.E. Ferruccio Ritossa's scientific legacy 50 years after his discovery of the heat shock response: A new view of biology, a new society, and a new journal. *Cell Stress Chaperones* **2012**, *17*, 139–143. [CrossRef] [PubMed]

14. Garbuz, D.G.; Astakhova, L.N.; Zatsepina, O.G.; Arkhipova, I.R.; Nudler, E.; Evgen'ev, M.B. Functional organization of *hsp70* cluster in camel (*Camelus dromedarius*) and other mammals. *PLoS ONE* **2011**, *6*, 27205. [CrossRef] [PubMed]

15. Lanneau, D.; Wettstein, G.; Bonniaud, P.; Garrido, C. Heat Shock Proteins: Cell Protection through Protein Triage. *Sci. World J.* **2010**, *10*, 1543–1552. [CrossRef] [PubMed]

16. Sung, Y.Y.; MacRae, T.H. Heat shock proteins and disease control in aquatic organisms. *J. Aquac. Res. Dev. S* **2011**, *2*. [CrossRef]

17. Wan, T.; Zhou, X.; Chen, G.; An, H.; Chen, T.; Zhang, W.; Liu, S.; Jiang, Y.; Yang, F.; Wu, Y.; et al. Novel heat shock protein HSP70L1 activates dendritic cells and acts as a Th1 polarizing adjuvant. *Blood* **2004**, *103*, 1747–1754. [CrossRef] [PubMed]

18. Juo, L.Y.; Liao, W.C.; Shih, Y.L.; Yang, B.Y.; Liu, A.B.; Yan, Y.T. HSPB7 interacts with dimerized FLNC and its absence results in progressive myopathy in skeletal muscles. *J. Cell Sci.* **2016**, *129*, 1661–1670. [CrossRef] [PubMed]

19. Dubé, V.; Grigull, J.; DeSouza, L.V.; Ghanny, S.; Colgan, T.J.; Romaschin, A.D.; Siu, K.M. Verification of endometrial tissue biomarkers previously discovered using mass spectrometry-based proteomics by means of immunohistochemistry in a tissue microarray format. *J. Proteom. Res.* **2007**, *6*, 2648–2655. [CrossRef] [PubMed]

20. Meyer, A.S.; Gillespie, J.R.; Walther, D.; Millet, I.S.; Doniach, S.; Frydman, J. Closing the folding chamber of the eukaryotic chaperonin requires the transition state of ATP hydrolysis. *Cell* **2003**, *113*, 369–381. [CrossRef]

21. Vidyasagar, A.; Wilson, N.A.; Djamali, A. Heat shock protein 27 (HSP27): Biomarker of disease and therapeutic target. *Fibrogenesis Tissue Repair* **2012**, *5*, 7. [CrossRef] [PubMed]

22. Li, J.; Qian, X.; Sha, B. Heat shock protein 40: Structural studies and their functional implications. *Protein Pept. Lett.* **2009**, *16*, 606–612. [CrossRef] [PubMed]

23. Belles, C.; Kuhl, A.; Nosheny, R.; Carding, S.R. Plasma membrane expression of heat shock protein 60 in vivo in response to infection. *Infect. Immun.* **1999**, *67*, 4191–4200. [PubMed]

24. Tuttle, J.A.; Castle, P.C.; Metcalfe, A.J.; Midgley, A.W.; Taylor, L.; Lewis, M.P. Downhill running and exercise in hot environments increase leukocyte Hsp72 (HSPA1A) and Hsp90α (HSPC1) gene transcripts. *J. Appl. Physiol.* **2015**, *118*, 996–1005. [CrossRef] [PubMed]

25. Krobitsch, S.; Brandau, S.; Hoyer, C.; Schmetz, C.; Hübel, A.; Clos, J. Leishmania donovani heat shock protein 100 characterization and function in amastigote stage differentiation. *J. Biol. Chem.* **1998**, *273*, 6488–6494. [CrossRef] [PubMed]

26. Zuo, D.; Subjeck, J.; Wang, X.Y. Unfolding the role of large heat shock proteins: New insights and therapeutic implications. *Front. Immunol.* **2016**, *7*, 75. [CrossRef] [PubMed]

27. Van Eden, W.; Van der Zee, R.; Prakken, B. Heat-shock proteins induce T-cell regulation of chronic inflammation. *Nat. Rev. Immunol.* **2005**, *5*, 318. [CrossRef] [PubMed]

28. Wu, Y.; Wan, T.; Zhou, X.; Wang, B.; Yang, F.; Li, N.; Chen, G.; Dai, S.; Liu, S.; Zhang, M.; et al. Hsp70-like Protein 1 fusion protein enhances induction of carcinoembryonic antigen–specific CD8+ CTL response by dendritic cell vaccine. *Cancer Res.* **2005**, *65*, 4947–4954. [CrossRef] [PubMed]

29. Colaco, C.A.; Bailey, C.R.; Walker, K.B.; Keeble, J. Heat shock proteins: Stimulators of innate and acquired immunity. *BioMed. Res. Int.* **2013**, *2013*. [CrossRef] [PubMed]

30. Ahmad, R.; Rasheed, Z.; Ahsan, H. Biochemical and cellular toxicology of peroxynitrite: Implications in cell death and autoimmune phenomenon. *Immunopharmacol. Immunotoxicol.* **2009**, *31*, 388–396. [CrossRef] [PubMed]

31. Wong, R.S. Apoptosis in cancer: From pathogenesis to treatment. *J. Exp. Clin. Cancer Res.* **2011**, *30*, 87. [CrossRef] [PubMed]

32. Elmore, S. Apoptosis: A review of programmed cell death. *Toxicol. Pathol.* **2007**, *35*, 495–516. [CrossRef] [PubMed]

33. Lowe, S.W.; Lin, A.W. Apoptosis in cancer. *Carcinogenesis* **2000**, *21*, 485–495. [CrossRef] [PubMed]

34. Beere, H.M. The stress of dying': The role of heat shock proteins in the regulation of apoptosis. *J. Cell Sci.* **2004**, *117*, 2641–2651. [CrossRef] [PubMed]

35. Wolf, B.B.; Green, D.R. Suicidal tendencies: Apoptotic cell death by caspase family proteinases. *J. Biol. Chem.* **1999**, *274*, 20049–20052. [CrossRef] [PubMed]

36. McIlwain, D.R.; Berger, T.; Mak, T.W. Caspase functions in cell death and disease. *Cold Spring Harb. Perspect. Biol.* **2013**, *5*, a008656. [CrossRef] [PubMed]

37. Novara, G.; Galfano, A.; Berto, R.B.; Ficarra, V.; Navarrete, R.V.; Artibani, W. Inflammation, apoptosis, and BPH: What is the evidence? *Eur. Urol. Suppl.* **2006**, *5*, 401–409. [CrossRef]

38. Takayama, S.; Reed, J.C.; Homma, S. Heat-shock proteins as regulators of apoptosis. *Oncogene* **2003**, *22*, 9041–9047. [CrossRef] [PubMed]

39. Jolly, C.; Morimoto, R.I. Role of the heat shock response and molecular chaperones in oncogenesis and cell death. *J. Natl. Cancer Inst.* **2000**, *92*, 1564–1572. [CrossRef] [PubMed]

40. Leung, A.M.; Redlak, M.J.; Miller, T.A. Role of heat shock proteins in oxygen radical–induced gastric apoptosis. *J. Surg. Res.* **2015**, *193*, 135–144. [CrossRef] [PubMed]

41. Bukau, B.; Weissman, J.; Horwich, A. Molecular chaperones and protein quality control. *Cell* **2006**, *125*, 443–451. [CrossRef] [PubMed]

42. Garrido, C.; Bruey, J.M.; Fromentin, A.; Hammann, A.; Arrigo, A.P.; Solary, E. HSP27 inhibits cytochrome c-dependent activation of procaspase-9. *FASEB J.* **1999**, *13*, 2061–2070. [PubMed]

43. Rane, M.J.; Pan, Y.; Singh, S.; Powell, D.W.; Wu, R.; Cummins, T.; Chen, Q.; McLeish, K.R.; Klein, J.B. Heat shock protein 27 controls apoptosis by regulating Akt activation. *J. Biol. Chem.* **2003**, *278*, 27828–27835. [CrossRef] [PubMed]

44. Ravagnan, L.; Gurbuxani, S.; Susin, S.A.; Maisse, C.; Daugas, E.; Zamzami, N.; Mak, T.; Jäättelä, M.; Penninger, J.M.; Garrido, C.; et al. Heat-shock protein 70 antagonizes apoptosis-inducing factor. *Nat. Cell Biol.* **2001**, *3*, 839–843. [CrossRef] [PubMed]

45. Goto, H.; Yano, S.; Matsumori, Y.; Ogawa, H.; Blakey, D.C.; Sone, S. Sensitization of tumor-associated endothelial cell apoptosis by the novel vascular-targeting agent ZD6126 in combination with cisplatin. *Clin. Cancer Res.* **2004**, *10*, 7671–7676. [CrossRef] [PubMed]

46. Samali, A.; Cai, J.; Zhivotovsky, B.; Jones, D.P.; Orrenius, S. Presence of a pre-apoptotic complex of pro-caspase-3, HSP60 and Hsp10 in the mitochondrial fraction of Jurkat cells. *EMBO J.* **1999**, *18*, 2040–2048. [CrossRef] [PubMed]

47. Gupta, S.; Knowlton, A.A. Cytosolic heat shock protein 60, hypoxia, and apoptosis. *Circulation* **2002**, *106*, 2727–2733. [CrossRef] [PubMed]

48. Lobo, V.; Patil, A.; Phatak, A.; Chandra, N. Free radicals, antioxidants and functional foods: Impact on human health. *Pharmacogn. Rev.* **2010**, *4*, 118. [CrossRef] [PubMed]

49. Ji, L. Oxidative stress during exercise: Implication of antioxidant nutrients. *Free Radic. Biol. Med.* **1995**, *18*, 1079–1086. [CrossRef]

50. Fubini, B.; Hubbard, A. Reactive oxygen species (ROS) and reactive nitrogen species (RNS) generation by silica in inflammation and fibrosis. *Free Radic. Biol. Med.* **2003**, *34*, 1507–1516. [CrossRef]

51. Uttara, B.; Singh, A.V.; Zamboni, P.; Mahajan, R.T. Oxidative stress and neurodegenerative diseases: A review of upstream and downstream antioxidant therapeutic options. *Curr. Neuropharmacol.* **2009**, *7*, 65–74. [CrossRef] [PubMed]

52. Alfadda, A.A.; Sallam, R.M. Reactive oxygen species in health and disease. *BioMed. Res. Int.* **2012**. [CrossRef] [PubMed]

53. Oyinloye, B.E.; Adenowo, A.F.; Kappo, A.P. Reactive oxygen species, apoptosis, antimicrobial peptides and human inflammatory diseases. *Pharmaceuticals* **2015**, *8*, 151–175. [CrossRef] [PubMed]

54. Lushchak, V.I. Free radicals, reactive oxygen species, oxidative stress and its classification. *Chem.-Biol. Int.* **2014**, *224*, 164–175. [CrossRef] [PubMed]

55. Finkel, T. Signal transduction by reactive oxygen species. *J. Cell. Biol.* **2011**, *194*, 7–15. [CrossRef] [PubMed]

56. Gonzalez, C.; Sanz-Alfayate, G.; Agapito, M.T.; Gomez-Nino, A.; Rocher, A.; Obeso, A. Significance of ROS in oxygen sensing in cell systems with sensitivity to physiological hypoxia. *Respir. Physiol. Neurobiol.* **2002**, *132*, 17–41. [CrossRef]

57. Scandalios, J.G. Oxidative stress responses-what have genome-scale studies taught us? *Genome Biol.* **2002**, *3*, 1019–1021. [CrossRef]

58. Mittler, R.; Vanderauwera, S.; Suzuki, N.; Miller, G.; Tognetti, V.B.; Vandepoele, K.; Gollery, M.; Shulaev, V.; Van Breusegem, F. ROS signaling: The new wave? *Trends Plant Sci.* **2011**, *16*, 300–309. [CrossRef] [PubMed]

59. Coyle, J.T.; Puttfarcken, P. Oxidative stress, glutamate, and neurodegenerative disorders. *Science* **1993**, *262*, 689–695. [CrossRef] [PubMed]

60. Schneeberger, K.; Czirják, G.Á.; Voigt, C.C. Inflammatory challenge increases measures of oxidative stress in a free-ranging, long-lived mammal. *J. Exp. Biol.* **2013**, *216*, 4514–4519. [CrossRef] [PubMed]

61. Lee, J.; Koo, N.; Min, D.B. Reactive oxygen species, aging, and antioxidative nutraceuticals. *Compr. Rev. Food Sci. Food Saf.* **2004**, *3*, 21–33. [CrossRef]

62. Hsieh, H.L.; Yang, C.M. Role of redox signaling in neuroinflammation and neurodegenerative diseases. *BioMed. Res. Int.* **2013**, *2013*. [CrossRef] [PubMed]

63. Mayer, M.P.; Bukau, B. Hsp70 chaperones: Cellular functions and molecular mechanism. *Cell. Mol. Life Sci.* **2005**, *62*, 670. [CrossRef] [PubMed]

64. Jacquier-Sarlin, M.R.; Fuller, K.; Dinh-Xuan, A.T.; Richard, M.J.; Polla, B.S. Protective effects of HSP70 in inflammation. *Cell. Mol. Life Sci.* **1994**, *50*, 1031–1038. [CrossRef]

65. Trott, A.; West, J.D.; Klaić, L.; Westerheide, S.D.; Silverman, R.B.; Morimoto, R.I.; Morano, K.A. Activation of heat shock and antioxidant responses by the natural product celastrol: Transcriptional signatures of a thiol-targeted molecule. *Mol. Biol. Cell.* **2008**, *19*, 1104–1112. [CrossRef] [PubMed]

66. Wu, C.-W.; Biggar, K.K.; Zhang, J.; Tessier, S.N.; Pifferi, F.; Perret, M.; Storey, K.B. Induction of antioxidant and heat shock protein responses during torpor in the gray mouse lemur, Microcebus murinus. *Genom. Proteom. Bioinform.* **2015**, *13*, 119–126. [CrossRef] [PubMed]

67. Ashley, N.T.; Weil, Z.M.; Nelson, R.J. Inflammation: Mechanisms, costs, and natural variation. *Ann. Rev. Ecol. Evol. Syst.* **2012**, *43*, 385–406. [CrossRef]

68. Ferrero-Miliani, L.; Nielsen, O.H.; Andersen, P.S.; Girardin, S.E. Chronic inflammation: Importance of NOD2 and NALP3 in interleukin-1β generation. *Clin. Exp. Immunol.* **2007**, *147*, 227–235. [CrossRef] [PubMed]

69. Villar, J.; Blanco, J.; Añón, J.M.; Santos-Bouza, A.; Blanch, L.; Ambrós, A.; Gandía, F.; Carriedo, D.; Mosteiro, F.; Basaldúa, S.; et al. The ALIEN study: Incidence and outcome of acute respiratory distress syndrome in the era of lung protective ventilation. *Intensive Care Med.* **2011**, *37*, 1932–1941. [CrossRef] [PubMed]

70. Ware, L.B.; Matthay, M.A. The acute respiratory distress syndrome. *N. Engl. J. Med.* **2000**, *342*, 1334–1349. [CrossRef] [PubMed]

71. Rubenfeld, G.D.; Caldwell, E.; Peabody, E.; Weaver, J.; Martin, D.P.; Neff, M.; Stern, E.J.; Hudson, L.D. Incidence and outcomes of acute lung injury. *N. Engl. J. Med.* **2005**, *353*, 1685–1693. [CrossRef] [PubMed]

72. Slutsky, A.S. Hot new therapy for sepsis and the acute respiratory distress syndrome. *J. Clin. Investig.* **2002**, *110*, 737. [CrossRef] [PubMed]

73. González-Reimers, E.; Santolaria-Fernández, F.; Martín-González, M.C.; Fernández-Rodríguez, C.M.; Quintero-Platt, G. Alcoholism: A systemic proinflammatory condition. *World J. Gastroenterol.* **2014**, *20*, 14660. [CrossRef] [PubMed]

74. Hirsh, M.I.; Junger, W.G. Roles of heat shock proteins and γδT cells in inflammation. *Am. J. Respir. Cell Mol. Biol.* **2008**, *39*, 509–513. [CrossRef] [PubMed]

75. Weiss, Y.G.; Bromberg, Z.; Raj, N.; Raphael, J.; Goloubinoff, P.; Ben-Neriah, Y.; Deutschman, C.S. Enhanced heat shock protein 70 expression alters proteasomal degradation of IκB kinase in experimental acute respiratory distress syndrome. *Crit. Care Med.* **2007**, *35*, 2128–2138. [CrossRef] [PubMed]

76. Chu, E.K.; Ribeiro, S.P.; Slutsky, A.S. Heat stress increases survival rates in lipopolysaccharide-stimulated rats. *Crit. Care Med.* **1997**, *25*, 1727–1732. [CrossRef] [PubMed]

77. Bromberg, Z.; Raj, N.; Goloubinoff, P.; Deutschman, C.S.; Weiss, Y.G. Enhanced expression of 70-kilodalton heat shock protein limits cell division in a sepsis-induced model of acute respiratory distress syndrome. *Crit. Care Med.* **2008**, *36*, 246. [CrossRef] [PubMed]

78. Smolen, J.S.; Breedveld, F.C.; Burmester, G.R.; Bykerk, V.; Dougados, M.; Emery, P.; Kvien, T.K.; Navarro-Compán, M.V.; Oliver, S.; Schoels, M.; et al. Treating rheumatoid arthritis to target: 2014 update of the recommendations of an international task force. *Ann. Rheum. Dis.* **2016**, *75*, 3–15. [CrossRef] [PubMed]

79. Aletaha, D.; Neogi, T.; Silman, A.J.; Funovits, J.; Felson, D.T.; Bingham, C.O.; Birnbaum, N.S.; Burmester, G.R.; Bykerk, V.P.; Cohen, M.D.; et al. 2010 rheumatoid arthritis classification criteria: An American College of Rheumatology/European League Against Rheumatism collaborative initiative. *Arthritis Rheum.* **2010**, *62*, 2569–2581. [CrossRef] [PubMed]

80. Klareskog, L.; Malmström, V.; Lundberg, K.; Padyukov, L.; Alfredsson, L. Smoking, citrullination and genetic variability in the immunopathogenesis of rheumatoid arthritis. *Semin. Immunol.* **2011**, *23*, 92–98. [CrossRef] [PubMed]

81. Millar, K.; Lloyd, S.M.; McLean, J.S.; Batty, G.D.; Burns, H.; Cavanagh, J.; Deans, K.A.; Ford, I.; McConnachie, A.; McGinty, A.; et al. Personality, socio-economic status and inflammation: Cross-sectional, population-based study. *PLoS ONE* **2013**, *8*, 58256. [CrossRef] [PubMed]

82. Callahan, L.F.; Pincus, T. Education, self-care, and outcomes of rheumatic diseases: Further challenges to the "biomedical model" paradigm. *Arthritis Rheum.* **1997**, *10*, 283–288. [CrossRef]

83. Schett, G.; Redlich, K.; Xu, Q.; Bizan, P.; Gröger, M.; Tohidast-Akrad, M.; Kiener, H.; Smolen, J.; Steiner, G. Enhanced expression of heat shock protein 70 (HSP70) and heat shock factor 1 (HSF1) activation in rheumatoid arthritis synovial tissue. Differential regulation of HSP70 expression and hsf1 activation in synovial fibroblasts by proinflammatory cytokines, shear stress, and antiinflammatory drugs. *J. Clin. Investig.* **1998**, *102*, 302–311. [PubMed]

84. Kang, E.H.; Kim, D.J.; Lee, E.Y.; Lee, Y.J.; Lee, E.B.; Song, Y.W. Downregulation of heat shock protein 70 protects rheumatoid arthritis fibroblast-like synoviocytes from nitric oxide-induced apoptosis. *Arthritis Res. Ther.* **2009**, *11*, 130. [CrossRef] [PubMed]

85. Van Roon, J.A.; van Eden, W.; van Roy, J.L.; Lafeber, F.J.; Bijlsma, J.W. Stimulation of suppressive T cell responses by human but not bacterial 60-kD heat-shock protein in synovial fluid of patients with rheumatoid arthritis. *J. Clin. Investig.* **1997**, *100*, 459–463. [CrossRef] [PubMed]

86. Pockley, A.G. Heat shock proteins as regulators of the immune response. *Lancet* **2003**, *362*, 469–476. [CrossRef]

87. Anderton, S.M.; Van Der Zee, R.; Prakken, B.; Noordzij, A.; Van Eden, W. Activation of T cells recognizing self 60-kD heat shock protein can protect against experimental arthritis. *J. Exp. Med.* **1995**, *181*, 943–952. [CrossRef] [PubMed]

88. Kaul, G.; Thippeswamy, H. Role of heat shock proteins in diseases and their therapeutic potential. *Indian J. Microbiol.* **2011**, *51*, 124–131. [CrossRef] [PubMed]

89. Salinthone, S.; Ba, M.; Hanson, L.; Martin, J.L.; Halayko, A.J.; Gerthoffer, W.T. Overexpression of human Hsp27 inhibits serum-induced proliferation in airway smooth muscle myocytes and confers resistance to hydrogen peroxide cytotoxicity. *Am. J. Physiol. Lung Cell. Mol. Physiol.* **2007**, *293*, 1194–1207. [CrossRef] [PubMed]

90. Lazaar, A.L.; Panettieri, R.A. Airway smooth muscle as a regulator of immune responses and bronchomotor tone. *Clin. Chest Med.* **2006**, *27*, 53–69. [CrossRef] [PubMed]

91. Chiappara, G.; Gagliardo, R.; Siena, A.; Bonsignore, M.R.; Bousquet, J.; Bonsignore, G.; Vignola, A.M. Airway remodelling in the pathogenesis of asthma. *Curr. Opin. Allergy Clin. Immunol.* **2001**, *1*, 85–93. [CrossRef] [PubMed]

92. Feigin, V. Global, regional, and national life expectancy, all-cause mortality, and cause-specific mortality for 249 causes of death, 1980–2015: A systematic analysis for the Global Burden of Disease Study 2015. *Lancet* **2016**, *388*, 1459–1544.

93. Vos, T.; Allen, C.; Arora, M.; Barber, R.M.; Bhutta, Z.A.; Brown, A.; Carter, A.; Casey, D.C.; Charlson, F.J.; Chen, A.Z.; et al. Global, regional, and national incidence, prevalence, and years lived with disability for 310 diseases and injuries, 1990–2015: A systematic analysis for the Global Burden of Disease Study 2015. *Lancet* **2016**, *388*, 1545–1602. [CrossRef]

94. Wolff, P.T.; Arison, L.; Rahajamiakatra, A.; Raserijaona, F.; Niggemann, B. High asthma prevalence and associated factors in urban malagasy schoolchildren. *J. Asthma* **2012**, *49*, 575–580. [CrossRef] [PubMed]

95. Adeloye, D.; Chan, K.Y.; Rudan, I.; Campbell, H. An estimate of asthma prevalence in Africa: A systematic analysis. *Croatian Med. J.* **2013**, *54*, 519–531. [CrossRef]

96. Bertorelli, G.; Bocchino, V.; Zhuo, X.; Chetta, A.; Del Donno, M.; Foresi, A.; Testi, R.; Olivieri, D. Heat shock protein 70 upregulation is related to HLA-DR expression in bronchial asthma. Effects of inhaled glucocorticoids. *Clin. Exp. Allergy* **1998**, *28*, 551–560. [CrossRef] [PubMed]

97. Changchun, H.; Haijin, Z.; Wenjun, L.; Zhenyu, L.; Dan, Z.; Laiyu, L.; Wancheng, T.; Shao-Xi, C.; Fei, Z. Increased heat shock protein 70 levels in induced sputum and plasma correlate with severity of asthma patients. *Cell Stress Chaperones* **2011**, *16*, 663–671. [CrossRef] [PubMed]

98. Vignola, A.M.; Chanez, P.; Polla, B.S.; Vic, P.; Godard, P.; Bousquet, J. Increased expression of heat shock protein 70 on airway cells in asthma and chronic bronchitis. *Am. J. Respir. Cell. Mol. Biol.* **1995**, *13*, 683–691. [CrossRef] [PubMed]

99. Polla, B.S.; Bachelet, M.; Dall'Ava, J.; Vignola, A.M. Heat shock proteins in inflammation and asthma: Dr Jekyll or Mr Hyde? *Clin. Exp. Allergy* **1998**, *28*, 527–529. [CrossRef] [PubMed]

100. Aron, Y.; Busson, M.; Polla, B.S.; Dusser, D.; Lockhart, A.; Swierczewski, E.; Favatier, F. Analysis of HSP70 gene polymorphism in allergic asthma. *Allergy* **1999**, *54*, 165–170. [CrossRef] [PubMed]

101. Wong, H.R.; Wispe, J.R. The stress response and the lung. *Am. J. Physiol. Lung Cell. Mol. Physiol.* **1997**, *273*, L1–L9.

102. Shingai, R.; Maeda, T.; Onishi, S.; Yamamoto, Y. Autoantibody against 70 kD heat shock protein in patients with autoimmune liver diseases. *J. Hepatol.* **1995**, *23*, 382–390. [CrossRef]

103. Xu, Q.; Kiechl, S.; Mayr, M.; Metzler, B.; Egger, G.; Oberhollenzer, F.; Willeit, J.; Wick, G. Association of serum antibodies to heat-shock protein 65 with carotid atherosclerosis. *Circulation* **1999**, *100*, 1169–1174. [CrossRef] [PubMed]

104. Salman, A.N. Serum Levels Evaluation of Heat Shock Protein70 during Gestation and Fetal Birth Weight in Asthmatic Women of Thi-QAR Province, Iraq. *J. Al-Nahrain Univ.* **2015**, *18*, 117–122. [CrossRef]

105. Schatz, M. Is maternal asthma a life or death issue for the baby? *Thorax* **2009**, *64*, 93–95. [CrossRef] [PubMed]

106. Yang, M.; Wu, T.; Cheng, L.; Wang, F.; Wei, Q.; Tanguay, R.M. Plasma antibodies against heat shock protein 70 correlate with the incidence and severity of asthma in a Chinese population. *Respir. Res.* **2005**, *6*. [CrossRef] [PubMed]

107. PeRIšIć, T.; Srećković, M.; Matić, G. Changes of antioxidant enzyme activity and heat shock protein content in lymphocytes of children with asthma. *Arch. Biol. Sci.* **2007**, *59*, 257–266. [CrossRef]

108. Tong, W.; Luo, W. Heat shock proteins' mRNA expression in asthma. *Respirology* **2000**, *5*, 227–230. [CrossRef] [PubMed]

109. Karin, M.; Greten, F.R. NF-[kappa] B: Linking inflammation and immunity to cancer development and progression. *Nat. Rev. Immunol.* **2005**, *5*, 749–759. [CrossRef] [PubMed]

110. Torre, L.A.; Bray, F.; Siegel, R.L.; Ferlay, J.; Lortet-Tieulent, J.; Jermal, A. Global cancer statistics 2012. *CA Cancer J. Clin.* **2015**, *65*, 87–108. [CrossRef] [PubMed]

111. Hanahan, D.; Weinberg, R.A. The hallmarks of cancer. *Cell* **2000**, *100*, 57–70. [CrossRef]

112. Calderwood, S.K.; Stevenson, M.A.; Murshid, A. Heat shock proteins, autoimmunity, and cancer treatment. *Autoimmun. Dis.* **2012**, *2012*, 486069. [CrossRef] [PubMed]

113. Kapoor, C.; Vaidya, S. Heat shock protein (HSP) and cancer: An overview. *Am. J. Med. Dent. Sci.* **2013**, *1*, 31–34.

114. Beere, H.M.; Green, D.R. Stress management–heat shock protein-70 and the regulation of apoptosis. *Trends Cell Biol.* **2001**, *11*, 6–10. [CrossRef]

115. Wu, J.; Liu, T.; Rios, Z.; Mei, Q.; Lin, X.; Cao, S. Heat shock proteins and cancer. *Trends Pharmacol. Sci.* **2017**, *38*, 226–256. [CrossRef] [PubMed]

116. Vergara, D.; Simeone, P.; del Boccio, P.; Toto, C.; Pieragostino, D.; Tinelli, A.; Acierno, R.; Alberti, S.; Salzet, M.; Giannelli, G.; et al. Comparative proteome profiling of breast tumor cell lines by gel electrophoresis and mass spectrometry reveals an epithelial mesenchymal transition associated protein signature. *Mol. BioSyst.* **2013**, *9*, 1127–1138. [CrossRef] [PubMed]

117. Shiota, M.; Bishop, J.L.; Nip, K.M.; Zardan, A.; Takeuchi, A.; Cordonnier, T.; Beraldi, E.; Bazov, J.; Fazli, L.; Chi, K.; et al. Hsp27 regulates epithelial mesenchymal transition, metastasis, and circulating tumor cells in prostate cancer. *Cancer Res.* **2013**, *73*, 3109–3119. [CrossRef] [PubMed]

118. Lianos, G.D.; Alexiou, G.A.; Mangano, A.; Mangano, A.; Rausei, S.; Boni, L.; Dionigi, G.; Roukos, D.H. The role of heat shock proteins in cancer. *Cancer Lett.* **2015**, *360*, 114–118. [CrossRef] [PubMed]

119. Jego, G.; Hazoumé, A.; Seigneuric, R.; Garrido, C. Targeting heat shock proteins in cancer. *Cancer Lett.* **2013**, *332*, 275–285. [CrossRef] [PubMed]

120. Chaiwatanasirikul, K.A.; Sala, A. The tumour-suppressive function of CLU is explained by its localisation and interaction with HSP60. *Cell Death Dis.* **2011**, *2*, e219. [CrossRef] [PubMed]

121. Ghosh, J.C.; Siegelin, M.D.; Dohi, T.; Altieri, D.C. Heat shock protein 60 regulation of the mitochondrial permeability transition pore in tumor cells. *Cancer Res.* **2010**, *70*, 8988–8993. [CrossRef] [PubMed]

122. Chalmin, F.; Ladoire, S.; Mignot, G.; Vincent, J.; Bruchard, M.; Remy-Martin, J.P.; Boireau, W.; Rouleau, A.; Simon, B.; Lanneau, D.; et al. Membrane-associated Hsp72 from tumor-derived exosomes mediates STAT3-dependent immunosuppressive function of mouse and human myeloid-derived suppressor cells. *J. Clin. Investig.* **2010**, *120*, 457–471. [CrossRef] [PubMed]

123. Trinh, D.L.; Elwi, A.N.; Kim, S.W. Direct interaction between p53 and Tid1 proteins affects p53 mitochondrial localization and apoptosis. *Oncotarget* **2010**, *1*, 396–404. [CrossRef] [PubMed]

124. Spooner, R.; Yilmaz, Ö. The role of reactive-oxygen-species in microbial persistence and inflammation. *Int. J. Mol. Sci.* **2011**, *12*, 334–352. [CrossRef] [PubMed]

125. Simon, H.U.; Haj-Yehia, A.; Levi-Schaffer, F. Role of reactive oxygen species (ROS) in apoptosis induction. *Apoptosis* **2000**, *5*, 415–418. [CrossRef] [PubMed]

126. Fischer, R.; Maier, O. Interrelation of oxidative stress and inflammation in neurodegenerative disease: Role of TNF. *Oxid. Med. Cell. Longev.* **2015**, *2015*, 610813. [CrossRef] [PubMed]

127. Nowsheen, S.; Yang, E.S. The intersection between DNA damage response and cell death pathways. *Exp. Oncol.* **2012**, *34*, 243–254. [PubMed]

128. Nita, M.; Grzybowski, A. The role of the reactive oxygen species and oxidative stress in the pathomechanism of the age-related ocular diseases and other pathologies of the anterior and posterior eye segments in adults. *Oxid. Med. Cell. Longev.* **2016**, *2016*, 3164734. [CrossRef] [PubMed]

129. Barnes, P.J. Reactive oxygen species and airway inflammation. *Free Radic. Biol. Med.* **1990**, *9*, 235–243. [CrossRef]

130. Henricks, P.A.; Nijkamp, F.P. Reactive oxygen species as mediators in asthma. *Pulm. Pharmacol. Ther.* **2001**, *14*, 409–421. [CrossRef] [PubMed]

131. Winrow, V.R.; McLean, L.; Morris, C.J.; Blake, D.R. The heat shock protein response and its role in inflammatory disease. *Ann. Rheum. Dis.* **1990**, *49*, 128–132. [CrossRef] [PubMed]

132. Chen, Y.; Voegeli, T.S.; Liu, P.P.; Noble, E.G.; Currie, R.W. Heat shock paradox and a new role of heat shock proteins and their receptors as anti-inflammation targets. *Inflamm. Allergy Drug Targets* **2007**, *6*, 91–100. [CrossRef] [PubMed]

133. Hauet-Broere, F.; Wieten, L.; Guichelaar, T.; Berlo, S.; Van der Zee, R.; Van Eden, W. Heat shock proteins induce T cell regulation of chronic inflammation. *Ann. Rheum. Dis.* **2006**, *65*, 65–68. [CrossRef] [PubMed]

134. Tóth, M.E.; Gombos, I.; Sántha, M. Heat shock proteins and their role in human diseases. *Acta Biol. Szeged.* **2015**, *59*, 121–141.

135. Arnal, M.E.; Lallès, J.P. Gut epithelial inducible heat-shock proteins and their modulation by diet and the microbiota. *Nutr. Rev.* **2016**, *74*, 181–197. [CrossRef] [PubMed]

136. Goldstein, M.G.; Li, Z. Heat-shock proteins in infection-mediated inflammation-induced tumorigenesis. *J. Hematol. Oncol.* **2009**, *2*. [CrossRef] [PubMed]

137. Hatfield, P.D.; Lovas, S. Role of Hsp70 in cancer growth and survival. *Protein Pept. Lett.* **2012**, *19*, 616–624. [CrossRef] [PubMed]

138. Chauhan, D.; Li, G.; Hideshima, T.; Podar, K.; Mitsiades, C.; Mitsiades, N.; Catley, L.; Tai, Y.T.; Hayashi, T.; Shringarpure, R.; et al. Hsp27 inhibits release of mitochondrial protein Smac in multiple myeloma cells and confers dexamethasone resistance. *Blood* **2003**, *102*, 3379–3386. [CrossRef] [PubMed]

139. Nylandsted, J.; Rohde, M.; Brand, K.; Bastholm, L.; Elling, F.; Jäättelä, M. Selective depletion of heat shock protein 70 (HSP70) activates a tumor-specific death program that is independent of caspases and bypasses Bcl-2. *Proc. Natl. Acad. Sci. USA* **2000**, *97*, 7871–7876. [CrossRef] [PubMed]

140. Zininga, T.; Shonhai, A. Are heat shock proteins druggable candidates? *Am. J. Biochem. Biotech.* **2014**, *8*, 427–432. [CrossRef]

141. Henstridge, D.C.; Febbraio, M.A.; Hargreaves, M. Heat shock proteins and exercise adaptations. Our knowledge thus far and the road still ahead. *J. Appl. Physiol.* **2016**, *120*, 683–691. [CrossRef] [PubMed]

142. Noble, E.G.; Shen, G.X. Impact of exercise and metabolic disorders on heat shock proteins and vascular inflammation. *Autoimmun. Dis.* **2012**, *2012*, 836519. [CrossRef] [PubMed]

143. Naughton, L.; Lovell, R.; Madden, L. Heat shock proteins in exercise: A review. *J. Exerc. Sci. Physiother.* **2006**, *2*, 13–26.

2

Proximal Pathway Enrichment Analysis for Targeting Comorbid Diseases via Network Endopharmacology

Joaquim Aguirre-Plans [1] ⓘ**, Janet Piñero** [1] ⓘ**, Jörg Menche** [2] ⓘ**, Ferran Sanz** [1]**, Laura I. Furlong** [1]**,
Harald H. H. W. Schmidt** [3]**, Baldo Oliva** [1] **and Emre Guney** [1,3,]* ⓘ

[1] Research Programme on Biomedical Informatics, the Hospital del Mar Medical Research Institute and
   Pompeu Fabra University, Dr. Aiguader 88, 08003 Barcelona, Spain; joaquim.aguirre@upf.edu (J.A.-P.);
   janet.pinero@upf.edu (J.P.); ferran.sanz@upf.edu (F.S.); laura.furlong@upf.edu (L.I.F.);
   baldo.oliva@upf.edu (B.O.)
[2] CeMM Research Center for Molecular Medicine of the Austrian Academy of Sciences, Lazarettgasse 14,
   AKH BT 25.3, A-1090 Vienna, Austria; JMenche@cemm.oeaw.ac.at
[3] Department of Pharmacology and Personalised Medicine, CARIM, FHML, Maastricht University,
   Universiteitssingel 50, 6229 ER Maastricht, The Netherlands; h.schmidt@maastrichtuniversity.nl
*   Correspondence: emre.guney@upf.edu

Abstract: The past decades have witnessed a paradigm shift from the traditional drug discovery shaped around the idea of "one target, one disease" to polypharmacology (multiple targets, one disease). Given the lack of clear-cut boundaries across disease (endo)phenotypes and genetic heterogeneity across patients, a natural extension to the current polypharmacology paradigm is to target common biological pathways involved in diseases via endopharmacology (multiple targets, multiple diseases). In this study, we present proximal pathway enrichment analysis (PxEA) for pinpointing drugs that target common disease pathways towards network endopharmacology. PxEA uses the topology information of the network of interactions between disease genes, pathway genes, drug targets and other proteins to rank drugs by their interactome-based proximity to pathways shared across multiple diseases, providing unprecedented drug repurposing opportunities. Using PxEA, we show that many drugs indicated for autoimmune disorders are not necessarily specific to the condition of interest, but rather target the common biological pathways across these diseases. Finally, we provide high scoring drug repurposing candidates that can target common mechanisms involved in type 2 diabetes and Alzheimer's disease, two conditions that have recently gained attention due to the increased comorbidity among patients.

Keywords: drug repurposing; proximal pathway enrichment analysis; network endopharmacology; systems medicine; comorbidity; autoimmune disorders; Alzheimer's disease; type 2 diabetes

1. Introduction

Following Paul Ehrlich's more-than-a-century-old proposition on magic bullets (one drug, one target, one disease), the drug discovery pipeline traditionally pursues a handful of leads identified in vitro based on their potential to bind to target(s) known to modulate the disease [1]. The success of the selected lead in the consequent clinical validation process relies on the prediction of a drug's effect in vivo. Although it is often more desirable to tinker the cellular network by targeting multiple proteins [2], this is hard to achieve in practice due to the interactions of the compound and its targets with other proteins and metabolites. As a result, the characterization of drug effect has been a daunting task, yielding high pre-clinical attrition rates for novel compounds [3,4].

The high attrition rates can be attributed to the immense response heterogeneity across patients, likely stemming from a polygenic nature of most complex diseases. Consequently, researchers have turned their attention to polypharmacology, where novel therapies aim to alter multiple targets involved in the pathway cross-talk pertinent to the disease pathology, rather than single proteins [5,6]. This has given rise to network-based approaches that predict the effects of individual drugs [7] as well as drug combinations [8], allowing for the repositioning of compounds for novel indications.

Over the past years, reusing existing drugs for conditions different from their intended indications has emerged as a cost effective alternative to traditional drug discovery. Various drug repurposing methods aim to mimic the most likely therapeutic and safety outcomes of candidate compounds based on similarities between compounds and diseases characterized by high-throughput omics data [9–11]. Most studies so far, however, have focused on repurposing drugs for a single condition of interest, failing to recognize the cellular, genetic and ontological complexity inherent to human diseases [12,13]. In reality, pathway cross-talk plays an important role in modulating the pathophysiology of diseases [14] and most comorbid diseases are interconnected to each other in the interactome through proteins belonging to similar pathways [15–19]. The pathway cross-talk is especially relevant for autoimmune disorders, which have been shown to share several biological functions involved in immune and inflammatory responses [20,21]. Autoimmune disorders affect around 15% of the population in the USA [22] and co-occur in the same patient more often than expected (i.e., comorbid) [23]. Recent evidence suggests that endophenotypes—shared intermediate pathophenotypes—[24], such as inflammasome, thrombosome, and fibrosome play essential roles in the progression of not only autoimmune disorders but also many other diseases [25].

Here, we propose a novel drug repurposing approach, **Proximal pathway Enrichment Analysis (PxEA)**, to specifically target intertangled biological pathways involved in the common pathology of complex diseases. We first identify pathways proximal to disease genes across various autoimmune disorders. Then we use PxEA to investigate whether the drugs promiscuously used in these disorders target specifically the pathways associated with one disease or the pathways shared across the diseases. We find several examples of anti-inflammatory drugs where the pathways proximal to the drug targets in the interactome correspond to the pathways shared between two autoimmune disorders. The observed lack of specificity among these drugs points to the existence of immune system related endophenotypes, motivating us to explore shared disease mechanisms for repurposing drugs. We demonstrate that PxEA is a powerful computational strategy for targeting multiple pathologies involving common biological pathways, such as type 2 diabetes (T2D) and Alzheimer's disease (AD). Based on these findings, we argue that PxEA paves the way for simultaneously targeting endophenotypes that manifest across various diseases, a concept which we refer to as *endopharmacology*.

2. Results

2.1. Pathway Proximity Captures the Similarities between Autoimmune Disorders

Conventionally, functional enrichment analysis relies on the significance of the overlap between a set of genes belonging to a condition of interest and a list of genes involved in known biological processes (pathways). Using known pathway genes, one can identify pathways associated with the disease via a statistical test (e.g., Fisher's exact test for the overlap between genes or z-score comparing the observed number of common genes to the number of genes one would have in common if genes were randomly sampled from the data set). We start with the observation that such an approach (hereafter referred as to *conventional* approach) often misses key biological processes involved in the disease due to the limited overlap between the disease and pathway genes. To show that this is the case, we focus on nine autoimmune disorders for which we obtain genes associated with the disease in the literature and we calculate p-values based on the overlap between these genes and the pathway genes for each of the 674 pathways in the Reactome database (Fisher's exact test, one-sided $p \leq 0.05$). Intriguingly, Table 1 demonstrates that this conventional approach yields less than ten pathways that are significantly enriched in five out of nine diseases, potentially underestimating the molecular underpinning of these diseases.

Table 1. Number of pathways enriched across nine autoimmune disorders based on the overlap between the pathway and disease genes (one-sided $p \leq 0.05$, assessed by a Fisher's exact test) and the proximity of the pathway genes to the disease genes in the interactome ($z \leq -2$, see Methods for details).

Disease	# of Pathways	
	Overlap	Proximity
celiac disease	7	143
Crohn's disease	5	116
diabetes mellitus, insulin-dependent	16	121
Graves' disease	3	92
lupus erythematosus, systemic	17	98
multiple sclerosis	12	138
psoriasis	5	50
rheumatoid arthritis	55	17
ulcerative colitis	6	138

Alternatively, the shortest distance between genes in the interactome can be used to find pathways closer than random expectation to a given set of genes [7,26], augmenting substantially the number of pathways relevant to the disease pathology. Using network-based proximity [7], we define the *pathway span* of a disease as the set of pathways significantly proximal to the disease ($z \leq -2$, see Methods). We show that the number of pathways involved in diseases increases substantially when proximity is used (Table 1).

To show the biological relevance of the identified pathways using interactome-based proximity, we check how well these pathways can highlight genetic and phenotypic relationships between nine autoimmune disorders. First, to serve as a background model, we build a disease network for the autoimmune disorders (diseasome) using the genes and symptoms shared between these diseases as well as the comorbidity information extracted from medical insurance claim records (see Methods). The autoimmune diseasome (Figure 1a) is extremely connected, covering 33 out of 36 potential links between nine diseases (with average degree $< k > = 7.3$ and clustering coefficient $CC = 0.93$). The three missing links are those between ulcerative colitis and rheumatoid arthritis, ulcerative colitis and Graves' disease, and Graves' disease and type 1 diabetes. On the other hand, several diseases such as celiac disease, Crohn's disease, systemic lupus erythematosus, and multiple sclerosis are connected to each other with multiple evidence types in the autoimmune diseasome based on genetic (shared genes) and phenotypic (shared symptoms and comorbidity) similarities, emphasizing the shared pathological components underlying these diseases.

We compare the autoimmune diseasome generated using shared genes, common symptoms and comorbidity, to the disease network in which the disease-disease connections are identified using the pathways they share. We identify the pathways enriched in the diseases using both the conventional and proximity approaches mentioned above and check whether the number of common pathways between two diseases is significant (two-tailed Fisher's exact test, $p < 0.05$). The disease network based on pathways shared across diseases using the overlap between the pathway and disease genes is markedly sparser than the original diseasome, containing 17 links (Figure 1b). None of the diseases share pathways with psoriasis and among the connections supported by multiple evidence in the original diseasome, the links between Crohn's disease and celiac disease as well as Crohn's disease and systemic lupus erythematosus are missing. On the contrary, the disease network based on shared pathways using proximity of the pathway genes to the disease genes consists of 34 links, where the only unconnected disease pairs are Crohn's disease and Graves' disease and type 1 diabetes and psoriasis, suggesting that it captures the connectedness of the original diseasome better than the conventional approach.

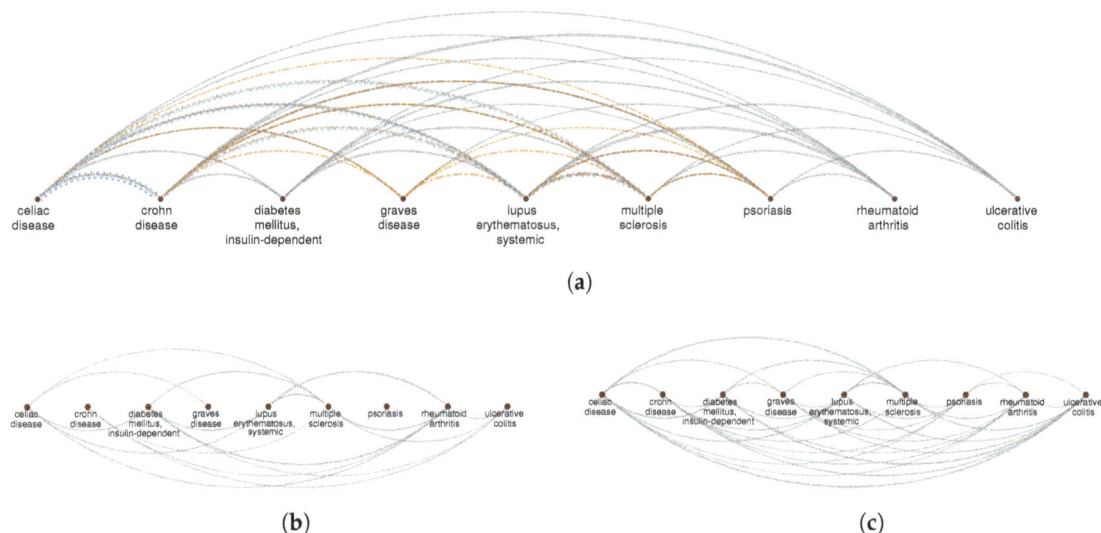

(a)

(b)   (c)

Figure 1. Genetic, phenotypic and functional overlap across autoimmune disorders. Disease relationships (links) based on (**a**) shared genes (gray solid lines), shared symptoms (orange dashed lines) and comorbidity (blue sinusoidal lines); (**b**) shared pathways (gray solid lines) using common disease and pathway genes, (**c**) shared pathways (gray solid lines) using the proximity of the pathway genes to the diseases genes in the interactome.

We next turn our attention to the shared pathways across diseases identified by both conventional and proximity based approaches and observe that most common pathways involve biological processes relevant to the immune system endophenotypes. In particular, we see that inflammasome-related pathways, such as signaling of cytokines (interferon gamma, interleukins like IL6, IL7) and lymphocytes (ZAP70, PD1, TCR, among others) are overrepresented. While conventional enrichment finds that most of these pathways are shared among only 4–5 diseases, proximity based enrichment points to the commonality of these pathways among almost all the diseases. Furthermore, the proximity based enrichment uncovers the involvement of additional interleukin (IL2, IL3, IL5) and lymphocyte (BCR) molecules ubiquitously in autoimmune disorders. These findings suggest that proximity-based pathway enrichment identifies biological processes relevant to the diseases, highlighting the common etiology across autoimmune disorders.

2.2. Diseases Targeted by the Same Drugs Exhibit Functional Similarities

Having observed that pathway proximity to diseases in the interactome captures the underlying biological mechanisms across diseases, we seek to investigate the potential implications of the connections between diseases for drug discovery. We hypothesize that a drug indicated for several autoimmune disorders would exert its effect by targeting the shared biological pathways across these diseases. To test this, we use 25 drugs that are indicated for two or more of the autoimmune disorders in Hetionet [27] and split disease pairs into two groups: (i) diseases for which a common drug exists and (ii) diseases for which no drugs are shared. We then count the number of pathways in common between two diseases for each pair in the two groups using pathway enrichment based on both the gene overlap and proximity in the interactome. We find that the diseases targeted by the same drugs tend to involve an elevated number of common pathways compared to the disease pairs that do not have any drug in common (Figure 2). The average number of pathways shared among diseases that are targeted by the same drug is 3.4 and 38 using overlap and proximity based enrichment, respectively, whereas, the remaining disease pairs share 2 and 31 pathways on average using the two enrichment approaches. We note that due to the relatively small sample size and potentially incomplete drug indication information, we interpret the elevated number of pathways as a trend rather than a general rule across all diseases ($p = 0.043$ and $p = 0.066$, assessed by one-tailed Mann-Whitney U test, for the overlap and proximity based approaches, respectively). Nevertheless, taken together with the high overall pathway level commonalities observed in the autoimmune disorders mentioned in the previous section, this result suggests that the drugs used for multiple indications are likely to target common pathways involved in these diseases.

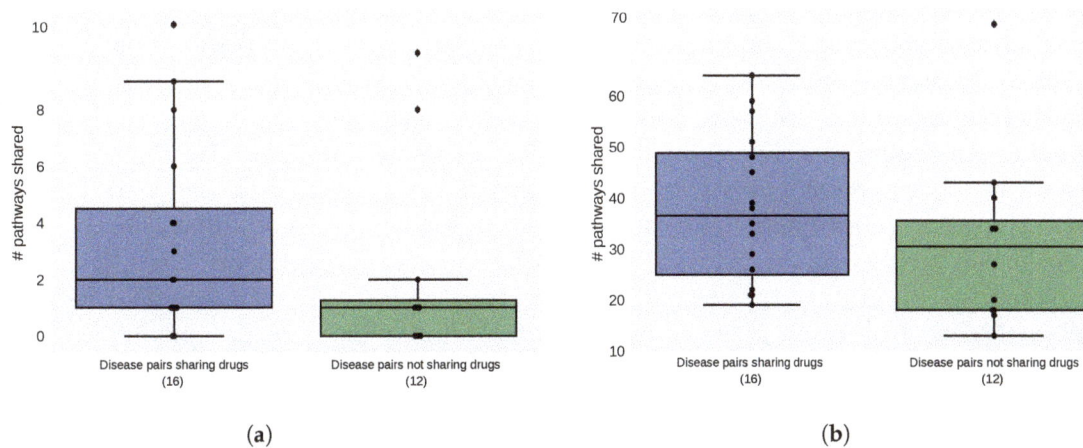

Figure 2. Number of shared pathways across disease pairs that are targeted by the same drug compared to the rest of the pairs. The pathway enrichment is calculated using (**a**) gene overlap and (**b**) proximity of genes in the interactome. The number of disease pairs in each group is given in the parenthesis below the group label in the x-axis.

2.3. Proximal Pathway Enrichment Analysis Reveals Drugs Targeting the Autoimmune Endophenotypes

The results indicating that the drugs used for multiple autoimmune disorders potentially target common pathways raise the following question: "Can pathway level commonalities between diseases be leveraged to quantify the impact of a given drug on these diseases?" To this end, we propose PxEA, a novel method for **P**roximal pathway **E**nrichment **A**nalysis that scores the likelihood of a set of pathways (e.g., targeted by a drug) to be represented among another set of pathways (e.g., disease pathways) based on the proximity of the pathway genes in the interactome. As opposed to the Gene Set Enrichment Analysis (GSEA) [28] which uses gene sets and the ranking of genes based on differential expression, PxEA uses pathway sets and the ranking of pathways based on proximity in the interactome. PxEA scores a drug based on whether or not the pathways targeted by the drug are proximal to a pathway set of interest, such as pathways shared across different diseases. For a given drug and a pair of diseases, we first identify the pathways in the pathway span of both of the diseases, then we rank the pathways with respect to the proximity of the drug targets to the pathway genes and finally we calculate a running sum statistics corresponding to the enrichment score between the drug and the disease pair (Figure 3, see Methods for details).

We employ PxEA to score 25 drugs indicated for at least two of the seven autoimmune disorders (there were no common drugs for celiac and Graves' diseases). For each disease, we first run PxEA using the pathways proximal to the disease and the proximity of the drugs used for that disease to these pathways. We then run PxEA for each disease pair, using the pathways proximal to both of the diseases in the pair and the drugs commonly used for the two diseases. We notice that several drugs indicated for multiple conditions score higher using common pathways between two diseases than using the pathways of the disease they are indicated for (Figure 4). This is not surprising considering that many of the drugs used for autoimmune disorders target common immune and inflammatory processes. For instance, sildenafil, a drug used for the treatment of erectile dysfunction and to relieve the symptoms of pulmonary arterial hypertension, is reported by Hetionet to show palliative effect on type 1 diabetes and multiple sclerosis. Actually, sildenafil is not specific to any of these two conditions and targets a number of the 57 pathways in common between type 1 diabetes and multiple sclerosis including but not limited to pathways mentioned in Table 2, such as "IL-3, 5 and GM CSF signaling" ($z = -1.6$), "regulation of signaling by CBL" ($z = -1.1$), "regulation of KIT signaling" ($z = -1.0$), "IL receptor SHC signaling" ($z = -1.0$), and "growth hormone receptor signaling" ($z = -1.0$).

Similarly, prednisone, a synthetic anti-inflammatory glucocorticoid agent that is indicated for six of the autoimmune disorders, is assigned a higher PxEA score using the pathways shared by Crohn's disease and systemic lupus erythematosus compared to using the pathways involved only in Crohn's disease, systemic lupus erythematosus, multiple sclerosis, psoriasis, rheumatoid arthritis, or ulcerative colitis. Thus, prednisone does not specifically target any of the six autoimmune disorders but rather acts on the endophenotypes that manifest across these diseases. We observe a similar trend in meloxicam, an anti-inflammatory drug that shows analgesic and antipyretic effects by inhibiting prostaglandin synthesis. Consistent with its known mechanism of action, meloxicam is proximal to "cholesterol biosynthesis" ($z = -3.5$), "fatty acid, triacylglycerol, and ketone body metabolism" ($z = -2.0$), and "prostanoid ligand receptors" ($z = -1.7$) pathways in the interactome. While meloxicam is originally indicated for rheumatoid arthritis and systemic lupus erythematosus, the higher PxEA score when common arthritis and lupus pathways are used suggests that it targets common inflammatory processes in these two diseases.

Table 2. Pathways shared by autoimmune disorders based on the overlap and proximity of genes (only pathways that appear most commonly across diseases are shown).

Pathway	# of Shared Diseases	
	Overlap	Proximity
interferon gamma signaling	5	8
costimulation by the CD28 family	5	7
cytokine signaling in immune system	5	7
translocation of ZAP-70 to immunological synapse	5	6
phosphorylation of CD3 and TCR zeta chains	5	6
PD1 signaling	5	4
IL-6 signaling	4	8
generation of second messenger molecules	4	6
TCR signaling	4	6
signaling by ILs	3	9
immune system	3	7
downstream TCR signaling	3	7
interferon signaling	3	7
adaptive immune system	3	3
regulation of KIT signaling	2	7
IL-7 signaling	2	6
CTLA4 inhibitory signaling	2	5
chemokine receptors bind chemokines	2	3
extrinsic pathway for apoptosis	2	3
MHC class II antigen presentation	2	2
IL receptor SHC signaling	-	9
IL-3, 5 and GM CSF signaling	-	9
signaling by the B cell receptor BCR	-	8
regulation of IFNG signaling	-	8
growth hormone receptor signaling	-	8
IL-2 signaling	-	8
regulation of signaling by CBL	-	8

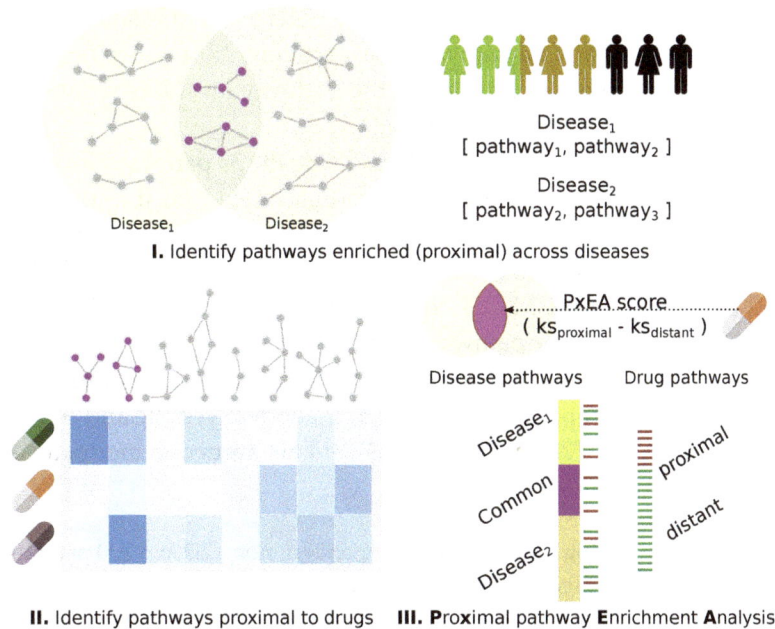

Figure 3. Schematic overview of proximal pathway enrichment analysis (PxEA). PxEA scores a drug with respect to its potential to target the pathways shared between two diseases. For a given drug and two diseases of interest, PxEA first identifies the common pathways between the two diseases and then uses the proximity-based ranking of the pathways (i.e., average distance in the interactome to the nearest pathway gene, normalized with respect to a background distribution of expected scores) to assign a score to the drug and the disease pair.

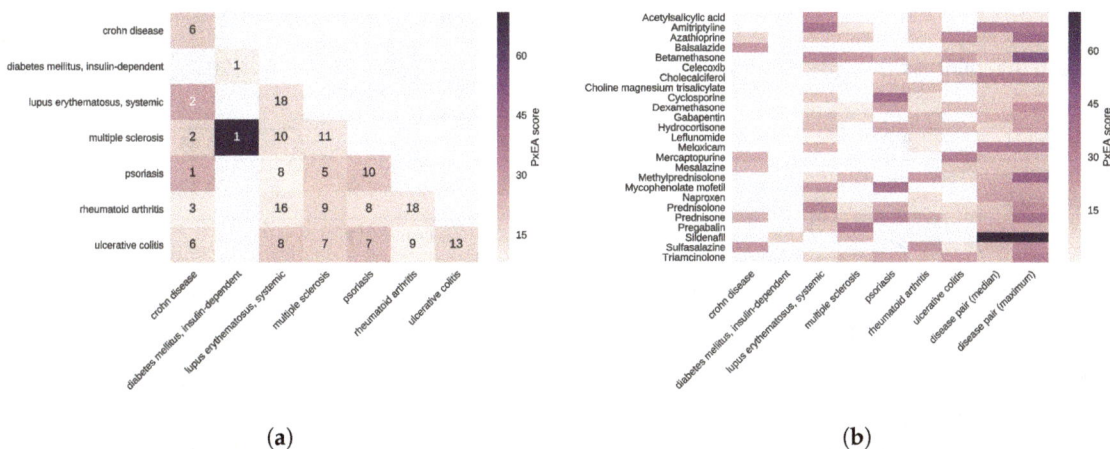

(a)   (b)

Figure 4. PxEA scores of drugs used in autoimmune disorders. (**a**) Disease-disease heatmap, in which for each disease pair, the common pathways proximal to the two diseases are used to run PxEA. Note that the diagonal contains the PxEA scores obtained when the proximal pathways for only that disease are used. The hue of the color scales with the PxEA score. (**b**) Drug-disease heatmap, in which the PxEA is run using the pathways proximal to the pathways of the disease in the column for the drugs in the rows (25 drugs that are used at least in two diseases). The last two columns show the median and maximum values of the PxEA scores obtained for the drug among all disease pairs the drug is indicated for.

2.4. Targeting the Common Pathology of Type 2 Diabetes and Alzheimer's Disease

T2D and AD, two diseases highly prevalent to an ageing society, are known to exhibit increased comorbidity [29,30]. Recently, repurposing anti-diabetic agents to prevent insulin resistance in AD has gained substantial attention due to the therapeutic potential it offers [31]. Indeed, the pathway spans of T2D and AD cover 170 and 82 pathways, respectively, 35 of which are shared between two diseases, linking significantly the two diseases at the pathway level (Fisher's exact test, two-sided $p = 2.2 \times 10^{-4}$).

We use PxEA to score 1466 drugs from DrugBank using the 35 pathways involved in the common pathology of T2D and AD. When we look at the drugs ranked on the top of the list (Table 3), we spot orlistat, a drug indicated for obesity and T2D in Hetionet. Interestingly, existing studies also suggest a role for this drug in the treatment of AD [32]. Orlistat targets extracellular communication (Ras-Raf-MEK-ERK, NOTCH, and GM-CSF/IL-3/IL-5 signaling) and lipid metabolism pathways (Figure 5). Several of the proteins in the pathways pertinent to the common T2D-AD pathology, such as APOA1, PSEN2, PNLIP, LPL, and IGHG1 are either Orlistat's targets themselves or are in the close vicinity of the targets. The next top scoring drugs are chenodeoxycholic and obeticholic acid, biliar acids that are in clinical trials for T2D (NCT01666223) and are argued to modulate cognitive changes in AD [33].

Table 3. Top ten drug repurposing opportunities to target common T2D and AD pathology, where the drugs that target the same proteins according to DrugBank are grouped together in the same row and the Anatomical Therapeutic Chemical (ATC) classification and indication information within the same group is marked with the first letter of the drug in the parenthesis (if applicable).

Drug	ATC	Hetionet Indication	DrugBank Indication	PxEA Score	Adjusted p-Value
orlistat	A08	obesity, type 2 diabetes	obesity	94.07	< 0.0001
obeticholic acid, chenodeoxycholic acid	A05	primary biliary cirrhosis (C)	liver disease (O), primary biliary cholangitis (O), gallbladders (C)	74.06	<0.0001
esmolol, practolol	C07	hypertension (E)	atrial fibrillation (E), noncompensatory sinus tachycardia (E), cardiac arrhythmias (P)	70.55	<0.0001
clenbuterol	R03	-	asthma	70.44	<0.0001
erythrityl tetranitrate	C01	-	angina	70.32	<0.0001
fenoterol, arbutamine, bupranolol	R03 (F), G02 (F) C01 (A), C07 (B)	-	asthma (F), coronary artery disease (A), hypertension (B), tachycardia (B), glaucoma (B)	68.97	<0.0001
dalfampridine	N07	multiple sclerosis	multiple sclerosis	68.44	<0.0001
magnesium sulfate	D11, V04, A06, B05, A12	-	eclampsia, acute nephritis, acute hypomagnesemia, uterine tetany	68.27	<0.0001
roflumilast, crisaborole	R03 (R)	chronic obstructive pulmonary disease (R)	chronic obstructive pulmonary disease (R), dermatitis (C), psoriasis (C)	66.33	<0.0001
montelukast	R03	chronic obstructive pulmonary disease, asthma, allergic rhinitis	asthma	65.94	<0.0001

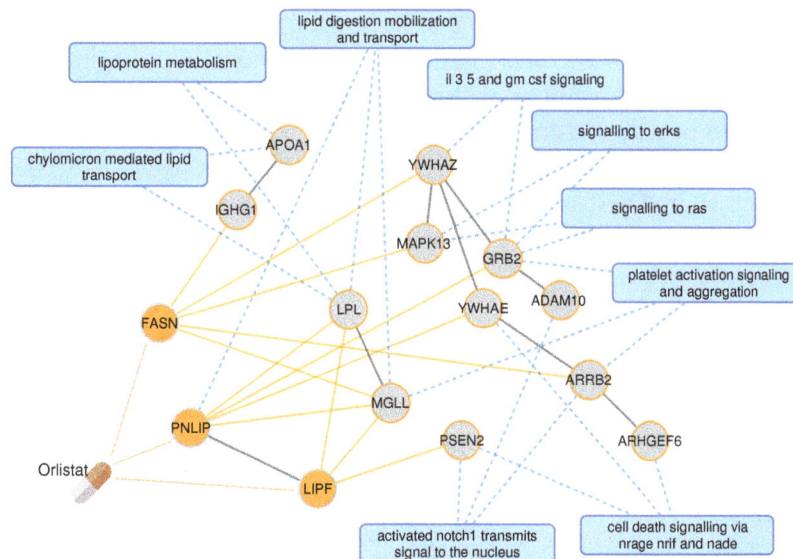

Figure 5. Orlistat from PxEA perspective. The subnetwork shows how the targets of Orlistat are connected to the nearest pathway protein for the pathways shared between T2D and AD. For clarity, only the pathways that are proximal to the drug are shown. Blue rectangles represent pathways, circles represent drug targets (orange) or proteins on the shortest path to the nearest pathway gene (gray). Blue dashed lines denote pathway membership, solid lines are protein interactions. The interactions between the drug and its targets are shown in dashed orange lines and the interactions between the drug targets and their neighbors are highlighted with solid orange lines.

It is noteworthy that the top scoring drugs belong to a diverse set of Anatomical Therapeutic Chemical (ATC) classes, covering alimentary tract and metabolism drugs (A05, A06, A08, A12), blood substitutes (B05), dermatologicals (D11) as well as cardiovascular (C01, C07), genito-urinary (G02), nervous (N07), and respiratory (R03) system drugs. The diversity of the ATC classes of top scoring drugs indicates that PxEA is not biased towards any particular ATC class. We also calculate the significance of the PxEA scores by permuting the ranking of the pathways. We find that the adjusted *p*-values (corrected for multiple hypothesis testing using Benjamini–Hochberg procedure) for the top candidates are all below 1×10^{-4}, the minimum possible value (due to the 10,000 permutations used in the calculation).

3. Discussion

The past decades have witnessed a substantial increase in human life expectancy owing to major breakthroughs in translational medicine. Yet, the increase on average age and changes in life style, have given rise to a spectra of problems challenging human health like cancer, neurodegenerative disorders and diabetes. These diseases do not only limit the life expectancy but also induce a high burden on public healthcare costs. In the US alone, more than 20 and 5 million people have been affected by T2D and AD, respectively, ranking these diseases among the most prevalent health problems [29].

Mainly characterized by hyperglycemia due to resistance to insulin, the disease mechanism of T2D involves a combination of multiple genetic and dietary factors. On the other hand, AD is relatively less understood and several hypotheses have been proposed for its cause: reduced synthesis of neurotransmitter acetylcholine, accumulation of amyloid beta plaques and/or tau protein abnormalities, giving rise to neurofibrillary tangles. Accordingly, most available treatments in AD are palliative (treating symptoms rather than the cause). Given the comorbidity between T2D and AD [29,30] several studies have recently suggested repurposing diabetes drugs for AD [31]. However, to our knowledge, currently there is no systematic method that can pinpoint drugs that could be useful to target common disease pathology such as the one between T2D and AD.

In this study, we first show that diseases that share drugs also tend to share biological pathways and hypothesize that these pathways can be targeted to exploit novel drug repurposing opportunities. We introduce PxEA, a method based on (i) pathways that are proximal to diseases and (ii) the ranking of the pathways targeted by a drug using the topology information encoded in the human interactome. We show that PxEA picks up whether drugs target specifically the pathways associated with a disease or common pathways shared across various conditions. We observe that many anti-inflammatory drugs are not specific to the condition they are used for and likely to target pathways involved in the autoimmune endophenotypes.

To further explore shared disease mechanisms for repurposing drugs, we use PxEA and rank drugs for their therapeutic potential in targeting the common disease pathology between T2D and AD. We identify orlistat, a semisynthetic derivative of lipstatin that inhibits lipase—a pancreatic enzyme that breaks down fat—as the top repurposing candidate. Orlistat inhibits hydrolysis of triglycerides, which in turn, reduces the absorption of monoaclglycerides and free fatty acids [34]. Recent evidence indicates that perturbations in unsaturated fatty acid metabolism are tightly coupled to neuritic plaque and neurofibrillary tangle formation in AD patients [35]. Thus, orlistat might help slowing down the plaque and tangle formation due to its effect on the fatty acid metabolism. Targeting of fatty acid metabolism for improving the cognitive performance presents a novel therapeutic approach and is further supported by experiments in mouse models [36].

PxEA can suggest rather counter-intuitive repositioning opportunities such as the use of clenbuterol, an asthmatic drug, in the treatment of metabolic and neurodegenerative diseases such as T2D and AD. In fact, the potential use of clenbuterol in these diseases is not too far fetched: it enhances cognitive performance in aging rats and monkeys [37], improves memory deficit in mice [38], and reduces the insulin resistance in obese rats [39]. On the flip side, while PxEA provides a cellular network based perspective to recommend drugs, it does not take into account dosage-related effects of drugs, potential adverse events, or the genetic background of the patients. For instance, practolol, a beta-adrenergic antagonist that stands out among the T2D-AD candidates, has been withdrawn from the market due to its high toxicity, limiting its potential therapeutic use in the clinical setting. Despite the limitations of PxEA, such as the incompleteness in the drug target, disease and pathway genes, lack of consideration of dosage-related effects or genetic heterogeneity, we believe PxEA is the first step towards achieving endopharmacology, that is, targeting endophenotypes involved across multiple diseases.

4. Materials and Methods

4.1. Protein Interaction Data and Interactome-Based Proximity

To define a global map of interactions between human proteins, we obtained the physical protein interaction data from a previous study that integrated various publicly available resources [16]. We downloaded the supplementary data accompanying the article to generate the human protein interaction network (interactome) containing data from MINT [40], BioGRID [41], HPRD [42], KEGG [43], BIGG [44], CORUM [45], and PhosphoSitePlus [46]. We used the largest connected component of the interactome in our analyses, which covered 141,150 interactions between 13,329 proteins (represented by ENTREZ gene ids).

Network-based proximity is a graph theoretic approach that incorporates the interactions of a set of genes (i.e., disease genes or drug targets) with other proteins in the human interactome and contextual information as to where the genes involved in pathways reside with respect to the original set of genes [7]. To quantify interactome-based proximity between two gene sets (such as drug targets, pathway genes or disease genes), we used the average shortest path length from the first set to the nearest protein in the second set following the definition in the original study [7]. Accordingly, the proximity from nodes S to nodes T in a network $G(V, E)$, is defined as

$$d(S, T) = \frac{1}{\|S\|} \sum_{u \in S} \min_{v \in T} d(u, v)$$

where $d(u, v)$ is the shortest path length between nodes u and v in G. We then calculated a z-score based on the distribution of the average shortest path lengths across random gene sets S_{random} and T_{random} ($d_{random}(S, T) = d(S_{random}, T_{random})$) as follows:

$$z(S, T) = \frac{d(S, T) - \mu_{d_{random}(S,T)}}{\sigma_{d_{random}(S,T)}}$$

where $\mu_{d_{random}(S,T)}$ and $\sigma_{d_{random}(T,S)}$ are the mean and the standard deviation of the $d_{random}(S, T)$, respectively, obtained using 1000 realizations of random sampling of gene sets that match the original sets in size and degree. We refer to the pathways that are significantly proximal ($z \leq -2$) to a disease as the *pathway span* of the disease throughout text.

Note that, instead of average shortest path distances, one can also use random-walk based distances to calculate proximity between gene sets [26]. However, random walks in the networks are inherently biased towards high-degree nodes [47,48] and require additional statistical adjustment [26,48]. Sampling based on size and degree matched gene sets has been shown to be robust against data-incompleteness in the interactome and in the known pathway annotations [7,48].

To investigate the effect of noise in the pathway data, following the procedure proposed in [49], we created a synthetic pathway data set, in which we defined pathways using a certain percentage k of known disease genes in T2D and AD ($k = 10, 25, 50, 75, 90$). Hence, for each value of k, we created 10 groups of genes, containing a random sampling of $k\%$ of the T2D-associated genes. We repeated the procedure using the AD-associated genes, yielding 100 gold standard pathways (10 for each disease across 5 different values of k) that were subsets of the known disease genes. For each gold standard pathway, we then generated so called control pathway, that is, randomly selected group of genes in the interactome that match the size of the gold standard pathway under consideration. Next, we assessed the shortest path distance based proximity between the gold standard pathways and the disease genes (proximity of the gold standard T2D pathways to the T2D disease genes and of the gold standard AD pathways to the AD disease genes) and compared it to the proximity of the control pathways to the same disease genes. We also calculated the proximity using random walk scores as proposed in a previous study [50]. We used the random walk implementation in GUILD software package [51] with the default parameters. As one would expect, the gold standard pathways were significantly more proximal ($z \leq -2$) to the disease genes than the control pathways using both proximity calculation approaches (Figure 6). On the other hand, the shortest path distance based proximity distinguished better the overlap between the gold standard pathway genes and the disease genes by providing lower values than the random walk based proximity as the noise in the pathway information decreased (higher values of k in the gold pathways).

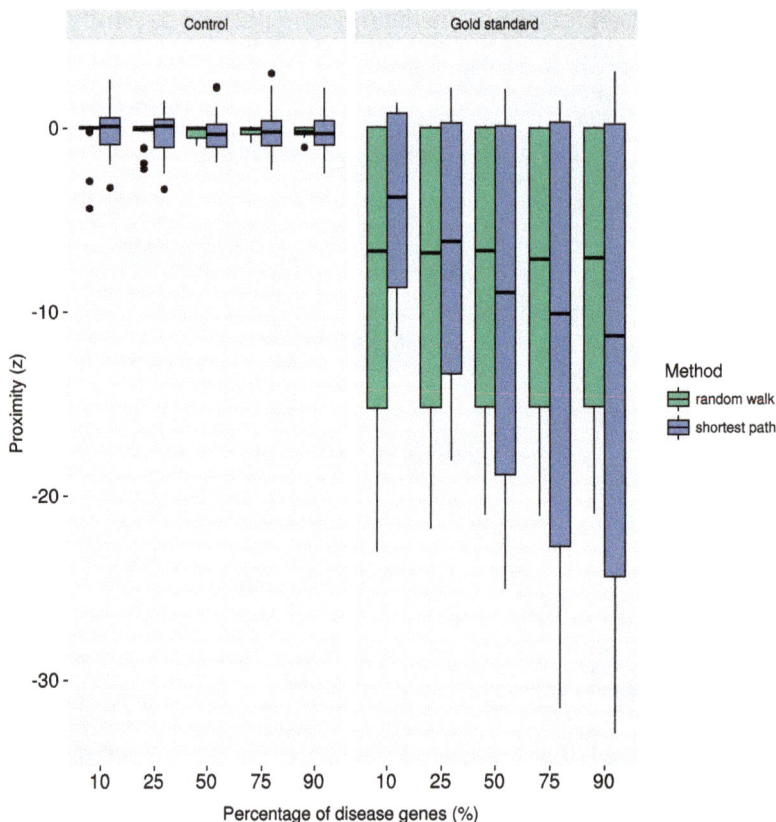

Figure 6. Effect of noise in the pathway data on the random walk and shortest path based proximity calculation. To assess the robustness of the interactome-based proximity in regards to noise in the pathway data, we generated synthetic gold standard pathways containing a certain proportion ($k\%$) of the known disease genes in T2D and AD (see text for details). We compared the proximity between these gold standard pathways and the disease genes to the proximity between the control pathways (random groups of gene in the interactome) and the disease genes. The proximity values using random walk and the shortest path for increasing k values are shown for the control and gold standard pathways.

4.2. Disease-Gene, Drug and Pathway Information

We compiled genes associated with nine autoimmune disorders listed in Table 4 using disease-gene annotations from DisGeNET [52]. We downloaded curated disease-gene associations from DisGeNET that contained infromation from UniProt [53], ClinVar [54], Orphanet [55], GWAS Catalog [56] and CTD [57]. To ensure that the disease-gene associations were of high confidence, we kept only the associations that were also provided in a previous large-scale analysis of human diseases [16].

We retrieved drug target information from DrugBank for 1489 drugs in the version 5.0.6 of the database [58], 1466 of which had at least a target in the interactome. UniProt ids from DrugBank were mapped to ENTREZ gene ids using UniProt id mapping file (retrieved on October 2017). We used drug indication information from Hetionet (compound treats or palliates disease edges) that compiled data from publicly available resources [27]. We focused on 78 drugs that were indicated for nine autoimmune disorders above. We created a subset of drugs used for two or more of the autoimmune disorders, yielding 25 drugs across seven conditions (there were no indications for celiac disease, and the two drugs used for Graves' disease were not used in any other disease).

The ENTREZ gene ids of the proteins involved in biological pathways were taken from the version 5.0 of MSigDB curated gene sets [59]. In our analysis, we used 674 Reactome [60] pathways and the genes associated with these pathways in the MSigDB.

Table 4. Disease-gene associations for the nine autoimmune disorders used in this study.

Disease	# of Genes	Genes
celiac disease	11	IL21 CCR4 HLA-DQA1 BACH2 RUNX3 ICOSLG SH2B3 CTLA4 MYO9B ZMIZ1 ETS1
Crohn's disease	19	DNMT3A IL12B IRGM IL10 CCL2 FUT2 SMAD3 TYK2 ATG16L1 BACH2 IL2RA NKX2-3 PTPN2 NOD2 TAGAP MST1 DENND1B IL23R ERAP2
diabetes mellitus, insulin-dependent	18	IL10 GLIS3 HLA-DQA1 HLA-DRB1 PTPN22 SLC29A3 INS BACH2 CLEC16A PAX4 HLA-DQB1 IL2RA CD69 IL27 HNF1A CTSH SH2B3 C1QTNF6
Graves' disease	4	RNASET2 CTLA4 FCRL3 TSHR
lupus erythematosus, systemic	29	IKZF1 CFB RASGRP3 PDCD1 RASGRP1 DNASE1 HLA-DRB1 PTPN22 ETS1 TNIP1 FCGR2B TNFSF4 IRF5 C2 PRDM1 PXK TLR5 TREX1 TNFAIP3 SLC15A4 PHRF1 HLA-DQA1 STAT4 ITGAX ITGAM BLK C4A BANK1 CR2
multiple sclerosis	15	CD58 CD6 IRF8 HLA-DQB1 CBLB HLA-DRA KIF1B IL2RA TNFSF14 VCAM1 IL7R HLA-DRB1 CD24 TNFRSF1A PTPRC
psoriasis	15	IL12B TNIP1 LCE3D IL13 IL23R TYK2 HLA-DQB1 HLA-C FBXL19 ERAP1 TRAF3IP2 TNFAIP3 TNF REL NOS2
rheumatoid arthritis	23	MIF CD40 ANKRD55 HLA-DRB1 PTPN22 RBPJ IL2RA AFF3 CCL21 REL SLC22A4 CCR6 IRF5 SPRED2 CTLA4 PADI4 TNFAIP3 NFKBIL1 HLA-DQA2 STAT4 IL6 BLK TRAF1
ulcerative colitis	24	IL12B JAK2 ICOSLG IL1R2 LSP1 CXCR2 IL10 IL7R CXCR1 DAP NKX2-3 CARD9 GNA12 IRF5 PRDM1 HNF4A CCNY SLC26A3 FCGR2A IL23R IL17REL MST1 TNFSF15 CDH3

4.3. Genetic, Phenotypic and Functional Relationships across Diseases

To identify relationships across disease pairs (autoimmune diseasome), we used the similarities between diseases in terms of the genes and symptoms they share. We assessed the significance of the overlap between genes (or symptoms) associated with two diseases using Fisher's exact test. An alpha value of 0.05 was set to deem the connections significant (two-sided test $p \leq 0.05$). The disease symptom information was taken from a previous study based on text mining of PubMed abstracts [61]. In this study, the number of times a symptom appears in a PubMed abstract was adjusted by the frequency of the symptom in the whole corpus using time frequency-inverse document frequency approach (TF-IDF). To ensure that the disease-symptom associations are of high quality, we considered associations with TF-IDF score higher than 3.5 as suggested in the original study.

Comorbidity relationships across diseases were inferred using data from medical insurance claims, where we assessed whether two diseases occurred more often in the same patient compared to the rest using the relative risk score [62]. Relative risk score relies on the relative occurrence frequencies of diseases across patients, adjusting for the prevalence of the diseases. We mapped the ICD9 codes to MeSH identifiers using the annotations provided by Disease Ontology [63] and we considered the disease pairs with a relative risk score higher than 1 as potential commorbidity links.

To identify pathways enriched in diseases, we used the significance (i) of the overlap between the pathway and disease genes assessed by a one-tailed Fisher's exact test and (ii) of the proximity between the pathway and disease genes in the interactome. We considered the pathways that had $p \leq 0.05$ and $z \leq -2$, respectively, as the pathways that were enriched in a given disease using the two approaches. The pathway information was taken from Reactome and the proximity was calculated as explained above.

4.4. PxEA: Proximal Pathway Enrichment Analysis

Toward the goal of pathway level characterization of the common pathology of diseases and to evaluate the therapeutic potential of drugs based on their impact on the common pathways, we developed **P**roximal pathway **E**nrichment **A**nalysis (PxEA), a novel method that scores drugs based on the proximity of drug targets to pathway genes in the interactome. PxEA uses a GSEA-like running sum score [28], where the pathways are ranked with respect to the proximity of drug targets to the pathways and each pathway is evaluated to see whether or not it appears among the pathways of interest (e.g., common pathways between two diseases). Given D, the pathways ranked with respect to their proximity to drug targets, p_i, the pathway in consideration within D, and C, the set of pathways of interest, the running score is defined as follows [64]:

$$ES(D,C) = \sum_{p_i \in D} X_i$$

where,

$$X_i = \{ \begin{array}{ll} \sqrt{\frac{|D|-|C|}{|C|}}, & if\ p_i \in C \\ -\sqrt{\frac{|C|}{|D|-|C|}}, & otherwise \end{array}$$

To calculate p-values for the case study, we repeat the procedure above 10,000 times, shuffling randomly D to calculate the expected enrichment score $ES(D^{random}, C)$. We then calculate the p-value for the enrichment using

$$P = \frac{|ES(D,C) < ES(D^{random}, C)|}{10,000}$$

The p-values were corrected for multiple hypothesis testing using Benjamini-Hochberg procedure [65].

4.5. Implementation Details and Code Availability

We used the toolbox Python package for running PxEA, available at github.com/emreg00/toolbox. The proximity was calculated using networkx package that implements Dijkstra's shortest path algorithm. The statistical tests were conducted in R (www.R-project.org) and Python (www.python.org). The network visualizations were generated using Cytoscape [66] and the plots were drawn using either Seaborn python package [67] or ggplot2 R package [68].

Author Contributions: Conceptualization, E.G.; Methodology, E.G.; Software, J.A.-P., J.P., E.G.; Validation, J.A.-P., J.P. and E.G.; Formal Analysis, J.A.-P. and E.G.; Investigation, J.A.-P., J.P. and E.G.; Resources, F.S., L.I.F., H.H.H.W.S., B.O. and E.G.; Data Curation, J.A.-P. and J.P.; Writing—Original Draft Preparation, J.A.-P. and E.G.; Writing—Review & Editing, J.A.-P., J.P., J.M., F.S., L.I.F, H.H.H.W.S., B.O. and E.G.; Visualization, J.A.-P., E.G.; Supervision, J.M., F.S., L.I.F., H.H.H.W.S., B.O., E.G.; Project Administration, E.G.; Funding Acquisition, J.M., F.S., L.I.F., H.H.H.W.S., B.O. and E.G.

Funding: The authors received funding from the Innovative Medicines Initiative 2 Joint Undertaking under grant agreement No. 116030. This Joint Undertaking receives support from the European Union's Horizon 2020 research and innovation programme and EFPIA. The authors also received support from EU H2020 Programme 2014–2020 under grant agreement No. 676559 (Elixir-Excelerate). E.G. was supported by EU-cofunded Beatriu de Pinós incoming fellowship from the Agency for Management of University and Research Grants (AGAUR) of Government of Catalunya and L.I.F. received support from ISCIII-FEDER (CPII16/00026). H.H.H.W.S. has received funding from from the European Union's Horizon 2020 research and innovation programme under grant agreement No. 777111 (Repotrial). The Research Programme on Biomedical Informatics (GRIB) is a member of the Spanish National Bioinformatics Institute (INB), PRB2-ISCIII and is supported by grant PT13/0001/0023, of the PE I+D+i 2013–2016, funded by ISCIII and FEDER. The DCEXS is a "Unidad de Excelencia María de Maeztu", funded by the MINECO (ref: MDM-2014-0370).

Abbreviations

The following abbreviations are used in this manuscript:

AD	Alzheimer's disease
ATC	Anatomical Therapeutic Chemical
GSEA	Gene set enrichment analysis
PxEA	Proximal pathway enrichment analysis
T2D	Type 2 diabetes
TF-IDF	Time frequency-inverse document frequency approach

References

1. Strebhardt, K.; Ullrich, A. Paul Ehrlich's magic bullet concept: 100 years of progress. *Nat. Rev. Cancer* **2008**, *8*, 473–480. [CrossRef] [PubMed]
2. Csermely, P.; Korcsmáros, T.; Kiss, H.J.; London, G.; Nussinov, R. Structure and dynamics of molecular networks: A novel paradigm of drug discovery: A comprehensive review. *Pharmacol. Ther.* **2013**, *138*, 333–408. [CrossRef] [PubMed]
3. Allison, M. Reinventing clinical trials. *Nat. Biotechnol.* **2012**, *30*, 41–49. [CrossRef] [PubMed]
4. Hay, M.; Thomas, D.W.; Craighead, J.L.; Economides, C.; Rosenthal, J. Clinical development success rates for investigational drugs. *Nat. Biotechnol.* **2014**, *32*, 40–51. [CrossRef] [PubMed]
5. Hopkins, A.L. Network pharmacology: The next paradigm in drug discovery. *Nat. Chem. Biol.* **2008**, *4*, 682–690. [CrossRef] [PubMed]
6. Pujol, A.; Mosca, R.; Farres, J.; Aloy, P. Unveiling the role of network and systems biology in drug discovery. *Trends Pharmacol. Sci.* **2010**, *31*, 115–123. [CrossRef] [PubMed]
7. Guney, E.; Menche, J.; Vidal, M.; Barábasi, A.L. Network-based in silico drug efficacy screening. *Nat. Commun.* **2016**, *7*, 10331. [CrossRef] [PubMed]
8. Jaeger, S.; Igea, A.; Arroyo, R.; Alcalde, V.; Canovas, B.; Orozco, M.; Nebreda, A.R.; Aloy, P. Quantification of Pathway Cross-talk Reveals Novel Synergistic Drug Combinations for Breast Cancer. *Cancer Res.* **2017**, *77*, 459–469. [CrossRef] [PubMed]
9. Jin, G.; Wong, S.T.C. Toward better drug repositioning: Prioritizing and integrating existing methods into efficient pipelines. *Drug Discov. Today* **2014**, *19*, 637–644. [CrossRef] [PubMed]
10. Hodos, R.A.; Kidd, B.A.; Shameer, K.; Readhead, B.P.; Dudley, J.T. In silico methods for drug repurposing and pharmacology. *Wiley Interdiscip. Rev. Syst. Biol. Med.* **2016**, *8*, 186–210. [CrossRef] [PubMed]
11. Vilar, S.; Hripcsak, G. The role of drug profiles as similarity metrics: Applications to repurposing, adverse effects detection and drug–drug interactions. *Brief. Bioinform.* **2016**, *18*, 670–681. [CrossRef] [PubMed]
12. Loscalzo, J.; Kohane, I.; Barabasi, A.L. Human disease classification in the postgenomic era: A complex systems approach to human pathobiology. *Mol. Syst. Biol.* **2007**, *3*, 124. [CrossRef] [PubMed]
13. Duran-Frigola, M.; Mateo, L.; Aloy, P. Drug repositioning beyond the low-hanging fruits. *Curr. Opin. Syst. Biol.* **2017**, *3*, 95–102. [CrossRef]
14. Li, Y.; Agarwal, P.; Rajagopalan, D. A global pathway crosstalk network. *Bioinformatics* **2008**, *24*, 1442–1447. [CrossRef] [PubMed]
15. Garcia-Garcia, J.; Guney, E.; Aragues, R.; Planas-Iglesias, J.; Oliva, B. Biana: A software framework for compiling biological interactions and analyzing networks. *BMC Bioinform.* **2010**, *11*, 56. [CrossRef] [PubMed]
16. Menche, J.; Sharma, A.; Kitsak, M.; Ghiassian, S.D.; Vidal, M.; Loscalzo, J.; Barabási, A.L. Disease networks. Uncovering disease-disease relationships through the incomplete interactome. *Science* **2015**, *347*, 1257601. [CrossRef] [PubMed]
17. Ko, Y.; Cho, M.; Lee, J.S.; Kim, J. Identification of disease comorbidity through hidden molecular mechanisms. *Sci. Rep.* **2016**, *6*, 39433. [CrossRef] [PubMed]
18. Rubio-Perez, C.; Guney, E.; Aguilar, D.; Piñero, J.; Garcia-Garcia, J.; Iadarola, B.; Sanz, F.; Fernandez-Fuentes, N.; Furlong, L.I.; Oliva, B. Genetic and functional characterization of disease associations explains comorbidity. *Sci. Rep.* **2017**, *7*, 6207. [CrossRef] [PubMed]
19. Cuadrado, A.; Manda, G.; Hassan, A.; Alcaraz, M.J.; Barbas, C.; Daiber, A.; Ghezzi, P.; León, R.; López, M.G.; Oliva, B.; et al. Transcription Factor NRF2 as a Therapeutic Target for Chronic Diseases: A Systems Medicine Approach. *Pharmacol. Rev.* **2018**, *70*, 348–383. [CrossRef] [PubMed]
20. Toro-Domínguez, D.; Carmona-Sáez, P.; Alarcón-Riquelme, M.E. Shared signatures between rheumatoid arthritis, systemic lupus erythematosus and Sjögren's syndrome uncovered through gene expression meta-analysis. *Arthritis Res. Ther.* **2014**, *16*, 489. [CrossRef] [PubMed]
21. Luan, M.; Shang, Z.; Teng, Y.; Chen, X.; Zhang, M.; Lv, H.; Zhang, R. The shared and specific mechanism of four autoimmune diseases. *Oncotarget* **2017**, *8*, 108355–108374. [CrossRef] [PubMed]
22. American Autoimmune Related Diseases Association. Autoimmune Disease Statistics. Available online: www.aarda.org/news-information/statistics (accessed on 13 June 2018).
23. Baranzini, S.E. Chapter 70—Autoimmune Disorders. In *Genomic and Personalized Medicine*, 2nd ed.; Ginsburg, G.S., Willard, H.F., Eds.; Academic Press: Cambridge, MA, USA, 2013; pp. 822–838. [CrossRef]

24. Gottesman, I.I.; Gould, T.D. The Endophenotype Concept in Psychiatry: Etymology and Strategic Intentions. *Am. J. Psychiatry* **2003**, *160*, 636–645. [CrossRef] [PubMed]

25. Ghiassian, S.D.; Menche, J.; Chasman, D.I.; Giulianini, F.; Wang, R.; Ricchiuto, P.; Aikawa, M.; Iwata, H.; Müller, C.; Zeller, T.; et al. Endophenotype Network Models: Common Core of Complex Diseases. *Sci. Rep.* **2016**, *6*, 27414. [CrossRef] [PubMed]

26. Glaab, E.; Baudot, A.; Krasnogor, N.; Schneider, R.; Valencia, A. EnrichNet: Network-based gene set enrichment analysis. *Bioinformatics* **2012**, *28*, i451–i457. [CrossRef] [PubMed]

27. Himmelstein, D.S.; Lizee, A.; Hessler, C.; Brueggeman, L.; Chen, S.L.; Hadley, D.; Green, A.; Khankhanian, P.; Baranzini, S.E. Systematic integration of biomedical knowledge prioritizes drugs for repurposing. *eLife* **2018**, *6*. [CrossRef]

28. Lamb, J.; Crawford, E.D.; Peck, D.; Modell, J.W.; Blat, I.C.; Wrobel, M.J.; Lerner, J.; Brunet, J.P.; Subramanian, A.; Ross, K.N.; et al. The Connectivity Map: Using Gene-Expression Signatures to Connect Small Molecules, Genes, and Disease. *Science* **2006**, *313*, 1929–1935. [CrossRef] [PubMed]

29. Sims-Robinson, C.; Kim, B.; Rosko, A.; Feldman, E.L. How does diabetes accelerate Alzheimer disease pathology? *Nat. Rev. Neurol.* **2010**, *6*, 551–559. [CrossRef] [PubMed]

30. Hiltunen, M.; Khandelwal, V.K.M.; Yaluri, N.; Tiilikainen, T.; Tusa, M.; Koivisto, H.; Krzisch, M.; Vepsäläinen, S.; Mäkinen, P.; Kemppainen, S.; et al. Increased risk of type 2 diabetes in Alzheimer disease. *J. Cell. Mol. Med.* **2012**, *16*, 1206–1222. [CrossRef] [PubMed]

31. Yarchoan, M.; Arnold, S.E. Repurposing Diabetes Drugs for Brain Insulin Resistance in Alzheimer Disease. *Diabetes* **2014**, *63*, 2253–2261. [CrossRef] [PubMed]

32. Du, J.; Wang, Z. Therapeutic potential of lipase inhibitor orlistat in Alzheimer's disease. *Med. Hypotheses* **2009**, *73*, 662–663. [CrossRef] [PubMed]

33. Mahmoudiandehkordi, S.; Arnold, M.; Nho, K.; Ahmad, S.; Jia, W.; Xia, G.; Louie, G.; Kueider, A.; Moseley, M.A.; Thompson, J.W.; et al. Altered Bile Acid Profile Associates with Cognitive Impairment in Alzheimer's Disease: An Emerging Role for Gut Microbiome. *bioRxiv* **2018**, 281956. [CrossRef]

34. Guerciolini, R. Mode of action of orlistat. *Int. J. Obes. Relat. Metab. Disord.* **1997**, *21*, S12–S23. [PubMed]

35. Snowden, S.G.; Ebshiana, A.A.; Hye, A.; An, Y.; Pletnikova, O.; O'Brien, R.; Troncoso, J.; Legido-Quigley, C.; Thambisetty, M. Association between fatty acid metabolism in the brain and Alzheimer disease neuropathology and cognitive performance: A nontargeted metabolomic study. *PLoS Med.* **2017**, *14*, e1002266. [CrossRef] [PubMed]

36. Daugherty, D.; Goldberg, J.; Fischer, W.; Dargusch, R.; Maher, P.; Schubert, D. A novel Alzheimer's disease drug candidate targeting inflammation and fatty acid metabolism. *Alzheimers Res. Ther.* **2017**, *9*, 50. [CrossRef] [PubMed]

37. Ramos, B.P.; Colgan, L.A.; Nou, E.; Arnsten, A.F. β2 adrenergic agonist, clenbuterol, enhances working memory performance in aging animals. *Neurobiol. Aging* **2008**, *29*, 1060–1069. [CrossRef] [PubMed]

38. Chai, G.S.; Wang, Y.Y.; Yasheng, A.; Zhao, P. Beta 2-adrenergic receptor activation enhances neurogenesis in Alzheimer's disease mice. *Neural Regener. Res.* **2016**, *11*, 1617–1624. [CrossRef]

39. Pan, S.J.; Hancock, J.; Ding, Z.; Fogt, D.; Lee, M.; Ivy, J.L. Effects of clenbuterol on insulin resistance in conscious obese Zucker rats. *Am. J. Physiol. Endocrinol. Metab.* **2001**, *280*, E554–E561. [CrossRef] [PubMed]

40. Ceol, A.; Aryamontri, A.C.; Licata, L.; Peluso, D.; Briganti, L.; Perfetto, L.; Castagnoli, L.; Cesareni, G. MINT, the molecular interaction database: 2009 update. *Nucleic Acids Res.* **2010**, *38*, D532–D539. [CrossRef] [PubMed]

41. Stark, C.; Breitkreutz, B.J.; Chatr-aryamontri, A.; Boucher, L.; Oughtred, R.; Livstone, M.S.; Nixon, J.; Van Auken, K.; Wang, X.; Shi, X.; et al. The BioGRID Interaction Database: 2011 update. *Nucleic Acids Res.* **2010**, *39*, D698–D704. [CrossRef] [PubMed]

42. Prasad, T.S.K.; Goel, R.; Kandasamy, K.; Keerthikumar, S.; Kumar, S.; Mathivanan, S.; Telikicherla, D.; Raju, R.; Shafreen, B.; Venugopal, A.; et al. Human Protein Reference Database—2009 update. *Nucleic Acids Res.* **2009**, *37*, D767–D772. [CrossRef] [PubMed]

43. Kanehisa, M.; Goto, S.; Hattori, M.; Aoki-Kinoshita, K.F.; Itoh, M.; Kawashima, S.; Katayama, T.; Araki, M.; Hirakawa, M. From genomics to chemical genomics: New developments in KEGG. *Nucleic Acids Res.* **2006**, *34*, D354–D357. [CrossRef] [PubMed]

44. Duarte, N.C.; Becker, S.A.; Jamshidi, N.; Thiele, I.; Mo, M.L.; Vo, T.D.; Srivas, R.; Palsson, B.O.

Global reconstruction of the human metabolic network based on genomic and bibliomic data. *Proc. Natl. Acad. Sci. USA* **2007**, *104*, 1777–1782. [CrossRef] [PubMed]

45. Ruepp, A.; Brauner, B.; Dunger-Kaltenbach, I.; Frishman, G.; Montrone, C.; Stransky, M.; Waegele, B.; Schmidt, T.; Doudieu, O.N.; Stümpflen, V.; et al. CORUM: The comprehensive resource of mammalian protein complexes. *Nucleic Acids Res.* **2008**, *36*, D646–D650. [CrossRef] [PubMed]

46. Hornbeck, P.V.; Kornhauser, J.M.; Tkachev, S.; Zhang, B.; Skrzypek, E.; Murray, B.; Latham, V.; Sullivan, M. PhosphoSitePlus: A comprehensive resource for investigating the structure and function of experimentally determined post-translational modifications in man and mouse. *Nucleic Acids Res.* **2012**, *40*, D261–D270. [CrossRef] [PubMed]

47. Leskovec, J.; Faloutsos, C. Sampling from Large Graphs. In Proceedings of the 12th ACM SIGKDD International Conference on Knowledge Discovery and Data Mining, Philadelphia, PA, USA, 20–23 August 2006; ACM: New York, NY, USA, 2006; pp. 631–636. [CrossRef]

48. Erten, S.; Bebek, G.; Ewing, R.; Koyuturk, M. DADA: Degree-Aware Algorithms for Network-Based Disease Gene Prioritization. *BioData Min.* **2011**, *4*, 19. [CrossRef] [PubMed]

49. Guney, E.; Oliva, B. Analysis of the Robustness of Network-Based Disease-Gene Prioritization Methods Reveals Redundancy in the Human Interactome and Functional Diversity of Disease-Genes. *PLoS ONE* **2014**, *9*, e94686. [CrossRef] [PubMed]

50. Guney, E. Investigating Side Effect Modules in the Interactome and Their Use in Drug Adverse Effect Discovery. In *Complex Networks VIII*; Springer: Cham, Switzerland, 2017; pp. 239–250. [CrossRef]

51. Guney, E.; Oliva, B. Exploiting Protein-Protein Interaction Networks for Genome-Wide Disease-Gene Prioritization. *PLoS ONE* **2012**, *7*, e43557. [CrossRef] [PubMed]

52. Piñero, J.; Bravo, A.; Queralt-Rosinach, N.; Gutiérrez-Sacristán, A.; Deu-Pons, J.; Centeno, E.; García-García, J.; Sanz, F.; Furlong, L.I. DisGeNET: A comprehensive platform integrating information on human disease-associated genes and variants. *Nucleic Acids Res.* **2017**, *45*, D833–D839. [CrossRef] [PubMed]

53. UniProt Consortium. UniProt: A hub for protein information. *Nucleic Acids Res.* **2015**, *43*, D204–D212. [CrossRef]

54. Landrum, M.J.; Lee, J.M.; Benson, M.; Brown, G.; Chao, C.; Chitipiralla, S.; Gu, B.; Hart, J.; Hoffman, D.; Hoover, J.; et al. ClinVar: Public archive of interpretations of clinically relevant variants. *Nucleic Acids Res.* **2016**, *44*, D862–D868. [CrossRef] [PubMed]

55. Rath, A.; Olry, A.; Dhombres, F.; Brandt, M.M.; Urbero, B.; Ayme, S. Representation of rare diseases in health information systems: The Orphanet approach to serve a wide range of end users. *Hum. Mutat.* **2012**, *33*, 803–808. [CrossRef] [PubMed]

56. Welter, D.; MacArthur, J.; Morales, J.; Burdett, T.; Hall, P.; Junkins, H.; Klemm, A.; Flicek, P.; Manolio, T.; Hindorff, L.; et al. The NHGRI GWAS Catalog, a curated resource of SNP-trait associations. *Nucleic Acids Res.* **2014**, *42*, D1001–D1006. [CrossRef] [PubMed]

57. Davis, A.P.; Grondin, C.J.; Lennon-Hopkins, K.; Saraceni-Richards, C.; Sciaky, D.; King, B.L.; Wiegers, T.C.; Mattingly, C.J. The Comparative Toxicogenomics Database's 10th year anniversary: Update 2015. *Nucleic Acids Res.* **2015**, *43*, D914–D920. [CrossRef] [PubMed]

58. Wishart, D.S.; Feunang, Y.D.; Guo, A.C.; Lo, E.J.; Marcu, A.; Grant, J.R.; Sajed, T.; Johnson, D.; Li, C.; Sayeeda, Z.; et al. DrugBank 5.0: A major update to the DrugBank database for 2018. *Nucleic Acids Res.* **2018**, *46*, D1074–D1082. [CrossRef] [PubMed]

59. Liberzon, A.; Subramanian, A.; Pinchback, R.; Thorvaldsdóttir, H.; Tamayo, P.; Mesirov, J.P. Molecular signatures database (MSigDB) 3.0. *Bioinformatics* **2011**, *27*, 1739–1740. [CrossRef] [PubMed]

60. Croft, D.; Mundo, A.F.; Haw, R.; Milacic, M.; Weiser, J.; Wu, G.; Caudy, M.; Garapati, P.; Gillespie, M.; Kamdar, M.R.; et al. The Reactome pathway knowledgebase. *Nucleic Acids Res.* **2014**, *42*, D472–D477. [CrossRef] [PubMed]

61. Zhou, X.; Menche, J.; Barabási, A.L.; Sharma, A. Human symptoms—Disease network. *Nat. Commun.* **2014**, *5*, 4212. [CrossRef] [PubMed]

62. Hidalgo, C.A.; Blumm, N.; Barabási, A.L.; Christakis, N.A. A Dynamic Network Approach for the Study of Human Phenotypes. *PLoS Comput. Biol.* **2009**, *5*, e1000353. [CrossRef] [PubMed]

63. Kibbe, W.A.; Arze, C.; Felix, V.; Mitraka, E.; Bolton, E.; Fu, G.; Mungall, C.J.; Binder, J.X.; Malone, J.; Vasant, D.; et al. Disease Ontology 2015 update: An expanded and updated database of human diseases for linking

biomedical knowledge through disease data. *Nucleic Acids Res.* **2015**, *43*, D1071–D1078. [CrossRef] [PubMed]

64. Clark, N.R.; Ma'ayan, A. Introduction to statistical methods for analyzing large data sets: Gene-set enrichment analysis. *Sci. Signal.* **2011**, *4*, tr4. [CrossRef] [PubMed]

65. Benjamini, Y.; Hochberg, Y. Controlling the False Discovery Rate: A Practical and Powerful Approach to Multiple Testing. *J. R. Stat. Soc. Ser. B (Methodol.)* **1995**, *57*, 289–300.

66. Shannon, P.; Markiel, A.; Ozier, O.; Baliga, N.S.; Wang, J.T.; Ramage, D.; Amin, N.; Schwikowski, B.; Ideker, T. Cytoscape: A software environment for integrated models of biomolecular interaction networks. *Genome Res.* **2003**, *13*, 2498–2504. [CrossRef] [PubMed]

67. VanderPlas, J. *Python Data Science Handbook*; O'Reilly Media, Inc.: Sebastopol, CA, USA, 2018.

68. Wickham, H. *ggplot2: Elegant Graphics for Data Analysis (Use R!)*; Springer: New York, NY, USA, 2009.

3

Heterodimer Binding Scaffolds Recognition via the Analysis of Kinetically Hot Residues

Ognjen Perišić [1,2]

[1] Big Blue Genomics, Vojvode Brane 32, 11000 Belgrade, Serbia; ognjen.perisic@gmail.com
[2] Department of Chemistry, New York University, 1001 Silver, 100 Washington Square East, New York, NY 10003, USA

Abstract: Physical interactions between proteins are often difficult to decipher. The aim of this paper is to present an algorithm that is designed to recognize binding patches and supporting structural scaffolds of interacting heterodimer proteins using the Gaussian Network Model (GNM). The recognition is based on the (self) adjustable identification of kinetically hot residues and their connection to possible binding scaffolds. The kinetically hot residues are residues with the lowest entropy, i.e., the highest contribution to the weighted sum of the fastest modes per chain extracted via GNM. The algorithm adjusts the number of fast modes in the GNM's weighted sum calculation using the ratio of predicted and expected numbers of target residues (contact and the neighboring first-layer residues). This approach produces very good results when applied to dimers with high protein sequence length ratios. The protocol's ability to recognize near native decoys was compared to the ability of the residue-level statistical potential of Lu and Skolnick using the Sternberg and Vakser decoy dimers sets. The statistical potential produced better overall results, but in a number of cases its predicting ability was comparable, or even inferior, to the prediction ability of the adjustable GNM approach. The results presented in this paper suggest that in heterodimers at least one protein has interacting scaffold determined by the immovable, kinetically hot residues. In many cases, interacting proteins (especially if being of noticeably different sizes) either behave as a rigid lock and key or, presumably, exhibit the opposite dynamic behavior. While the binding surface of one protein is rigid and stable, its partner's interacting scaffold is more flexible and adaptable.

Keywords: protein-protein interactions; normal mode analysis; Gaussian Network Model; protein decoys

1. Introduction

The revolutions in biotechnology of the past two decades opened an unprecedented ability to analyze and organize biological information. The advent of the next generation sequencing technologies and accompanying software tools enables the sequencing and analysis of complete genomes, not only of whole species but of individual specimens also, often at a single cell level [1–3]. More than 90 million protein sequences have been deciphered so far, and that number grows at an enormous rate [4], but the sequencing data alone is not sufficient to fully grasp the biological process on the molecular level. The detailed information on structural and physical interactions of biological molecules is of the utmost importance for the understanding of biological processes and their proper treatment. However, the capacity to generate and adequately connect structural data, i.e., protein, DNA, and RNA structures, to biological processes is diminutive in comparison to the sequencing yield or even to diagnostic abilities. The analysis of human proteome reveals that almost half of human genes and more than 60% of metabolic enzymes are expressed in majority of tissues [5], but for the majority of them roles and interactions are still unknown. An even more pressing issue, and one that is very related to structural and sequencing information, is the high attrition rate in drug development, a conclusion drawn in 2004 [6]. The past decade did not rectify this issue, as explained in [7]. New approaches, such as the one described in this manuscript, or the analysis of ligand binding behavior within a framework of chemico-biological space [8], may be a way toward a much better compound filtering during preclinical trials and thus toward a more efficient drug design.

To fully comprehend the biological process on the molecular level we first have to understand the physical laws that govern the interactions of biological polymers. Protein-DNA and protein-lipid interactions had been successfully addressed [9–13], but the problems of protein folding [14,15] and protein-protein interactions [16–21] are issues that still require the full attention of the research community. Many attempts were made to develop a comprehensive protein-protein interaction theory. The recognition of binding residues using an analysis of sequential and structural properties of heteromeric, transient protein-protein interactions produced very good overall results, as shown by Neuvirth et al. [22]. Chen and Zhou [23] used sequence profiles, as well as solvent accessibility of spatially neighboring surface residues fed to neural networks to develop a successful binding sites recognition protocol. By applying a linear combination of the energy score, interface propensity, and residue conservation score, Liang et al. [24] achieved decent coverage and accuracy. Zhang et al. focused their effort on the interface conservation across structure space [25], while Saccà et al. introduced multilevel (protein, domain, and residue) binding recognition using the Semantic Based Regularization Machine Learning framework [26]. It was shown that the three-dimensional structural information, either based on data from PDB [27] or obtained from homology modeling, produces a robust and efficient prediction of protein-protein interactions when applied with information on structural neighbors of queried proteins and Bayesian classifiers [28]. The protein (co)expression also attracts researchers' attention. For instance, Bhardwaj and Lu [29] showed that the complexity of co-expression profiles in protein networks rises with the increase of the interactions/connectedness of the networks.

The application of coarse-grained force fields in the analysis of protein-protein associations also attracted the attention of the research community [19,30]. Basdevant, Borgis, and Ha-Duong analyzed the dimer association using the coarse-grained SCORPION force field model of protein and solvent [31]. The force field model was able to recognize near native decoys of three different protein complexes (out of thousands of analyzed decoys) and to efficiently simulate the dynamics of recognition of a protein complex starting from different initial structures. A similar approach, in a combination with a push-pull-release sampling strategy, was applied by Ravikumar, Huang, and Yang to examine protein-protein association in a number of complexes [32]. M. Zacharias combined bonded atomistic with coarse-grained, non-bonded interactions in his force-field model to simulate peptide-protein docking and refinement from different stating geometries with acceptable accuracy [33]. Solernou and Fernandez-Recio developed pyDockCG [34], a coarse-grained potential for protein-protein docking scoring and refinement, based on the earlier UNRES model developed for the protein structure prediction [35]. A coarse-grained approach (one pseudo atom per every three residues) by Frembgen-Kesner and Elcock showed an ability to reproduce the absolute association rate constants of wild-type and mutant protein pairs via Brownian motion simulations when hydrodynamic interactions between diffusing proteins are included [36]. Chou and collaborators used Pseudo Amino Acid Composition (PseAAC) and Wavelet Transforms as inputs to predict algorithms based on Random forests, as well as Support Vector Machines to recognize protein binding sites [37–43].

The elucidation of physical interactions of proteins is appealing to the pharmaceutical industry as well [44], with an emphasis on small molecule inhibitors of protein-protein interactions [45,46]. The interest of the pharmaceutical industry is not surprising, because mutations, which disrupt the three-dimensional structure, can be cancer drivers [47].

The aim of this paper is to address the physical interactions between individual protein chains that form protein dimers. The approach described here uses the structural information only and the theory of phantom networks through its Gaussian network model (GNM) implementation [48–59].

The GNM produces a set of vibrational modes via the eigenvalues and eigenvectors of the protein Kirchhoff contact matrix. The fastest modes (with larger eigenvalues λ) are more localized and have steeper energy walls with a larger decrease in entropy. They are, therefore, referred to as kinetically hot residues. For more details, see the Supplementary Materials and [56].

The connection between kinetically hot residues and interface residues has been established already [60]. The methodology described here moves forward and introduces a self-adjusting approach that is aimed at recognizing binding surfaces and corresponding structural scaffolds (contact and neighboring first-layer residues; that approach was initially given in [61,62]). The results depicted here show that at least one of the proteins that forms a heterodimer has its contacting scaffold surrounded or bounded through its kinetically hot residues. One of the partners (usually the longer one) has binding areas and corresponding binding scaffolds defined by its kinetically hot residues, while its partner is presumably more flexible. It may pass through structural adjustments, which means that the recognition of its binding residues could be difficult with the coarse-grained methodology based on the distribution of kinetically hot residues only. A similar difficulty is encountered in heterodimers composed of similarly sized proteins (with similar chain lengths). Furthermore, with smaller proteins, the adjustable GNM approach may be less precise, because the small protein size easily produces many false positives. However, the fact that at least one of the binding partners has binding areas defined by its kinetically hot residues (and thus is less movable than other residues) may suggest that the heterodimer protein formation is entropically driven, i.e., that the protein chains often interact in an attempt to increase the overall entropy (i.e., increase the entropy of rigid binding scaffolds).

The term "kinetically hot residues" is similar to the term "hot spots" that is often used in protein science, but these terms have much more in common than linguistics. Residues that often appear in structurally preserved interfaces (in more than 50% of cases) are termed hot spots. The hot spots are important, because they are general contributors to the binding free energy. They are screened using the alanine-scanning mutagenesis and are therefore defined as spots where alanine mutation increases the binding free energy at least 2.0 kcal/mol [63–69]. Bogan and Thorn [63] showed that hot spot residues are enriched in tryptophan, tyrosine, and arginine, and that they are surrounded with residues whose role is to occlude solvent from the hot spots (O-ring residues hypothesis). They also observed that "(n)either the change in total side-chain solvent-accessible surface area on complex formation (ΔASA) nor the sidechain ΔASA of hydrophobic atoms is well correlated to the change in free energy" [63]. They concluded that solvent occlusion is a necessary but not sufficient condition for a residue to be a hot spot. The hot spots have been addressed using various computational methods [65]. Tuncbag et al. used information on conservation, the solvent accessibility area, and the statistical pairwise residue potentials of the interface residues to computationally determine hot spots. Their combined approach achieved both accuracy and precision between 64% and 73% of the Alanine Scanning Energetics and Binding Interface Databases. They observed that "conservation does not have significant effect in hot spot prediction as a single feature". However, their results indicate that the "residue occlusions from solvent and pairwise potentials are found to be the main discriminative features in hot spot prediction". Lise et al. [66,67] combined machine learning and energy-based methods to predict hot spot residues. They applied standard energy terms (Van der Waals potentials, solvation energy, hydrogen bonds, and Coulomb electrostatics) as input features to Support Vector Machine (SVM) and Gaussian Processes learning protocols. They also attempted to predict the change in binding free energy $\Delta\Delta G$ upon alanine substitution but achieved only a limited success. Den et al. [70] also used Support Vector Machines with Random Forest selection and Sequential Backward feature elimination to predict hot spots. They used various molecular attributes (local structural entropy, side chain energy score, four-body pseudo-potential, weighted relative surface area burial) as feature vector elements, as well as the residue neighborhood defined via the Euclidian distances between residues/heavy atoms, with Voronoi diagram/Delaunay triangulation employed to describe residue's neighbors. They ended with 38 features, which the SVM protocol utilized to predict hot spots very efficiently. Kozakov et al. [68] analyzed druggable hot-spots via a computational method that places small organic molecules—probes (16 of them)—on a grid around target protein. The spots on the surface of the target protein that favorably interact with a number of probes are clustered, and those clusters are ranked according to the average free energy. The consensus regions (the regions that bind many probes) are taken to be hot spots. Their method is able to recognize hot spots even in unbound cases. The authors concluded that according to their protocol, the hot spots *"possess a general tendency to bind organic compounds with a variety of structures, including key side chains of the partner protein"*. This sentence is emphasized, because the results depicted in this paper also show that the binding interface of large host proteins is often determined by their own structure only. That may imply that host proteins are receptive for other proteins and/or small molecules besides their usually encountered binding partners. The method depicted here is also able to distinguish dimer decoys that were created with structures of unbound chains (see Testing set analysis in this paper). Similarly, Tuncbag et al. [69] observed that *"globally different protein structures can interact via similar architectural motifs"*. They employed that fact through the PRISM algorithm that *"utilizes rigid-body structural comparisons of target proteins to known template protein-protein interfaces and flexible refinement using a docking energy function."*

To develop a really useful prediction method for a biological system as demonstrated in a series of recent publications (see, e.g., [71–85]), and especially in a set of publications relevant to the topic of protein-protein, protein-ligand, and protein-drug interactions [37–43], one should observe and possibly follow the 5-step methodology [86]; (I) how to construct or select a valid benchmark dataset to train and test the predictor; (II) how to formulate a set of biological sequences or structure samples with an effective mathematical expression that can truly reflect an intrinsic correlation with the targets to be predicted; (III) how to introduce or develop a powerful algorithm (or engine) to operate the prediction; (IV) how to properly perform cross-validation tests to objectively evaluate the anticipated accuracy of the predictor; (V) how to establish a user-friendly web-server for the predictor that is accessible to the public.

This paper follows the above-described 5-step methodology. It starts with an overview of methods and tools (a short overview of the theoretical background of the Gaussian network model is given in the Supplementary Materials). The definition of target residues, as well as the short description of training and testing sets, is given after that. The first simple prediction protocol that is based on the five fastest modes and the sequential influence of the hot residues only is given in the third chapter. The same chapter describes a prediction approach that uses the modes that correspond to the upper 10% of the eigenvalues range. After that, the paper offers a brief description of the behavior of dimers with different sequence lengths of their protein constituents and introduces a significant improvement in the prediction based on the adjustable number of fast modes. After that, the paper describes an adjustable prediction protocol based on the 3D influence of hot residues, as well as the combination of sequential and spatial approaches. Finally, the paper describes an evaluation of adjustable protocols on the Sternberg [87] and Vakser decoy sets [88]. While doing so, the paper compares the adjustable GNM to the Lu and Skolnick's detailed, residue-level statistical potential approach to contact residues recognition [89]. The paper ends with the Conclusion.

2. Materials and Methods

2.1. GNM Code

The software for the Adjustable Gaussian Network Model code is composed of several different programs. The first program calculates contact maps and the corresponding eigenvectors and eigenvalues [90] for both protein chains that form a protein dimer (given as a PDB file). To accomplish that, the program first calculates the Kirchhoff contact matrix Γ for each protein. The matrix Γ calculation is based on the distances between C_α atoms only, and those distances have to be less than or equal to 7 Å to consider two residues in a contact [54–56]. The code then calculates and sorts Γ matrix eigenvalues and eigenvectors. The eigenvectors are sorted according to their corresponding eigenvalues. Those eigenvalues and eigenvectors are used in the second part that (iteratively) calculates the weighted sum of modes [57] as

$$\langle (\Delta \mathbf{R}_i)^2 \rangle_{k_1-k_2} = (k_B T/\gamma) \sum_{k_1}^{k_2} \lambda_k^{-1} [\mathbf{u}_k]_i^2 / \sum_{k_1}^{k_2} \lambda_k^{-1} \tag{1}$$

This equation, normalized by dividing the sum by , produces mean square fluctuations of each residue by a given set of modes (k_1 to k_2). The equation produces an estimate of a kinetic contribution of each residue for a given set of modes. The above equation is very similar to the singular value decomposition method [91] used in the linear least squares optimization method. For details on the phantom networks and the Gaussian Network Model, see a short overview in the Supplementary Materials. An additional code extracts contact and first-layer residues. Finally, the third set of routines extracts neighboring residues and their distances for each residue per protein chain. That information is later used in the spatial spreading of the influence of kinetically hot residues.

2.2. Targets

The aim of the methods presented here is to recognize contact patches on protein surfaces and the corresponding scaffolds in the protein interiors. The first aim is to recognize contact residues. These are amino acid residues in which at least one atom is at the maximum distance of 4.5 Å from one or more atoms from the surface of the other chain. The distance of 4.5 Å corresponds to the size of one water molecule. The second aim is to recognize the first-layer residues (FLR), i.e., residues in contact with contact patches, but which are not contacts themselves. Therefore, those are neighboring residues from the same protein (at the maximum atom-atom distance of 4.5 Å from contact residues). They form scaffolds that surround contact residues (for a visual description of contact and first-layer residues, see Figure S1 in the Supplementary Materials).

2.3. Training Set

The training set is comprised of 433 protein dimer complexes (see Supplementary Materials for the full list of dimers; this set is inspired by the Chen dimer set). It is separated into heterodimer and homodimers, using two criteria: (1) If the ratio of protein lengths (protein sequence length is the number of its amino acid residues) in a dimer complex is greater than 2, that complex is considered to be heterodimer; (2) If the ratio of protein lengths is smaller than 2, the Smith-Waterman sequence alignment algorithm [92] is applied to recognize and separate dimers in which proteins sequences are highly similar. This approach was applied following the homology modeling principle that says that high sequence similarity implies structural similarity [93–96]. In some cases, proteins were considered to be heterodimers, although they have a high sequence similarity due to large sequence gaps (1IAI and 1EKI). Therefore, the first group contains dimers in which constituents do not bear obvious structural similarity, while the second group has members that are sequentially and structurally highly similar. The dimers were separated into two groups, because heterodimers and homodimers may exhibit different binding mechanisms. Different behaviors of these two groups may imply that their kinetically hot residues may not be have the same role in protein binding. This approach was used because the Gaussian Network Model is based on structural organization of residues, i.e., on the spatial distribution of C_α atoms in proteins.

Of 433 dimers, 139 are heterodimers, and the rest are homodimers. Majority of proteins in our training set have sequences shorter than 300 residues, but we also have a number of proteins longer than 400 residues. The distribution of chain lengths is shown in Figure S2 in the Supplementary Materials.

2.4. Testing Sets

The Sternberg [87] and Vakser [88] decoy sets are numerically created decoy sets created for testing and evaluation of protein binding prediction protocols. Each decoy set is based on a naturally occurring protein dimer complex with a known structure. Each individual decoy from a set is a protein complex numerically created by joining two (or more) individual proteins based on the corresponding non-bound structures.

The Sternberg decoys sets [87] are comprised of 100 decoys each with first four being near native structures and the first one being the native structure itself. The decoys are generated using unbound structures of the chains that form native dimer structures. In this work only dimer sets were used (10 sets). The adjustable GNM algorithms were applied independently to both proteins per decoy.

Every Vakser set contains 110 decoys. Certain number of those decoys are near native structures (in most cases, 10 of decoys in a set are near native, as determined by their root mean square deviations from the native structure(s)). Only dimer sets (41 of the 61 decoy sets) were used in this research.

3. Results and Discussion

3.1. Simplest 1D Prediction (Sequential Neighbors Influence only) Based on 5 Fastest Modes

The first attempted method is based on the approach of Demirel et al. [57], which used five fastest modes to recognize kinetically hot residues in proteins. With a direct implementation of their scheme, the first step was the calculation of the weighted sum (Equation (1)). With normalized sum, only residues with the normalized amplitude higher than 0.05 (hot residues) were tested against extracted contact and first-layer residues. The number of hot residues is usually smaller than the number of contact or first-layer residues. To account for that, the influence of hot residues was spread to their sequential neighbors using sequence information obtained from their structure PDB files (to account for possible missing residues). The influence of hot residues was spread linearly, to sequential neighbors only, because proteins are polymer chains with physically connected residues. That implies that sequentially neighboring residues should exhibit correlated behavior. For chains longer than 100 amino acids, hot residues and 8 their sequential neighbors upstream and downstream were labeled as predictions (four upstream, four downstream). For shorter chains, the influence was spread to 6 neighboring residues only. The labeled residues are assumed to be either contact or first-layer residues. This approach was used on all 433 dimers regardless of the sequence length or the nature (hetero or homodimer) of a particular dimer complex.

Figure 1a shows the algorithm output for all 866 proteins (433 dimers). The ratio (percentage) of true predictions versus ratio of false prediction per protein is depicted on a two dimensional Cartesian plane, i.e., as a scatterplot. The ratio of true predictions per protein is the number of true predictions over the total number of targets (contact and first-layer residues). They are true positives. The ratio of false predictions per protein is the number of residues falsely predicted as being either contact or FLR over the total number of non-target residues, and they treated as false positives. The Cartesian plane is separated into two parts by a diagonal going from the lover left to the upper right quadrant. The proteins above the diagonal are considered as satisfying prediction, because the ratio of their true positives over false positives is over 1. The proteins under the diagonal are, obviously, unsatisfying, i.e., they are considered bad predictions. The chains (i.e., predictions) in the upper left quadrant we define as good predictions (the ratio of true positives is above 0.5, and the ratio of false positives lower or equal to 0.5). In addition, very bad predictions are taken to be the ones that fall into the lower left quadrant (the ratio of false positives is over 0.5, and the ratio of true positives lower or equal than 0.5). Henceforth, these two measures, percentage of good predictions and percentage of bad predictions, besides true positives mean, and false positives mean, will be used as measures of the quality of the prediction methods. There are obviously better definitions of good and bad prediction. The two used in this research were applied primarily for the algorithm tuning, because they are easy to interpret and implement.

Figure 1a clearly shows that satisfying and unsatisfying predictions are almost equally distributed. The true and false means are 43.09% and 40.78%, respectively. The percentage of good predictions (22.17%) is higher than the percentage of very bad predictions (12.70%), but the amount of good predictions is still not good enough for the general purpose application. However, the distribution of good and bad predictions is not uniform over the protein chain lengths, as the histogram in Figure S3 in the Supplementary Materials nicely depicts. The prediction method based on the five fastest modes is much more successful with shorter (and thus less voluminous) proteins than with longer ones. With proteins longer than 100 residues, but shorter than 200, the prediction algorithm was not satisfying at all, because it put more predictions in the lower right quadrant than in upper left. However, with proteins shorter than 100 residues, it put much more predictions in the upper left (good predictions) than in lower right quadrant, which means that 5 modes may be only good for smaller proteins.

To test the assumption that heterodimers behave differently from homodimers, the above-described method was applied on heterodimers only (278 chains). Figure 1b depicts the results of that analysis. It is obvious that more predictions are in the upper left quadrant than in the lower right. That indicates that hot residues and their neighbors, recognized using only five fastest modes, are much closer to binding patches on the surface and in the interior of heterodimer chains. On average, there are 50.74% of true positives and 42.68% of false positives. The distribution of good and very bad predictions is better than with the complete set (see Figure S4 in Supplementary Materials) but is still not satisfactory enough, because there is only 31.29% of good predictions (87 chains in the upper left quadrant) and 11.15% of bad ones (31 proteins are in the lower right quadrant).

Figure S5 in the Supplementary Materials depicts the example of this initial approach on four different protein chains. It shows the weighted sums for those four proteins, their contact and first later residues (expressed as the ratio of atoms per the total number of atoms in residue), and the predictions. It is clearly visible that, for the longer proteins (chain P from 1BVN in particular), five fastest modes fail at predicting the target residues. For shorter chains (2SNI chain E, 1UDI chain E, and 1CXZ chain A), five modes are better at connecting the kinetically hot residues to contact and FLR patches, but the overall prediction is still not very favorable, because the percent of the accurately predicted contact and FLR residues is comparatively small.

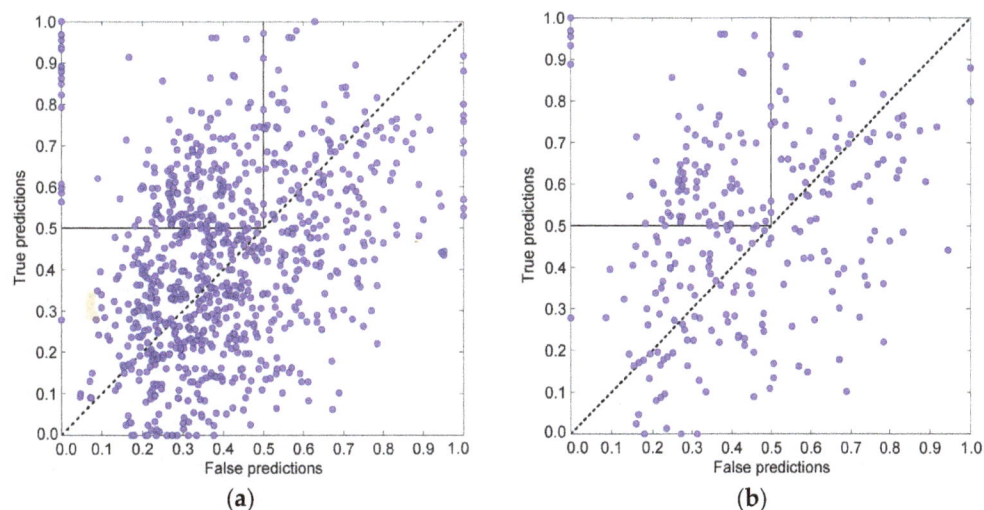

Figure 1. *Cont.*

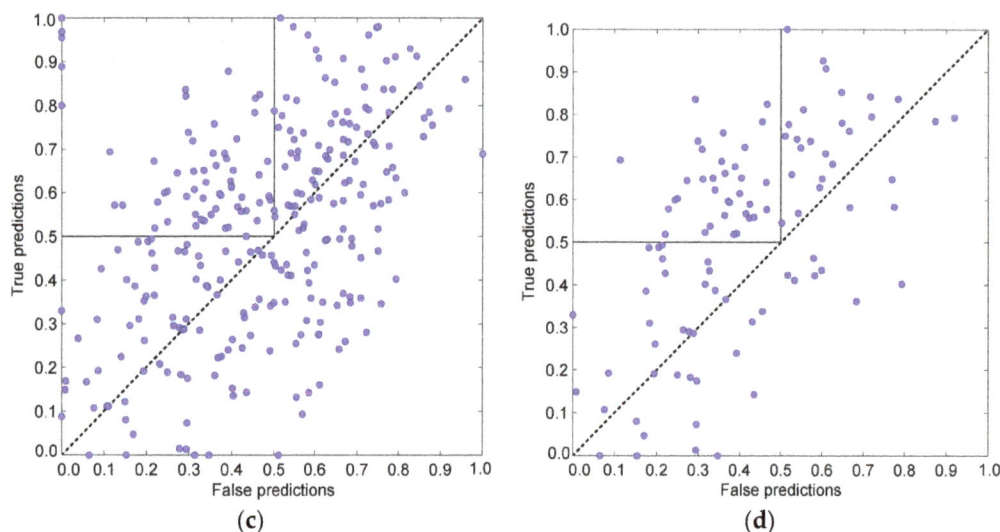

Figure 1. (**a**) Prediction output (ratio of true vs. false predictions depicted as a scatterplot) for a simple prediction approach based on the 5 fastest modes, for each protein chain in our list (433 dimers in total). The diagonal line separates area where true positives outpace false positives from the area where false positives are dominant. The square in the upper left quadrant is the area of good predictions (ratio of true predictions is greater than 0.5, and ratio of bad predictions is lass or equal than 0.5). The true positives mean is 43.09%, and the false positives mean is 40.77%. There is 22.17% of good predictions (192 chains, they are in the upper left quadrant) and 12.70% of very bad predictions (110 chains). The very bad predictions are in the lower right quadrant, which is not depicted as rectangle to emphasize the importance of good predictions. (**b**) Prediction output for 278 heterodimers chains only, for the basic approach based on the 5 fastest modes. The true positives mean is 50.74%, and the false positives mean is 42.68%. There is 31.29% of good predictions (87 chains) and 11.15% of very bad predictions (31 chains). (**c**) Prediction output for the simple approach based on the fastest 10% of modes per chain for all heterodimers (278 chains). The true positives mean is 52.52%, and the false positives mean is 46.27%. There is 23.02% of good predictions (64 chains) and 14.39% of very bad predictions (40 chains). (**d**) Prediction output for the simple approach based on the modes that correspond to top 10% of the eigenvalues range, for heterodimer chains with high sequence length ratios (the chain length ratio >2, the individual chain lengths longer than 80 residues). The true positives mean is 52.03%, and the false positives mean is 40.67%. There is 33.01% of good predictions (34 chains) and 6.80% of very bad predictions (7 chains).

3.2. First Attempt to Improve the Prediction

3.2.1. Prediction Based on the Fast Modes That Corresponds to Top 10% of the Eigenvalues

The previous analysis and the corresponding distribution of good and bad predictions over the protein sequence lengths indicate that the weighted sum based on five modes only is not able to decipher the contact patterns on the surface and in the interior of proteins. With shorter protein chains (up to 100 residues), the weighted sum of five fastest modes is able to give a satisfying prediction of binding and first-layer residues, but with longer chains, the prediction efficiency fails (Figures S3 and S4 in the Supplementary Materials). Therefore, it can be assumed that the number of modes should be adapted to each individual protein. That number would be difficult to determine knowing only the length of a protein chain, because, when sorted, the distribution of the mode intensities (eigenvalues) is not a linear function of the mode index (see Figure S6 in the Supplementary Materials). The distribution of eigenvalues depends on the chain's length, as well as on the protein's three-dimensional configuration. Therefore, a new approach with a variable number of modes that corresponds to the top 10% of the eigenvalues span for every protein was attempted. Figure S6 nicely depicts that top ten percent of eigenvalues are covered by five modes for the protein 1ETT chain H, itself made of 231 amino acid residues. The protein chain P from dimer 1BVN (496 residues) has 14 modes covering top 10%, and the protein chain A from 1QGK (876 residues) has 29 fastest modes covering the top 10% of eigenvalues. There is a correlation between the number of residues and the number of fast modes, but it is not strictly linear.

When this approach is applied to heterodimers, the amount of true positives becomes increased. That can be observed with the four protein chains analyzed previously (Figure S7 in the Supplementary Materials). However, the percentage of false positives also gets increased. With the whole set of heterodimers (278 protein chains), the overall improvement is miniscule, the true positives mean is 52.52%, and the false positives mean of 46.27% (Figure 1c). The increase of the false positives mean corresponds to the decrease of the number of good predictions to 23.02% of the total number of proteins (64 proteins), as well as the increase of the very bad prediction to 14.39% (40). The distribution of good and very bad predictions over the chain lengths shows that this approach is not ideal for all protein chains (Figure S8 in the Supplementary Materials). The bad predictions are dominant for proteins longer than 100 residues and shorter than 200 residues. However, this approach is able to accurately access contact and first-layer residues in a protein with very high number of residues (876, chain A from 1QGK).

3.2.2. Analysis of Heterodimers with Very Different Sequence Lengths

Heterodimers are protein complexes composed of two protein chains with no apparent sequential and structural similarity. What forms such entities? What kind of attraction forces two or more different protein chains to from a stable structure? In protein-DNA or protein-lipid interactions, electrostatic forces are often the key binding factors, but with protein interactions such forces usually have a small or negligible influence.

When a protein dimer is analyzed, one may wonder whether its two constituents evolved separately, or whether they created by a mutation that broke a single protein chain into two separate parts. If we expand this premise, we can assume that such mutation can more easily survive if a point of separation is close to the terminal ends of the initial, single chain (single mutation is, of course, a euphemism for a much more complex random biological process). In that case, a longer sub-chain has a higher probability of preserving its fold and function, because it will be highly homologous to the initial chain (homology implies similar folding patterns, see [93–96]). The probability of surviving is much higher than with mutations that break a protein into constituents of similar sizes. Namely, a protein produced by an asymmetric breaking will more easily preserve its fold and have more of a chance of surviving evolutionary pressures. That may also imply that a protein with longer sequence (more voluminous protein), produced by that single mutation, when interacting with its shorter partner (if that partner survived throughout evolution), may preserve its fold during (and upon) the binding. Similarly, if dimer constituents evolved separately, longer partners may be less prone to significant structural changes during the binding due to their sheer size. All this may imply that kinetically hot residues may determine the shape and the position of a scaffold that determines binding spots in individual heterodimer chains.

To test this assumption, the previously analyzed heterodimers were divided into two groups according to the length ratios of their constituents. The heterodimers with sequence length ratios higher than two were analyzed separately from the rest of heterodimers. Figure S9 in the Supplementary Materials depicts the analysis of the heterodimer chain lengths. The panel (a) depicts the sequence length for each monomer, with longer monomers given via the green line and shorter via the blue line. The panel (b) depicts the corresponding sequence length ratios. The vertical line separates heterodimers into heterodimers with sequence length ratios higher than two from heterodimers with smaller sequence length ratios. The chains with sequence lengths shorter than 80 were eliminated from this group to reduce the occurrence of chains with high percentage of both true and false positives.

Figure 1d depicts the results of the analysis of heterodimers with high sequence length ratios of constituents. In the analysis, only modes that corresponded to top 10% of eigenvalues range were used. This approach, although based on a smaller subset of proteins, shows a visible improvement. It is obvious that the number of proteins with badly characterized target residues (proteins in which the ratio of true positives vs. false positives is less than 1) is reduced. The true positive mean is 52.03%, and the false positive mean is 40.67%. Although only 6.80% of predictions are characterized as very bad (7 proteins), the method is still not satisfactory, because only 33.01% of all chains (34 proteins) are in the upper left quadrant (good predictions). The distribution of good vs. very bad predictions (Figure S10 in the Supplementary Materials) shows much better behavior of this prediction method over the protein sequence lengths than the previous two attempts.

The same analysis, performed on proteins forming heterodimers with low sequence length ratios (for proteins with more than 80 residues), reveals a different picture (Figure S11 in the Supplementary Materials). There is only 13.64% of good predictions (18 proteins out of 132) versus 20.45% of very bad predictions (27 proteins). The true positives mean is 52.75%, a value very similar to the true negatives mean of 53.18%. The distribution of good vs. very bad predictions (Figure S12 in Supplementary Materials) is also not very favorable to good predictions and indicates a negative correlation between kinetically hot residues and binding scaffolds in heterodimers of similar size.

3.3. Prediction Based on the Adjustable Number of Modes

The previous attempts to recognize contact and first-layer residues via the Gaussian Network Model were based on a static approach in which protein dimer structures were analyzed using either 5 fastest normal modes or modes that corresponded to the top 10% of the eigenvalues range. Those approaches showed that kinetically hot residues may play a role in protein-protein interactions, but they did not offer enough proof for that assertion. With some protein chains they produced excellent results, but with some they failed. More importantly, the percentage of good predictions (the amount of chains with more than 50% of true positives and less than 50% of false positives) was comparatively small (always less than 40% of all the chains analyzed). Many of the proteins had a very high percentage of both true positives and false positives. In addition, a significant number of proteins had a very small percentage of both true and false predictions. All of this implied that prediction algorithm had to be improved.

The analysis of the average percentage of targets per sequence length reveals that the amount of targets and the chain length are inversely proportional. Larger proteins with longer sequences have a smaller percentage of contact and first-layer residues than shorter chains. Figure 2 depicts the distribution of targets over the protein sequence lengths. It clearly shows that small proteins (shorter sequence lengths) have much higher ratio of contact and first-layer residues than larger proteins (longer amino acid sequence lengths).

The information on the targets distribution can be used to improve the prediction approach. The prediction can be adjusted to each particular protein chain through a comparison of the current prediction output, i.e., current ratio of predictions (the total number of residues assigned to be either contact or first-layer residues by the algorithm) over the total number of residues, to the expected, i.e., average, percentage of targets for that protein's sequence length class. The improvement of the prediction algorithm can be performed as follows:

–   If the overall percentage of predictions is too large for that protein's sequence length class (for example, if the percentage of predictions is larger than 60% of the total number of residues), the number of fast modes should be reduced by one, and the whole prediction procedure should be repeated (Equation (1)).

–   If the percentage of predictions is too small for the protein's sequence length class (e.g., less than 20% of all residues), the number of fast modes should be increased by one, and the whole prediction procedure should be repeated (Equation (1)).

–   The procedure should be repeated until the percentage of predictions does not fit between the maximum and minimum amount of predictions for a given sequence length.

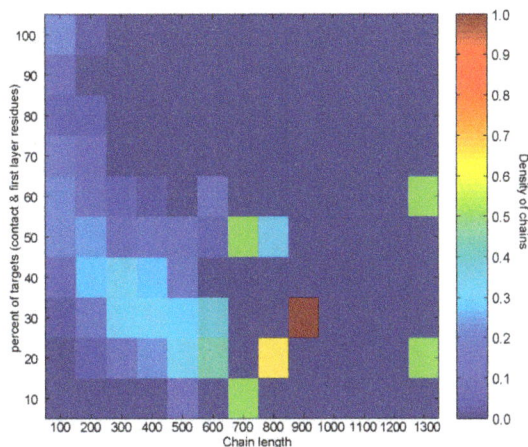

Figure 2. Distribution of targets per sequence length for 414 dimers that belong to the training set depicted as a heat map. The burgundy square designates a length/percent pair with a highest concentration of chains. Yellow and light green squares are length/percent pairs with a medium number of chains. The dark blue squares are length/percent pairs with low occupancy. The navy areas designate zero chain occupancy. It is obvious that the percent of targets is a decreasing function of the sequence length.

3.3.1. One-Dimensional Linear Prediction

A simple strategy adjusts the number of modes for each particular chain: if the number of residues in a chain is less than or equal to 300, too many predictions are taken to be 60%. In that case, i.e., if the amount of predictions is over 60% of all residues, the number of modes is reduced by one, and the prediction procedure is repeated (Equation (1)). Similarly, if the number of residues is greater than 300, too many predictions are taken to be 50%. Furthermore, if the chain length is less or equal to 500 residues, too few predictions are taken to be 40%. For cases like that, the number of modes is increased by one, and the whole procedure is repeated. For longer chains, too few predictions are 20%. To avoid infinite loops, only one increase followed by a decrease is allowed, and vice versa. The prediction procedure itself spreads the influence of kinetically hot residues linearly upstream and downstream along the sequence, as with the previously described methods. The procedure starts with a number of modes that correspond to the top 10% of eigenvalues range for the protein being analyzed. This approach ensures that longer proteins have enough predictions, and that shorter ones are not saturated with too many false positives.

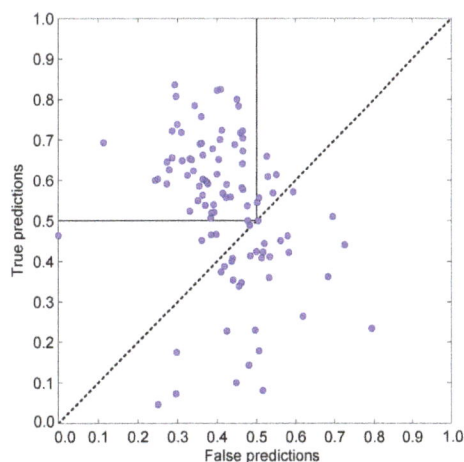

(a)

Figure 3. *Cont.*

(b)

(c)

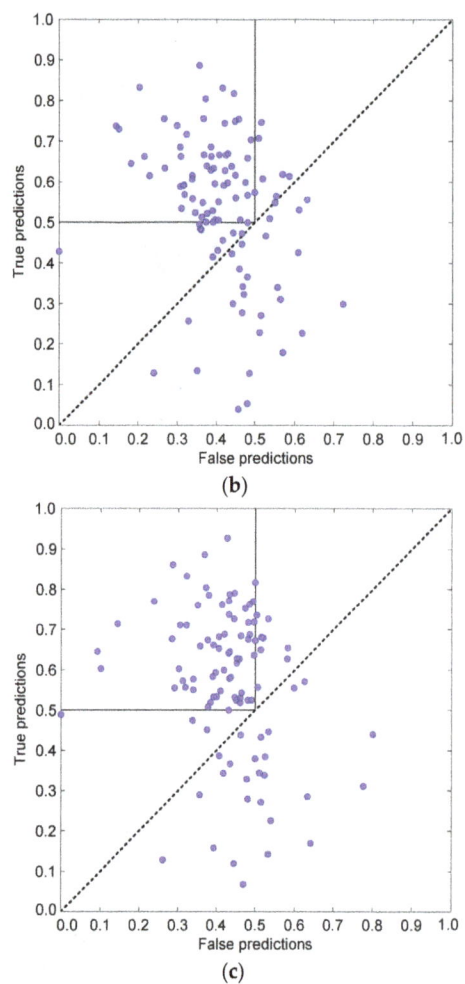

Figure 3. (**a**) Algorithm output for the prediction based on the adjustable number of fastest modes per chain and sequential influence of hot residues, for high sequence-length ratio dimer chains (length ratio greater than two, chain length greater than 80 residues). The true positives mean true is 53.27%, and the false positives mean is 42.05%. There is 56.31% of good predictions (58 of 103 chains) and only 14.56% of very bad predictions (15 chains). (**b**) Algorithm output for the prediction based on the adjustable number of fastest modes per chain and the variable 3D influence per hot residue (the influence of a hot residue is spread to spatial neighbors closer than 6 or 8 Å), for chains in dimers with high sequence length ratios (Length ratio > 2, length > 80 residues). The true positives mean true is 53.77%, and false positives mean is 41.29%. There is 56.31% of good predictions (58 chains) and 8.74% of very bad predictions (9 chains). (**c**) Algorithm output for the prediction based on the adjustable number of fastest modes per chain and combined 1D & 3D influences of hot residues, for chains in dimers with high sequence length ratio (Length ratio > 2, length > 80 residues). The true positives mean is 56.77%, and the false positives mean is 43.21%. There is 63.11% of good predictions (65 chains) and 11.65% of very bad predictions (12 chains).

Figure 3a shows how this adaptable approach works with heterodimers with high sequence length ratios (the length ratio larger than two and chain lengths longer than 80). The statistical analysis shows a remarkable improvement over the previous prediction attempts. The true positives mean is 53.27%, and the false positives mean is 42.05%. There is 56.31% of good predictions (58 proteins) and only 14.56% of very bad predictions (15 proteins). The distribution of good and very bad predictions over the chain lengths is also very favorable (Figure S13 in the Supplementary Materials).

The analysis performed on the four chains used previously to describe the prediction procedure confirms the above results (Figure S14 in the Supplementary Materials). For the three longest protein chains, 1BVN chain P, 2SNI chain E, and 1UDI chain E, the percent of true positives is over 50%, and the percent of false positives is less than 50%. The protein chain E of 1UDI has a highest difference between the true and false positives, which is an indication of a high correlation between the kinetically hot residues and contact scaffolds for that chain. Only the shortest example, 1CXZ chain A, has both true and false positives over 50%.

When this approach is applied to heterodimer proteins with low sequence length ratios (with the chains longer than 80 residues), the results are less than satisfactory (Figure S15 in the Supplementary Materials). The true positives mean is 50.39%, and the false positives mean is 49.53%. The amount of good and bed predictions is very close, namely, there is 34.85% of good predictions (upper left quadrant, 46 of 132 proteins) and 27.27% of very bad predictions (lower left quadrant, 36 proteins). The distribution of good and bad predictions is also not favorable (Figure S16 in the Supplementary Materials).

3.3.2. 3D Spatial Prediction—Variable Influence of Hot Residues

The adjustable algorithm introduced in the previous chapter uses sequential neighbors only to spread the influence of hot residues. It produces good predictions of contact and first-layer residues but offers a room for improvement. The prediction can be improved if spatial neighbors, instead of sequential ones, are used to spread the influence of hot residues. This approach is much closer to the true nature of the GNM algorithm that uses only spatial distances between C_α atoms and disregards any sequential/connectivity information. To apply this approach, the maximum cutoff C_α-C_α distance from the center of a hot residue was introduced, from which its influence can be spread. The cutoff distance of 6 Å was applied with for shorter protein chains (for sequence lengths shorter than 250), and the cutoff of 8 Å was applied for longer protein chains. All residues that are within the sphere centered at the C_α atom of the hot residue and within the assigned cutoff distance are considered to be "predictions", i.e., they are assumed to be either contact or first-layer residues. All other residues are rejected (for that particular hot residue). The two cutoff values were estimated empirically. To extract spatial neighbors, distances between residues (C_α-C_α distances) were calculated for each particular protein and sorted in ascending order.

Figure 3b depicts the algorithm output for the heterodimers with the sequence length ratios higher than two for protein chains with a chain length longer than 80 residues. The true positives mean is 53.77%, and false positives mean is 41.29%. There is 56.31% of good predictions (58 proteins) and only 8.74% of very bad predictions (8 proteins). There is also a noticeable number of predictions with a very favorable ratio of true positives vs. false positives, which are outside the upper left quadrant and thus do not belong to the good predictions as we defined them. Figure S17 in the Supplementary Materials shows the distribution of good and very bad predictions. Figure S18 in the Supplementary Materials shows the predictions for the four examples used previously.

With proteins from low sequence length ratio dimers, the results are not as good. The true positives mean is 52.22%, and the false positives mean is 48.81%. There is 42.42% of good predictions (56 proteins) and 27.27% of very bad predictions (36 proteins). See Figures S19 and S20 in the Supplementary Materials.

3.3.3. Combining the Sequential and Spatial Approaches

The two methods described previously base their prediction on the adjustable number of modes. The first method spreads the influence of hot residues linearly, i.e., to sequential neighbors only, while the second method spreads the influence to spatial neighbors within a sphere of a given cutoff radius. The first method treats a protein chain as a set of amino acids that are chained together. The second method only sees the spatial-3D neighborhood of a hot residue and rejects the fact that the protein is an ordered set of amino acids that are physically connected. This chapter introduces the combination of the sequential and 3D spatial approaches in attempt to boost the overall prediction. By combining the one-dimensional linear approach with the three-dimensional one, the residue connectivity information is included into the structure based method, which thus takes into account the chain-like nature of proteins (GNM method disregards chain connectivity and uses only physical distances between C_α atoms to calculate the protein connectivity matrix). In this combined approach, the influence of a hot residue is first spread linearly to its sequential neighbors (upstream and downstream along the sequence). After that, the influence is spread to the hot residue's spatial neighbors whose C_α atoms are within a sphere of a given cutoff radius with a center in the hot residue's C_α atom (the radius is 6 or 8 Å, depending on the sequence length).

Figure 3c shows the effects of the combined approach. When applied to the set of heterodimers with a high sequence length ratio, this approach produces an increase in the true positives mean (56.77%) without a significant increase in the false positives mean (43.21%). More importantly, the combined approach puts 63.11% of proteins in the upper left quadrant (good predictions, 65 proteins), but keeps very bad predictions at a reasonably low 11.65% (12 proteins). The number of good predictions for sequence lengths between 200 and 300 is slightly increased, as well as the number of predictions for sequence lengths between 400 and 500 (see Figure S21 in the Supplementary Materials). This change may indicate that method based on the variable influence of hot residues on their spatial neighborhood works better with longer protein chains. That may be expected, because bigger proteins with longer sequences have more modes and offer finer resolution with the weighted sum than smaller proteins with shorter sequences. See also Figure S22 for the four examples used previously.

With the proteins from low sequence-length ratio dimers, the situation is, as expected, not as good. The true positives mean is 51.57% to the false positives of 50.00%. There is 37.88% of predictions in the upper left quadrant (50 out of 132 proteins) to 29.55% in the lower right quadrant (39 proteins), see Figures S23 and S24 in the Supplementary Materials.

When both proteins per dimer are addressed as a pair using the combined approach (adjustable GNM, plus 1D & 3D influence of kinetically hot residues), the analysis confirms that heterodimers with high sequence length ratios often behave quite differently from heterodimers with low sequence length ratios (see Figure 4). In majority of cases belonging to the former group, at least one protein has contact and first-layer residues gathered around its kinetically hot residues (as recognized by the adjustable GNM). Figure 4a shows that 85.29% of the high sequence length ratio dimers has at least one chain in the upper left quadrant (32.35% of those dimers has both chains in the upper left quadrant, and 53% only one chain), as opposed to 58.46% of the low sequence length dimers (only 18.46% of them have both chains in the upper left quadrant). Only 8.82% of the high sequence length ratio dimers has none of the chains above the diagonal, as opposed to 27.69% of the low sequence length dimers (Figure 4b). In 47% of cases, the high sequence length ratio dimers have both chains above the diagonal (44.12% of high sequence dimers has only one). On the other hand, 29.23% of the low sequence length ratio dimers have both chains above the diagonal (43.08% of low sequence heterodimers has only one chain above the diagonal). This analysis suggests that proteins that form high sequence-length ratio heterodimers (sequence length ration higher than 2) often behave like a rigid lock and key. They have at least one rigid interfacial surface (often both surfaces are rigid). Chains forming low sequence-length ratio dimers are presumably more flexible in that respect and more often than not have one of the chains more flexible than the other. That protein chain adjusts its conformations for a tighter fit. This should not be a general conclusion because smaller (sequentially shorter) protein chains have a large number of false positives, simply because they have relatively large total number of targets (contact and first-layer residues, see Figure 2). A similar observation was made by Martin and Lavery [97]. They concluded that the surface of a small chain easily gets saturated with contacts when bound to a larger partner. With larger proteins, contact residues are highly localized. They also observed that docking hits tend to accumulate closer to the geometrical center of the protein. That observation is in concordance with the approach presented here, which, besides contact residues, also uses first-layer residues to enhance the prediction. Residues in the geometrical center are surrounded with a large number of neighbors and have higher packing density. They are, therefore, more stable and thus emphasized by the fast modes.

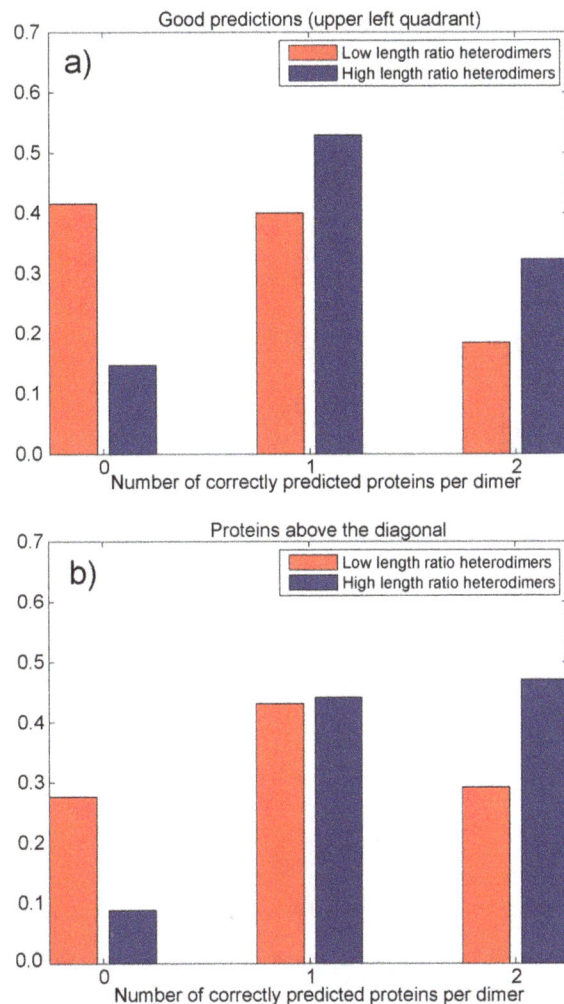

Figure 4. Number of correctly predicted chains per heterodimer using the combined (1D and 3D) adjustable approach, for dimers in which both chains are longer than 80 residues. Two cases are analyzed: heterodimers with long sequence length ratios (>2) and heterodimers with short sequence length ratio (≤2). (**a**) Number of chains per dimer in the upper left quadrant. (**b**) Number of chains per heterodimer above the main diagonal (the diagoanal that passes through the lower left and upper right quadrants).

3.4. Prediction Algorithms Comparison

In the previous chapters a number of methods for the contact and first-layer residues prediction were presented. The presentation started with a very simple approach based on the fixed number of modes (5) and ended with a protocol that adjusts the number of modes to the analyzed chain and spreads the influence of a hot residue in the adaptable fashion using the sequential and spatial influence of hot residues. The true evaluation of these protocols can be done only through a direct comparison of their prediction efficiencies. The comparison of the true positives mean vs. the false positives mean and comparison of their good vs. very bad predictions are obvious measures of the quality of the prediction, and we used them here (see Figure 5). As the figure shows, the true prediction improvement is achieved only with the adjustable number of modes (prediction protocol **d** in the Figure 5a,b). Additional improvements are achieved with the full 3D influence spread (protocol **e** in Figure 5a,b), as well as with the combination of sequential (1D) and spatial (3D) approaches (protocol **f** in Figure 5a,b).

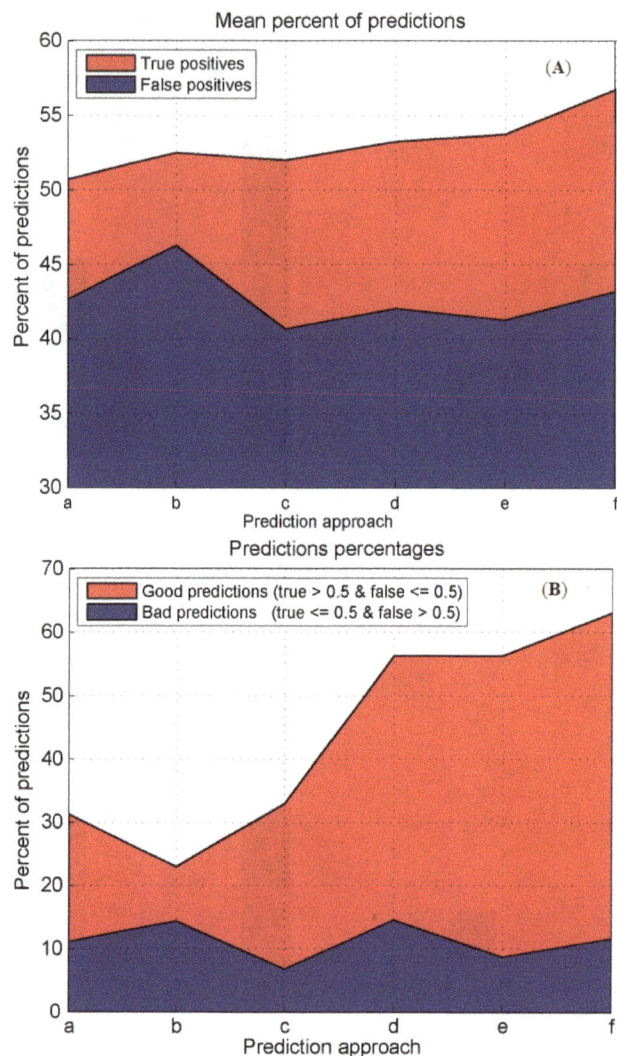

Figure 5. (**A**) Prediction algorithms comparison expressed as a plot of the true positives mean and the false positives mean percentages for each algorithm described previously. The first two algorithms were applied on all heterodimer chains. In all other cases, algorithms were applied on the heterodimer chains with high sequence-length ratios. The algorithms are (a) all heterodimers, 5 fastest modes; (b) all heterodimers, fastest modes corresponding to top 10% of eigenvalues range; (c) high sequence length ratio, fastest modes corresponding to top 10% of eigenvalues range; (d) adjustable number of modes, 1D influence; (e) adjustable modes, 3D influence, within a sphere with a radius of 6 or 8 Å; and (f) algorithms **d** and **e** combined. (**B**) Prediction algorithms comparison expressed as a percentage of good and very bad chains. The first two algorithms were applied on all heterodimer chains. In all other cases, algorithms were applied on the chains with high sequence-length ratios. The algorithms are (a) all heterodimers, 5 fastest modes; (b) all heterodimers, with fastest modes corresponding to top 10% of eigenvalues range; (c) high sequence length ratio, with fastest modes corresponding to top 10% of eigenvalues range; (d) adjustable number of modes, 1D influence; (e) adjustable modes, 3D influence, within a sphere with a radius of 6 or 8 Å; (f) algorithms **d** and **e** combined.

Figure 6 illustrates the ability of the adjustable approach (1D and 3D influences combined) to recognize binding scaffolds. It nicely depicts than in some cases, the adjustable GNM very accurately predicts the binding scaffolds.

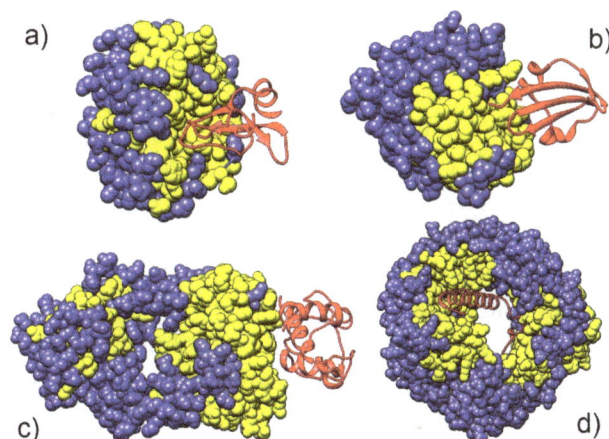

Figure 6. Ability of the adjustable 1D&3D GNM algorithm to predict binding scaffolds. It is depicted via four heterodimers (PDB ID codes 1BRC, 1DTD, 1WEJ, and 1QGK). The analyzed chains are blue, depicted using the whole atom representation, with the adjustable GNM predictions colored yellow. Partnering chains are red and depicted as ribbons. (**a**) Chains E and I from the protein 1BRC. The chain E was analyzed with the adjustable GNM. This is a very good prediction. There is 75.29% true positives, with 47.41% false positives. (**b**) Chains A and B from the protein 1DTD. The chain A was analyzed with the adjustable GNM. This is a very good prediction. There is 71.08% true positives, and only 30.45% false positives. For the chain A, only residues 363 to 665 are given in the PDB file. There is a Zinc atom and four water molecules embedded in the interface (not shown). The binding interface is defined only using the weighted sum (Equation (1)). (**c**) Chains L and F from the protein 1WEJ. The chain L was analyzed with the adjustable GNM. This is a very good prediction. There is 92.73% true positives, and 42.67% false positives. (**d**) Chains A and B from 1QGK. The chain A was analyzed with the adjustable GNM. This is a very good prediction. There is 88.58% true positives, and only 36.83% false positives.

The analysis of the relationship between the number of modes and sequence length (Table S1 and Figure S25 in the Supplementary Materials) reveals an interesting trend. For protein chains shorter than 600 residues, with accurately predicted contact and first-layer residues via the combined approach, the relationship between the number of fast modes n and the sequence length s is roughly linear ($m = 2.1831 + 0.014254 \times s$, i.e., $m \approx 2.1831 + (1/70) \times s$). However, when longer chains are included, the relationship becomes quadratic ($m = 3.4794 + (0.00030756) \times s + (2.8381 \times 10^{-5}) \times s^2$). Those relationships are strongly influenced by the distribution of chains in the training set (Figure S1 in the Supplementary Materials). A more uniform distribution will probably change the shapes/slopes of these two lines. It should be noted that two relationships are close to each other for chains shorter than 600 residues; Figure S25 in the Supplementary Materials nicely depicts those trends. Haliloglu et al. [60] used a cutoff of 15% of the number of residues to establish a number of modes used in kinetically hot residues recognition. Our results show that the number of fast modes is generally smaller.

3.5. Vakser and Sternberg Decoy Sets

Previous chapters dealt with the development of the contact residues recognition protocol. This chapter depicts how the adjustable protocol behaves with the Vakser [88] and Sternberg decoy sets [87]. Those decoy sets are numerically created protein structure sets created with the intention of evaluating the quality of protein binding prediction protocols. To properly evaluate the adjustable GNM protocols, for each decoy in both sets, contact and first-layer residues were calculated for each protein that formed a dimer. All adjustable GNM algorithms were tested, and the 3D adjustable approach showed the best overall results.

For each decoy pair, the binding energy was calculated using the statistical potential of Lu and Skolnick [89]. That energy was used to compare and evaluate the adjustable GNM prediction protocol against a residue level statistical potential. The residue-residue based approach of Lu and Skolnick assesses the strength of each decoy (taking both chains together) using an empirical statistical potential (given as a 20 × 20 matrix). The binding affinity of each decoy is expressed as a potential energy of binding. The lower that energy is, the more probable the decoy is, according to the statistical potential method.

Figure 7 depicts the behavior of decoys on the true/false scatter plot used in previous chapters via two decoy subsets (1CHO and 2SIC). The standing of each protein chain is calculated as its Cartesian distance from the point with coordinates (0, 1), i.e., the standing of a protein is its "distance" from a point with 0% of false predictions and 100% true predictions. Figure 8 depicts the behavior of the adjustable GNM in combination with the statistical potential using the same two decoy subsets.

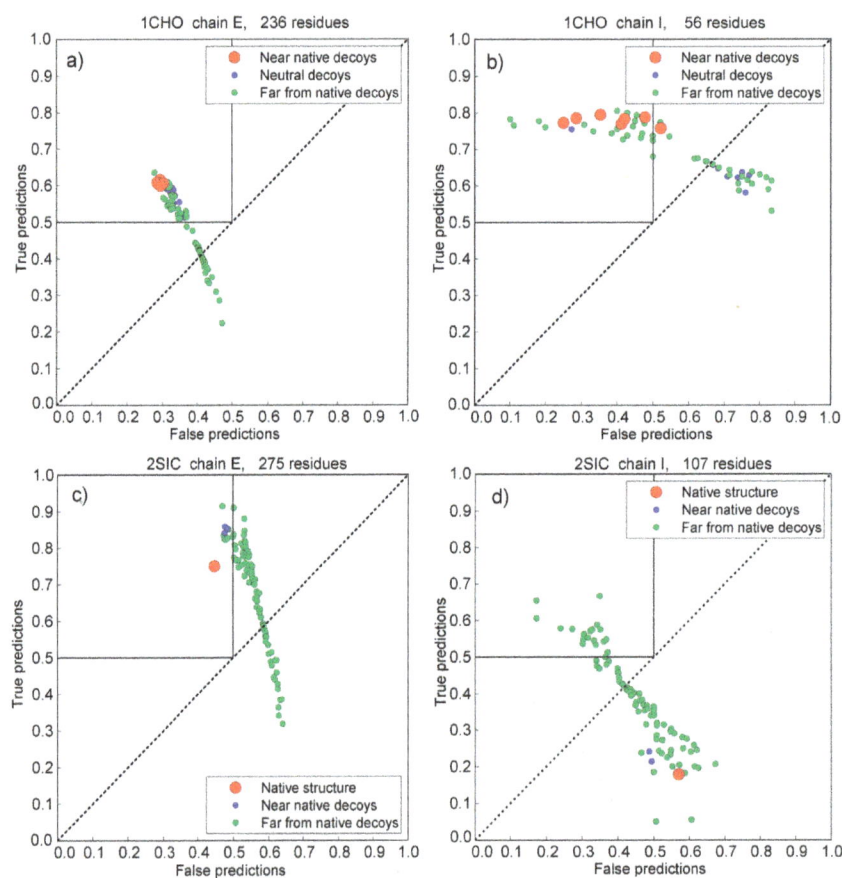

Figure 7. Protein dimer decoys recognition using the adjustable GNM protocol. The influence of hot residues is spread to spatial neighbors closer than 6 or 8 Å. Subplots (**a**) and (**b**) are from the Vakser decoy sets (PDB ID 1CHO). Blue circles depict neutral decoys regardless (neither native nor far from it). Decoys far from native structure are green, and near native ones are red. Subplots (**c**) and (**d**) are from the Sternberg decoy sets (PDB ID 2SIC). Green dots depict far from native decoys. Near native decoys are blue, and the native structure is a red circle.

The quality of the assessment of both methods (adjustable GNM and statistical potential) is expressed via two scores: the best status of a near native decoy among the all decoys, and the coverage, i.e., the number of near native decoys among the best n decoys, in which n is the number of near native decoys. Those two evaluations are depicted in Tables S2 and S3, and in Figures S26 and S27 in the Supplementary Materials. The combination of the two approaches is given in the last 6 columns of the Tables S2 and S3. The combined standing is given as a Cartesian distance of a chain with two scores between 1 and 110 (100 for Vakser) from the point with coordinates (1, 1). The point (1, 1) corresponds to a structure that should be first according to the both methods.

Our analysis reveals that in 19 out of 41 Vakser decoys sets (1AVW_AV, 1BUI_AC, 1BVN_PT, 1CHO_EI, 1EWY_AC, 1FM9_DA, 1GPQ_DA, 1HE1_CA, 1MA9_AB, 1OPH_AB, 1PPF_EI, 1UGH_EI, 1WQ1_GR, 1YVB_AI, 2BKR_AB, 2FI4_EI, 2SNI_EI, 3SIC_EI, 2BTF_AP), and in 4 out of 10 Sternberg decoys sets (1BRC, 1UGH, 1WQ1, 2SIC), either one or both chains are properly accessed by the adjustable GNM method. Those observations are even more significant if decoy sets badly characterized by both methods (adjustable GNM and statistical potential) are removed from the analysis (Vakser sets 1F6M_AC, 1G6V_AK, 1GPQ_DA, 1TX6_AI, and Sternberg set 1AVZ). The chains that form these dimers probably experience significant structural rearrangements during or upon the binding. In most cases, the longer chain is better assessed through the adjustable GNM than its shorter partner, which was to be expected following the assumption of the opposite behavior of binding partners, but in some cases (Vakser sets 1BVN_PT, 1GPQ_DA, 1HE1_CA, 1MA9_AB, 2BKR_AB, 2BTF_AP) the shorter partner has a higher score. The adjustable GNM protocol is fairly successful in predicting near native structures. That information should be taken in the light of fact that near native decoys are based on nonbound structures, which makes the protocol even more successful. Similar ability was reported by Kozakov et al. [68]. The statistical potential produces much better overall results, but in some cases (Vakser set 1PPF_EI, for example) the structural evaluation of the decoys set was better than the evaluation using the empirical statistical potential.

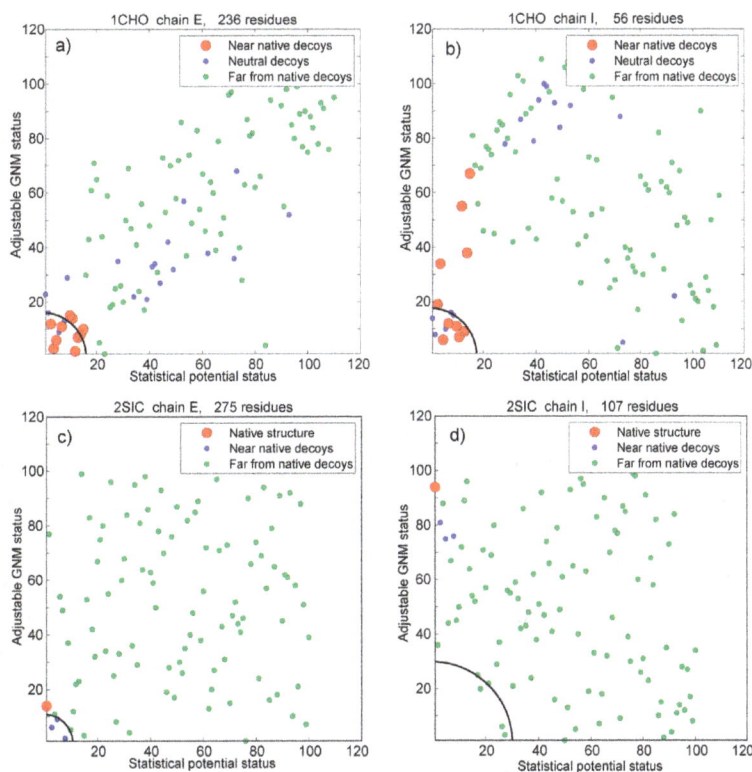

Figure 8. Comparison of the abilities of the adjustable spatial GNM approach and the statistical potential to distinguish near native decoys/structures from false decoys. Blue dots depict neutral decoys. Decoys far from native structure are green, and near native ones are red. Two decoys sets are depicted (1CHO from Vakser set, and 2SIC from Sternberg set), with two chains per example. The left plot in each example corresponds to the longer chain, and the right plot to its shorter pair. The circular segments in the lower left corners correspond to the distances of the n-th best chain according to the combined approach of the adjustable GNM and the statistical potential, in which n is the number of near native structures. It is a good measure of the concordance between the two methods.

4. Conclusions

This paper addresses the physical interactions of proteins, which is an important issue in molecular biology and biophysics. It depicts a method based on the theory of phantom networks [48,49,52] and its Gaussian Network Model expansion [54–57,60]. The described methodology attempts to relate the stable, kinetically hot residues, together with residues in their direct neighborhood (together termed binding scaffolds), to the binding residues on the surface and in the interior of the proteins forming protein dimers. As the number of residues emphasized by GNM is usually smaller than the number of target residues, an improvement of GNM was developed to spread the influence of each kinetically hot residue to its neighbors in an adjustable fashion. The paper first describes a method based on a small and fixed number of fast modes and a similar approach that uses the fast modes that correspond to the upper 10% of the eigenvalues span. Both approaches offer only a limited ability to correlate the kinetically hot residues and the binding scaffolds. A limited improvement was achieved with heterodimers with a significant difference in chain length. The true improvement was produced when the number of modes was allowed to fluctuate until the number of predictions matched the expected number of targets for a given sequence length. The combination of sequential and spatial influence was shown to have the best ability to recognize the target residues. That may imply that connectivity information, although not explicit in the Gaussian Network Model, partially determines the kinetic behavior of residues. Therefore, it should be used together with the graph representation of protein structure in the analysis of the behavior of proteins and their contact patterns.

The adjustable GNM protocols were tested on Sternberg [87] and Vakser [88] decoy sets. With both sets, the adjustable GNM approach with the spatial spread only achieved a noticeable success in predicting target residues. The combined approach using both the adjustable GNM and the statistical potential of Lu and Skolnick [89] improved the prediction in comparison to the pure adjustable approach.

The approach described here can be an excellent guide to a more efficient drug design, especially for the design of small molecule inhibitors of protein-protein interactions [44–47]. The algorithm(s) depicted here can help in filtering "in-house" databases [45] and thus facilitate the drug screening process.

As pointed out in [98] and demonstrated in a series of recent publications (see, e.g., [71–73,75,79,82,83,85,99–102]), user-friendly and publicly accessible web-servers represent the future direction for developing more useful and practical prediction methods. Actually, many practically useful web-servers have had an increasing impact on medical science [103], driving medicinal chemistry into an unprecedented revolution. We shall make efforts in our future work to provide a web-server for the prediction method presented in this paper.

The adjustable approach, although able to dynamically connect the kinetically hot residues and binding patches and the corresponding structural scaffolds, still has a space for improvement. For instance, the application of surface area descriptors may reduce the false positives rate. A better estimation of the number of expected target residues may also improve the prediction. The application of the latest protein-protein and protein-ligand databases [46] may also help in that regard.

This work was primarily focused on the behavior of heterodimers. Homodimers were not explored in detail. Their behavior should be addressed more thoroughly, for example, by using a combination of slow and fast modes [30]. Furthermore, the slow modes describe global motions of chain segments and may lead toward a better understanding of the conformational changes that proteins undergo during and upon binding. Those changes still lack proper quantification [104].

The importance of this work is twofold. First, it gives an efficient algorithm that is able to decipher individual protein-protein interactions, and it offers a theoretical insight into the mechanism of protein binding. Second, it shows that a simple approach based only on the statistic of residue-residue interactions may lead to overfitting; thus, the shape of partnering protein chains, as well as the absolute and relative size of the interacting proteins (molecules), should be also taken into account.

The fact that in heterodimers, at least one of the proteins has its binding scaffold determined by the kinetically hot residues may imply that protein-protein interactions are, at least partially, entropically driven [105]. Highly organized pockets delineated by kinetically hot residues attract physically smaller partnering proteins in an attempt to increase the total entropy of the system (i.e., to decrease the structural order defined by unmovable, kinetically hot residues). This observation opens an area for further research.

Supplementary Materials: The following are available online at http://www.mdpi.com/1424-8247/11/1/29/s1, Figure S1: An illustration of the targets, Figure S2: Protein chain lengths distribution for both heterodimers and homodimers, Figure S3: Prediction histogram based on the analysis of all chains over the sequence lengths for the simple prediction approach based on five fastest modes, Figure S4: Prediction histogram for heterodimer chains only, for the simple prediction approach based on the 5 fastest modes, Figure S5: An example of the one dimensional, i.e., sequential approach to prediction, for 4 different chains (1BVN chain P, 2SNI chain E, 1UDI chain E and 1CXZ chain A), Figure S6: Distributions of eigenvalues for three different protein chains (dimer 1ETT chains H, dimer 1BVN chain P and dimer 1QGK chain A), Figure S7: An example of the 1D prediction (sequential neighbors influence only) based on the fastest 10% of modes per chain, for 4 different chains (1BVN chain P, 2SNI chain E, 1UDI chain E and 1CXZ chain A), Figure S8: Prediction histogram for heterodimer chains only, for the prediction approach based on the modes that correspond to top 10% of the eigenvalues span, Figure S9: Dimer chain lengths for the set of 139 different heterodimers, Figure S10: Prediction histogram, for chains in heterodimers with high sequence length ratios for the prediction approach based on the modes which correspond to top 10% of eigenvalues span, Figure S11: Prediction output for chains in heterodimers with low sequence length ratios for the prediction approach based on modes corresponding to top 10% of eigenvalues range, Figure S12: Prediction histogram over the sequence lengths for the simple prediction approach based on the fastest 10% of modes for each chain, for chains in heterodimers with low sequence length ratios, Figure S13: Histogram of predictions over the sequence lengths for the prediction approach based on the adjustable number of fast modes, with the 1D influence of hot residues, for chains in dimers with high sequence length ratio, Figure S14: Examples of the prediction based on the adjustable number of fast modes and the sequential influence of hot residues, Figure S15: Prediction output based on the approach that uses an adjustable number of fastest modes per chain and sequential influence of hot residues, for low sequence-length ratio dimer chains, Figure S16: Prediction histogram over the sequence lengths for the prediction approach based on the adjustable number of fast modes, for the 1D influence of hot residues, for chains in dimers with low sequence length ratio, Figure S17: Prediction histogram over the sequence lengths for the prediction approach based on the adjustable number of fast modes and variable 3D influence per hot residue, for chains in dimers with high sequence length ratio, Figure S18: Examples of the prediction based on the adjustable number of fast modes and the sequential influence of hot residues, Figure S19: Prediction output for the prediction approach based on the adjustable number of fastest modes per chain and the variable 3D influence per hot residue, for chains in dimers with low sequence length ratios, Figure S20: Prediction histogram over the sequence lengths for the prediction approach based on the adjustable number of fast modes and the variable 3D influence per hot residue, for chains in dimers with low sequence length ratio, Figure S21: Prediction histogram over the sequence lengths for the prediction approach based on the adjustable number of fast modes and combined 1D & fixed 3D influence per hot residue for chains in dimers with high sequence length ratio (length ratio higher than 2, length > 80 residues), Figure S22: Examples of the prediction based on the adjustable number of fast modes and combined 1D & 3D influence per hot residue, Figure S23: Prediction output for the prediction approach based on the adjustable number of fastest modes per chain and combined 1D & 3D influences of hot residues, for chains in dimers with low sequence length ratio, Figure S24: Prediction histogram over the sequence lengths for the prediction approach based on the adjustable number of fast modes and combined 1D & fixed 3D influence per hot residue for chains in dimers with low sequence length ratio, Figure S25: Linear and quadratic relationships of the number of modes per chain, for successfully characterized heterodimer chains from dimers with high sequence length ratios, Figure S26: Comparison of the abilities of the adjustable 3D GNM approach, the statistical potential and their combination to distinguish near native decoys from the false decoys, Figure S27, Comparison of the abilities of the adjustable 3D GNM approach, the statistical potential and their combination to distinguish near native decoys from the false decoys, Table S1: The summary of good predictions, Table S2: The efficiency of the adjustable prediction algorithm (3D algorithm with variable number of modes) with the Vakser decoy sets, Table S3: The efficiency of the adjustable prediction algorithm (3D algorithm with variable number of modes) with the Sternberg decoy sets.

Acknowledgments: The author is indebted to Dr. Hui Lu for suggesting him to work on the problem of heterodimer interactions and for advising him to use the first-layer residues to boost up the prediction.

References

1. Mardis, E.R. The impact of next-generation sequencing technology on genetics. *Trends Genet.* **2008**, *24*, 133–141. [CrossRef] [PubMed]

2. Quail, M.A.; Smith, M.; Coupland, P.; Otto, T.D.; Harris, S.R.; Connor, T.R.; Bertoni, A.; Swerdlow, H.P.; Gu, Y. A tale of three next generation sequencing platforms: Comparison of Ion Torrent, Pacific Biosciences and Illumina MiSeq sequencers. *BMC Genom.* **2012**, *13*, 341. [CrossRef] [PubMed]

3. Pabinger, S.; Dander, A.; Fischer, M.; Snajder, R.; Sperk, M.; Efremova, M.; Krabichler, B.; Speicher, M.R.; Zschocke, J.; Trajanoski, Z. A survey of tools for variant analysis of next-generation genome sequencing data. *Brief. Bioinform.* **2014**, *15*, 256–278. [CrossRef] [PubMed]

4. The UniProt Consortium. UniProt: A hub for protein information. *Nucleic Acids Res.* **2015**, *43*, D204–D212.

5. Uhlén, M.; Faqerberg, L.; Hallstrom, B.M.; Lindskog, C.; Oksvold, P.; Mardinoqlu, A.; Sivertsson, A.; Kampf, C.; Sjostedt, E.; Asplund, A.; et al. Tissue-based map of the human proteome. *Science* **2015**, *347*, 1260419. [CrossRef] [PubMed]

6. Kola, I.; Landis, J. Can the pharmaceutical industry reduce attrition rates? *Nat. Rev. Drug Discov.* **2004**, *3*, 711–716. [CrossRef] [PubMed]

7. Hutchinson, L.; Kirk, R. High drug attrition rates-where are we going wrong? *Nat. Rev. Clin. Oncol.* **2011**, *8*, 189–190. [CrossRef] [PubMed]

8. Abad-Zapatero, C.; Perišić, O.; Wass, J.; Bento, A.P.; Overington, J.; Al-Lazikani, B.; Johnson, M.E. Ligand efficiency indices for an effective mapping of chemico-biological space: The concept of an atlas-like representation. *Drug Discov. Today* **2010**, *15*, 804–811. [CrossRef] [PubMed]

9. Bhardwaj, N.; Langlois, R.E.; Zhao, G.; Lu, H. Kernel-based machine learning protocol for predicting DNA-binding proteins. *Nucleic Acid Res.* **2005**, *30*, 6486–6493. [CrossRef] [PubMed]

10. Langlois, R.E.; Carson, M.B.; Bhardwaj, N.; Lu, H. Learning to Translate Sequence and Structure to Function: Identifying DNA Binding and Membrane Binding Proteins. *Ann. Biomed. Eng.* **2007**, *35*, 1043–1052. [CrossRef] [PubMed]

11. Bhardwaj, N.; Stahelin, R.V.; Zhao, G.; Cho, W.; Lu, H. MeTaDoR: A comprehensive resource for membrane targeting domains and their host proteins. *Bioinformatics* **2007**, *23*, 3110–3112. [CrossRef] [PubMed]

12. Carson, M.B.; Langlois, R.; Lu, H. NAPS: A residue-level nucleic acid-binding prediction server. *Nucleic Acid Res.* **2010**, *38*, W431–W435. [CrossRef] [PubMed]

13. Bhardwaj, N.; Gerstein, M.; Lu, H. Genome-wide sequence-based prediction of peripheral proteins using a novel semi-supervised learning technique. *BMC Bioinform.* **2010**, *11*, S6. [CrossRef] [PubMed]

14. Piana, S.; Lindorff-Larsen, K.; Shaw, D.E. Atomistic Description of the Folding of a Dimeric Protein. *J. Phys. Chem. B* **2013**, *117*, 12935–12942. [CrossRef] [PubMed]

15. Piana, S.; Klepeis, J.L.; Shaw, D.E. Assessing the accuracy of physical models used in protein-folding simulations: Quantitative evidence from long molecular dynamics simulations. *Curr. Opin. Struct. Biol.* **2014**, *24*, 98–105. [CrossRef] [PubMed]

16. Shoemaker, B.A.; Panchenko, A.R. Deciphering Protein-Protein Interactions. Part I. Experimental Techniques and Databases. *PLoS Comput. Biol.* **2007**, *3*. [CrossRef] [PubMed]

17. Shoemaker, B.A.; Panchenko, A.R. Deciphering Protein-Protein Interactions. Part II. Computational Methods to Predict Protein and Domain Interaction Partners. *PLoS Comput. Biol.* **2007**, *3*. [CrossRef] [PubMed]

18. Moal, I.H.; Moretti, R.; Baker, D.; Fernandez-Recio, J. Scoring functions for protein-protein interactions. *Curr. Opin. Struct. Biol.* **2013**, *23*, 862–867. [CrossRef] [PubMed]

19. Baaden, M.; Marrink, S.J. Coarse-grain modelling of protein-protein interactions. *Curr. Opin. Struct. Biol.* **2013**, *23*, 878–886. [CrossRef] [PubMed]

20. Wodak, S.J.; Vlasblom, J.; Turinsky, A.L.; Pu, S. Protein-protein interaction networks: The puzzling riches. *Curr. Opin. Struct. Biol.* **2013**, *23*, 941–953. [CrossRef] [PubMed]

21. Mosca, R.; Pons, T.; Céol, A.; Valencia, A.; Aloy, P. Towards a detailed atlas of protein-protein interactions. *Curr. Opin. Struct. Biol.* **2013**, *23*, 929–940. [CrossRef] [PubMed]

22. Neuvirth, H.; Raz, R.; Schreiber, G. ProMate: A Structure Based Prediction Program to Identify the Location of Protein-Protein Binding Sites. *J. Mol. Biol.* **2004**, *338*, 181–199. [CrossRef] [PubMed]

23. Chen, H.; Zhou, HX. Prediction of interface residues in protein-protein complexes by a consensus neural network method: Test against NMR data. *Proteins Struct. Funct. Bioinform.* **2005**, *61*, 21–35. [CrossRef] [PubMed]

24. Liang, S.; Zhang, C.; Liu, S.; Zhou, Y. Protein binding site prediction using an empirical scoring function. *Nucleic Acid Res.* **2006**, *34*, 3698–3707. [CrossRef] [PubMed]

25. Zhang, Q.C.; Petrey, D.; Norel, R.; Honig, B.H. Protein interface conservation across structure space. *Proc. Natl. Acad. Sci. USA* **2010**, *107*, 10896–10901. [CrossRef] [PubMed]

26. Saccà, C.; Teso, S.; Diligenti, M.; Passerini, A. Improved multi-level protein-protein interaction prediction with semantic-based regularization. *BMC Bioinform.* **2014**, *15*, 103. [CrossRef] [PubMed]

27. Berman, H.M.; Westbrook, J.; Feng, Z.; Gilliland, G.; Bhat, T.N.; Weissig, H.; Shindyalov, I.N.; Bourne, P.E. The Protein Data Bank. *Nucleic Acids Res.* **2000**, *28*, 235–242. [CrossRef] [PubMed]

28. Zhang, Q.C.; Petrey, D.; Deng, L.; Qiang, L.; Shi, Y.; Thu, C.A.; Bisikirska, B.; Lefebvre, C.; Accili, D.; Hunter, T.; et al. Structure-based prediction of protein-protein interactions on a genome-wide scale. *Nature* **2012**, *490*, 556–560. [CrossRef] [PubMed]

29. Bhardwaj, N.; Lu, H. Co-expression among constituents of a motif in the protein-protein interaction network. *J. Bioinform. Comput. Biol.* **2009**, *7*, 1–17. [CrossRef] [PubMed]

30. Bahar, I.; Rader, A.J. Coarse-grained normal mode analysis in structural biology. *Curr. Opin. Struct. Biol.* **2005**, *15*, 586–592. [CrossRef] [PubMed]

31. Basdevant, N.; Borgis, D.; Ha-Duong, T. Modeling Protein-Protein Recognition in Solution Using the Coarse-Grained Force Field SCORPION. *J. Chem. Theory Comput.* **2012**, *9*, 803–813. [CrossRef] [PubMed]

32. Ravikumar, K.M.; Huang, W.; Yang, S. Coarse-Grained Simulations of Protein-Protein Association: An Energy Landscape Perspective. *Biophys. J.* **2012**, *103*, 837–845. [CrossRef] [PubMed]

33. Zacharias, M. Combining coarse-grained nonbonded and atomistic bonded interactions for protein modeling. *Proteins Struct. Funct. Bioinform.* **2013**, *81*, 81–92. [CrossRef] [PubMed]

34. Solernou, A.; Fernandez-Recio, J. pyDockCG: New Coarse-Grained Potential for Protein-Protein Docking. *J. Phys. Chem. B* **2011**, *115*, 6032–6039. [CrossRef] [PubMed]

35. Ołdziej, S.; Czaplewski, C.; Liwo, A.; Chinchio, M.; Nanias, M.; Vila, J.A.; Khalili, M.; Jagielska, Y.A.A.A.; Makowski, M.; Schafroth, H.D.; et al. Physics-based protein-structure prediction using a hierarchical protocol based on the UNRES force field: Assessment in two blind tests. *Proc. Natl. Acad. Sci. USA* **2005**, *102*, 7547–7552. [CrossRef] [PubMed]

36. Frembgen-Kesner, T.; Elcock, A.H. Absolute Protein-Protein Association Rate Constants from Flexible, Coarse-Grained Brownian Dynamics Simulations: The Role of Intermolecular Hydrodynamic Interactions in Barnase-Barstar Association. *Biophys. J.* **2010**, *99*, L75–L77. [CrossRef] [PubMed]

37. Min, J.-L.; Xiao, X.; Chou, K.-C. iEzy-Drug: A Web Server for Identifying the Interaction between Enzymes and Drugs in Cellular Networking. *BioMed Res. Int. (BMRI)* **2013**, *2013*, 701317. [CrossRef] [PubMed]

38. Xiao, X.; Min, J.-L.; Wang, P.; Chou, K.-C. iGPCR-Drug: A Web Server for Predicting Interaction between GPCRs and Drugs in Cellular Networking. *PLoS ONE* **2013**, *8*, e72234. [CrossRef] [PubMed]

39. Xiao, X.; Min, J.-L.; Wang, P.; Chou, K.-C. Predict Drug-Protein Interaction in Cellular Networking. *Curr. Top. Med. Chem.* **2013**, *13*, 1707–1712. [CrossRef] [PubMed]

40. Fan, Y.-N.; Xiao, X.; Min, J.-L.; Chou, K.-C. iNR-Drug: Predicting the Interaction of Drugs with Nuclear Receptors in Cellular Networking. *Int. J. Mol. Sci. (IJMS)* **2014**, *15*, 4915–4937. [CrossRef] [PubMed]

41. Xiao, X.; Min, J.-L.; Lin, W.-Z.; Liu, Z.; Cheng, X.; Chou, K.-C. iDrug-Target: Predicting the interactions between drug compounds and target proteins in cellular networking via benchmark dataset optimization approach. *J. Biomol. Struct. Dyn.* **2015**, *33*, 2221–2233. [CrossRef] [PubMed]

42. Jia, J.; Liu, Z.; Xiao, X.; Liu, B.; Chou, K.-C. iPPI-Esml: An ensemble classifier for identifying the interactions of proteins by incorporating their physicochemical properties and wavelet transforms into PseAAC. *J. Theor. Biol.* **2015**, *377*, 47–56. [CrossRef] [PubMed]

43. Jia, J.; Liu, Z.; Xiao, X.; Liu, B.; Chou, K.-C. Identification of protein-protein binding sites by incorporating the physicochemical properties and stationary wavelet transforms into pseudo amino acid composition. *J. Biomol. Struct. Dyn.* **2016**, *34*, 1946–1961. [CrossRef] [PubMed]

44. Mullard, A. Protein-protein interaction inhibitors get into the groove. *Nat. Rev. Drug Discov.* **2012**, *11*, 173–175. [CrossRef] [PubMed]

45. Morelli, X.; Bourgeas, R.; Roche, P. Chemical and structural lessons from recent successes in protein-protein interaction inhibition (2P2I). *Curr. Opin. Chem. Biol.* **2011**, *15*, 475–481. [CrossRef] [PubMed]

46. Basse, M.J.; Betzi, S.; Bourgeas, R.; Bouzidi, S.; Chetrit, B.; Hamon, V.; Morelli, X.; Roche, P. 2P2Idb: A structural database dedicated to orthosteric modulation of protein-protein interactions. *Nucleic Acids Res.* **2013**, *41*, D824–D827. [CrossRef] [PubMed]

47. Porta-Pardo, E.; Hrabe, T.; Godzik, A. Cancer3D: Understanding cancer mutations through protein structures. *Nucleic Acids Res.* **2014**, *43*, D968–D973. [CrossRef] [PubMed]

48. James, H.M.; Guth, E. Theory of the Increase in Rigidity of Rubber during Cure. *J. Chem. Phys.* **1947**, *15*, 669–683. [CrossRef]

49. Flory, P.J. Statistical thermodynamics of random networks. *Proc. R. Soc. A* **1976**, *351*, 351–380. [CrossRef]

50. Karplus, M.; Kushick, J. Method for estimating the configurational entropy of macromolecules. *Macromolecules* **1981**, *14*, 325–332. [CrossRef]

51. Levy, R.M.; Karplus, M.; Kushick, J.; Perahia, D. Evaluation of the configurational entropy for proteins: Application to molecular dynamics simulations of an α-helix. *Macromolecules* **1984**, *17*, 1370–1374. [CrossRef]

52. Flory, P.J. Molecular Theory of Rubber Elasticity. *Polym. J.* **1985**, *17*, 1–12. [CrossRef]

53. Tirion, M.M. Large Amplitude Elastic Motions in Proteins from a Single-Parameter, Atomic Analysis. *Phys. Rev. Lett.* **1995**, *77*, 1905–1908. [CrossRef] [PubMed]

54. Haliloglu, T.; Bahar, I.; Erman, B. Gaussian Dynamics of Folded Proteins. *Phys. Rev. Lett.* **1997**, *79*, 3090–3093. [CrossRef]

55. Bahar, I.; Atilgan, A.R.; Erman, B. Direct evaluation of thermal fluctuations in proteins using a single-parameter harmonic potential. *Fold. Des.* **1997**, *2*, 173–181. [CrossRef]

56. Bahar, I.; Atilgan, A.R.; Demirel, M.C.; Erman, B. Vibrational Dynamics of Folded Proteins. *Phys. Rev. Lett.* **1998**, *80*, 2733–2736. [CrossRef]

57. Demirel, M.C.; Atilgan, A.R.; Jernigan, R.L.; Erman, B.; Bahar, I. Identification of kinetically hot residues in proteins. *Protein Sci.* **1998**, *7*, 2522–2532. [CrossRef] [PubMed]

58. Bahar, I.; Erman, B.; Jernigan, R.L.; Atilgan, A.R.; Covell, D.G. Collective motions in HIV-1 reverse transcriptase: Examination of flexibility and enzyme function. *J. Mol. Biol.* **1999**, *285*, 1023–1037. [CrossRef] [PubMed]

59. Yang, L.; Eyal, E.; Chennubhotla, C.; Jee, J.; Gronenborn, A.M.; Bahar, I. Insights into Equilibrium Dynamics of Proteins from Comparison of NMR and X-Ray Data with Computational Predictions. *Structure* **2007**, *15*, 741–749. [CrossRef] [PubMed]

60. Haliloglu, T.; Keskin, O.; Ma, B.; Nussinov, R. How Similar Are Protein Folding and Protein Binding Nuclei? Examination of Vibrational Motions of Energy Hot Spots and Conserved Residues. *Biophys. J.* **2005**, *88*, 1552–1559. [CrossRef] [PubMed]

61. Perišić, O. Contact and first layer residues prediction in protein dimers using the Gaussian Network model with adjustable number of fast modes. *arXiv*, **2013**, arXiv:1312.7376v1.

62. Perišić, O. Heterodimer binding scaffolds recognition via the analysis of kinetically hot residues. *arXiv*, **2016**, arXiv:1609.06556.

63. Bogan, A.A.; Thorn, K.S. Anatomy of hot spots in protein interfaces. *J. Mol. Biol.* **1998**, *280*, 1–9. [CrossRef] [PubMed]

64. Moreira, I.S.; Fernandes, P.A.; Ramos, M.J. Hot spots-A review of the protein-protein interface determinant amino-acid residues. *Proteins Struct. Funct. Bioinform.* **2007**, *68*, 803–812. [CrossRef] [PubMed]

65. Tuncbag, N.; Gursoy, A.; Keskin, O. Identification of computational hot spots in protein interfaces: Combining solvent accessibility and inter-residue potentials improves the accuracy. *Bioinformatics* **2009**, *25*, 1513–1520. [CrossRef] [PubMed]

66. Lise, S.; Archambeau, C.; Pontil, M.; Jones, D.T. Prediction of hot spot residues at protein-protein interfaces by combining machine learning and energy-based methods. *BMC Bioinform.* **2009**, *10*, 365. [CrossRef] [PubMed]

67. Lise, S.; Buchan, D.; Pontil, M.; Jones, D.T. Predictions of Hot Spot Residues at Protein-Protein Interfaces Using Support Vector Machines. *PLoS ONE* **2011**, *6*, e16774. [CrossRef] [PubMed]

68. Kozakov, D.; Hall, D.R.; Chuang, G.-Y.; Cencic, R.; Brenke, R.; Grove, L.E.; Beglov, D.; Pelletier, J.;

Whitty, A.; Vajda, S. Structural conservation of druggable hot spots in protein-protein interfaces. *Proc. Natl. Acad. Sci. USA* **2011**, *108*, 13528–13533. [CrossRef] [PubMed]

69. Tuncbag, N.; Gursoy, A.; Nussinov, R.; Keskin, O. Predicting protein-protein interactions on a proteome scale by matching evolutionary and structural similarities at interfaces using PRISM. *Nat. Protoc.* **2011**, *6*, 1341–1354. [CrossRef] [PubMed]

70. Deng, L.; Guan, J.; Wei, X.; Yi, Y.; Zhang, Q.C.; Zhou, S. Boosting Prediction Performance of Protein-Protein Interaction Hot Spots by Using Structural Neighborhood Properties. *J. Comput. Biol.* **2013**, *20*, 878–891. [CrossRef] [PubMed]

71. Chen, W.; Tang, H.; Ye, J.; Lin, H.; Chou, K.-C. iRNA-PseU: Identifying RNA pseudouridine sites. *Mol. Ther. Nucleic Acids* **2016**, *5*, e332. [PubMed]

72. Chenga, X.; Xiaoa, X.; Chou, K.-C. pLoc-mVirus: Predict subcellular localization of multi-location virus proteins via incorporating the optimal GO information into general PseAAC. *Gene* **2017**, *628*, 315–321. [CrossRef] [PubMed]

73. Feng, P.; Ding, H.; Yang, H.; Chen, W.; Lin, H.; Chou, K.-C. iRNA-PseColl: Identifying the Occurrence Sites of Different RNA Modifications by Incorporating Collective Effects of Nucleotides into PseKNC. *Mol. Ther. Nucleic Acids* **2017**, *7*, 155–163. [CrossRef] [PubMed]

74. Cheng, X.; Xiao, X.; Chou, K.-C. pLoc-mPlant: Predict subcellular localization of multi-location plant proteins by incorporating the optimal GO information into general PseAAC. *Mol. BioSyst.* **2017**, *13*, 1722–1727. [CrossRef] [PubMed]

75. Liu, B.; Wang, S.; Long, R.; Chou, K.-C. iRSpot-EL: Identify recombination spots with an ensemble learning approach. *Bioinformatics* **2017**, *33*, 35–41. [CrossRef] [PubMed]

76. Xiao, X.; Cheng, X.; Su, S.; Mao, Q.; Chou, K.-C. pLoc-mGpos: Incorporate Key Gene Ontology Information into General PseAAC for Predicting Subcellular Localization of Gram-Positive Bacterial Proteins. *Nat. Sci.* **2017**, *9*, 330–349. [CrossRef]

77. Qiu, W.-R.; Sun, B.-Q.; Xiao, X.; Xua, Z.-C.; Jia, J.-H.; Chou, K.-C. iKcr-PseEns: Identify lysine crotonylation sites in histone proteins with pseudo components and ensemble classifier. *Genomics* **2017**. [CrossRef] [PubMed]

78. Cheng, X.; Xiao, X.; Chou, K.-C. pLoc-mGneg: Predict subcellular localization of Gram-negative bacterial proteins by deep gene ontology learning via general PseAAC. *Genomics* **2017**. [CrossRef] [PubMed]

79. Cheng, X.; Zhao, S.-G.; Lin, W.-Z.; Xiao, X.; Chou, K.-C. pLoc-mAnimal: Predict subcellular localization of animal proteins with both single and multiple sites. *Bioinformatics* **2017**, *33*, 3524–3531. [CrossRef] [PubMed]

80. Cheng, X.; Xiao, X.; Chou, K.-C. pLoc-mEuk: Predict subcellular localization of multi-label eukaryotic proteins by extracting the key GO information into general PseAAC. *Genomics* **2018**, *110*, 50–58. [CrossRef] [PubMed]

81. Ehsan, A.; Mahmood, K.; Khan, Y.D.; Khan, S.A.; Chou, K.-C. A Novel Modeling in Mathematical Biology for Classification of Signal Peptides. *Sci. Rep.* **2018**, *8*, 1039. [CrossRef] [PubMed]

82. Feng, P.; Yang, H.; Ding, H.; Lin, H.; Chen, W.; Chou, K.-C. iDNA6mA-PseKNC: Identifying DNA N^6-methyladenosine sites by incorporating nucleotide physicochemical properties into PseKNC. *Genomics* **2018**. [CrossRef] [PubMed]

83. Liu, B.; Yang, F.; Huang, D.S.; Chou, K.-C. iPromoter-2L: A two-layer predictor for identifying promoters and their types by multi-window-based PseKNC. *Bioinformatics* **2018**, *34*, 33–40. [CrossRef] [PubMed]

84. Song, J.; Li, F.; Takemoto, K.; Haffari, G.; Akutsu, T.; Chou, K.-C.; Webb, G.I. PREvaIL, an integrative approach for inferring catalytic residues using sequence, structural, and network features in a machine-learning framework. *J. Theor. Biol.* **2018**, *443*, 125–137. [CrossRef] [PubMed]

85. Cheng, X.; Xiao, X.; Chou, K.-C. pLoc-mHum: Predict subcellular localization of multi-location human proteins via general PseAAC to winnow out the crucial GO information. *Bioinformatics* **2018**. [CrossRef] [PubMed]

86. Chou, K.-C. Some remarks on protein attribute prediction and pseudo amino acid composition (50th Anniversary Year Review). *J. Theor. Biol.* **2011**, *273*, 236–247. [CrossRef] [PubMed]

87. Sternberg Decoy Sets. Available online: http://www.sbg.bio.ic.ac.uk/docking/ (accessed on 8 March 2018).

88. Liu, S.; Gao, Y.; Vakser, I.A. DOCKGROUND protein-protein docking decoy set. *Bioinformatics* **2008**, *24*, 2634–2635. [CrossRef] [PubMed]

89. Lu, H.; Skolnick, J. Development of Unified Statistical Potentials Describing Protein-Protein Interactions. *Biophys. J.* **2003**, *84*, 1895–1901. [CrossRef]

90. Press, W.H.; Teukolsky, S.A.; Vetterling, W.T.; Flannery, B.P. *Numerical Recipes in C++*; Cambridge University Press: Cambridge, UK, 2002.

91. Weisstein, E.W. Singular Value Decomposition at mathworld.wolfram.com. Available online: http://mathworld.wolfram.com/SingularValueDecomposition.html (accessed on 8 March 2018).

92. Smith, T.F.; Waterman, M.S. Identification of Common Molecular Subsequences. *J. Mol. Biol.* **1981**, *147*, 195–197. [CrossRef]

93. Abagyan, R.A.; Batalov, S. Do Aligned Sequences Share the Same Fold? *J. Mol. Biol.* **1997**, *273*, 355–368. [CrossRef] [PubMed]

94. Wood, T.C.; Pearson, W.R. Evolution of Protein Sequences and Structures. *J. Mol. Biol.* **1999**, *291*, 977–995. [CrossRef] [PubMed]

95. Gan, H.H.; Perlow, R.A.; Roy, S.; Ko, J.; Wu, M.; Huang, J.; Yan, S.; Nicoletta, A.; Vafai, J.; Sun, D.; et al. Analysis of Protein Sequence/Structure Similarity Relationships. *Biophys. J.* **2002**, *83*, 2781–2791. [PubMed]

96. Eswar, N.; Marti-Renom, M.A.; Webb, B.; Madhusudhan, M.S.; Eramian, D.; Shen, M.; Pieper, U.; Sali, A. Comparative Protein Structure Modeling With MODELLER. *Curr. Protoc. Bioinform.* **2006**. [CrossRef]

97. Martin, J.; Lavery, R. Arbitrary protein-protein docking targets biologically relevant interfaces. *BMC Biophys.* **2012**, *5*, 7. [CrossRef] [PubMed]

98. Chou, K.-C.; Shen, H.-B. Recent advances in developing web-servers for predicting protein attributes. *Nat. Sci.* **2009**, *1*, 63–92. [CrossRef]

99. Lin, H.; Deng, E.-Z.; Ding, H.; Chen, W.; Chou, K.-C. iPro54-PseKNC: A sequence-based predictor for identifying sigma-54 promoters in prokaryote with pseudo k-tuple nucleotide composition. *Nucleic Acids Res.* **2014**, *42*, 12961–12972. [CrossRef] [PubMed]

100. Liu, B.; Yang, F.; Chou, K.-C. 2L-piRNA: A Two-Layer Ensemble Classifier for Identifying Piwi-Interacting RNAs and Their Function. *Mol. Ther. Nucleic Acids* **2017**, *7*, 267–277. [CrossRef] [PubMed]

101. Liu, B.; Long, R.; Chou, K.-C. iDHS-EL: Identifying DNase I hypersensitive sites by fusing three different modes of pseudo nucleotide composition into an ensemble learning framework. *Bioinformatics* **2016**, *32*, 2411–2418. [CrossRef] [PubMed]

102. Liu, B.; Fang, L.; Long, R.; Lan, X.; Chou, K.-C. iEnhancer-2L: A two-layer predictor for identifying enhancers and their strength by pseudo k-tuple nucleotide composition. *Bioinformatics* **2016**, *32*, 362–369. [CrossRef] [PubMed]

103. Chou, K.-C. Impacts of Bioinformatics to Medicinal Chemistry. *Med. Chem.* **2015**, *11*, 218–234. [CrossRef] [PubMed]

104. Kastritis, P.L.; Bonvin, A.M.J.J. Molecular origins of binding affinity: Seeking the Archimedean point. *Curr. Opin. Struct. Biol.* **2013**, *23*, 868–877. [CrossRef] [PubMed]

105. London, N.; Raveh, B.; Schueler-Furman, O. Peptide docking and structure-based characterization of peptide binding: From knowledge to know-how. *Curr. Opin. Struct. Biol.* **2013**, *23*, 894–902. [CrossRef] [PubMed]

4

The Role of TRP Channels in the Metastatic Cascade

Benedikt Fels *, Etmar Bulk, Zoltán Pethő and Albrecht Schwab

Institut für Physiologie II, Robert-Koch-Str. 27b, 48149 Münster, Germany; ebulk@uni-muenster.de (E.B.); pethoe@uni-muenster.de (Z.P.); aschwab@uni-muenster.de (A.S.)
* Correspondence: b_fels01@uni-muenster.de

Abstract: A dysregulated cellular Ca^{2+} homeostasis is involved in multiple pathologies including cancer. Changes in Ca^{2+} signaling caused by altered fluxes through ion channels and transporters (the transportome) are involved in all steps of the metastatic cascade. Cancer cells thereby "re-program" and "misuse" the cellular transportome to regulate proliferation, apoptosis, metabolism, growth factor signaling, migration and invasion. Cancer cells use their transportome to cope with diverse environmental challenges during the metastatic cascade, like hypoxic, acidic and mechanical cues. Hence, ion channels and transporters are key modulators of cancer progression. This review focuses on the role of transient receptor potential (TRP) channels in the metastatic cascade. After briefly introducing the role of the transportome in cancer, we discuss TRP channel functions in cancer cell migration. We highlight the role of TRP channels in sensing and transmitting cues from the tumor microenvironment and discuss their role in cancer cell invasion. We identify open questions concerning the role of TRP channels in circulating tumor cells and in the processes of intra- and extravasation of tumor cells. We emphasize the importance of TRP channels in different steps of cancer metastasis and propose cancer-specific TRP channel blockade as a therapeutic option in cancer treatment.

Keywords: metastatic cascade; TRP channels; tumor microenvironment; transportome

1. Introduction

Metastasis is the most important factor determining patient prognosis because most cancer patients die from the consequences of metastases [1]. This is particularly relevant for cancers which are usually asymptomatic in early stages and for which no easy screening tools are available such as the determination of prostate-specific antigen (PSA) levels in the plasma for prostate cancer. Thus, pancreatic ductal adenocarcinoma (PDAC) and non-small cell lung cancer (NSCLC) are two examples for cancers that are frequently diagnosed only in an advanced stage when macroscopic metastases have already developed. Accordingly, the prognosis of these cancers is extremely poor with 5-year survival rates of only 5% and 13% for European PDAC [2] and NSCLC patients [3], respectively. Disappointingly, the enormous gain of knowledge with respect to molecular and genetic mechanisms underlying these cancers has not yet led to therapeutic success. Thus, there still remains an unmet need for better understanding the pathophysiology of these diseases. Given the crucial role of metastasis for patient prognosis, it is particularly important to develop new concepts in the understanding of the mechanisms underlying metastasis.

Such a new concept, namely the involvement of ion-conducting transporters in neoplastic diseases has been emerging in recent years. Proteins involved in ion transport (the transportome) were found to contribute to essentially all "hallmarks of cancer" [4]. In this context, it is important to keep in mind that the transportome is the "working horse" of epithelial cells that are the origin of ~90% of all malignant tumors. The transportome is "misused" by cancer cells and regulates, among others, processes such as tumor cell proliferation, apoptosis, senescence, migration, invasion, metabolism and growth factor signaling. This is in part due to the dysregulated expression and function of transportome members in many tumors. Moreover, dysregulated expression frequently correlates with patient prognosis (see [5] for a series of reviews, e.g., [6–9]). The consistent presence of dysregulated ion channel expression and function in all cancers studied so far [10] has recently led to the provocative question of whether cancer hallmarks can be viewed as oncochannelopathies [11].

In the present review, we will focus on the contribution of transportome members to steps of the so-called metastatic cascade, i.e., on the mechanisms underlying the hematogenous or lymphatic spread of tumor cells from the primary tumor to distant organs. The literature on the cancer transportome has grown exponentially during the last years so that we will limit our discussion primarily to transient receptor potential (TRP) channels (see Table 1). The steps of the metastatic cascade are well defined. After leaving the primary tumor cancer cells invade into and migrate through the neighboring tissue to reach blood or lymph vessels that may have been newly formed (tumor angiogenesis). Following intravasation they are swept away with the bloodstream or the lymph. Within the bloodstream, circulating tumor cells (CTCs) interact with different blood cells such as platelets [12]. Platelet-CTC interactions seem to increase CTC survival, extravasation and metastasis [13,14]. Surviving CTCs adhere to endothelial cells lining the vessels, migrate intravascularly and penetrate the endothelial cell layer (extravasation). Alternatively, individual cancer cells or cell clusters may be trapped mechanically in small capillaries. Finally, the cells expand to form metastases in different parts of the body, and new vessels are formed to supply them with nutrients [1,15]. The extravasation of tumor cells bears many similarities with the recruitment of immune cells [16]. For example, some of the relevant adhesion molecules required for immune cell recruitment, such as LFA-1 or ICAM-1, have also been found in lung adenocarcinoma cells [17,18].

TRP channels are a large family of cation channels all showing sequence homology to the *Drosophila* TRP protein. Its subfamilies present in mammals are: the ankyrin subfamily TRPA, the canonical subfamily TRPC, the melastatin subfamily TRPM, the mucolypin subfamily TRPML, the polycystin subfamily TRPP and the vanilloid subfamily TRPV. They have varying selectivity ranging from nonselective cation channels to highly selective channels (e.g., for Ca^{2+}). Their gating is also quite heterogeneous, as they can be gated by e.g., ligands, temperature or mechanical stimuli. [19,20]. TRP channels are involved in a wide variety of cellular processes. Some examples include Ca^{2+} homeostasis, nociception, inflammation, phagocytosis, or cell motility (e.g., reviewed in [21–24]). Their function can be described in very general terms as that of "cellular sensors". Thereby, TRP channels confer the ability onto metastasizing cancer cells to respond to ambient physico-chemical signals. Microenvironmental stimuli are of central importance throughout the metastatic cascade. During the metastatic cascade cancer cell behavior is shaped by a wide variety of (harsh) microenvironmental stimuli [1]. Examples of such stimuli along the metastatic cascade and how their potential impact on TRP channel activity can regulate tumor and stromal cell behavior will be the main focus of this review.

There are numerous studies showing a clear correlation between cancer patient survival and TRP channel expression, e.g., TRPC1, TRPM2 and TRPV4 in breast cancer [25–27], TRPM7 in PDAC [28], TRPM8 in bladder cancer and osteosarcoma [29,30] and TRPV2 in breast and esophageal cancer [31,32] to name just a few examples (see also Table 2). Since cancer patients usually die from the consequences of metastases, the multitude of these observations strongly indicates that TRP channels have a significant share in the processes underlying the metastatic cascade. Thus, studying the role of TRP channels in steps of the metastatic cascade is a clinically relevant undertaking and bears great therapeutic potential.

Table 1. TRP channels and their impact in malignant phenotypes.

Channel	Cancer Type	Cell line/Tissue	Function/Phenotype	Ref.
TRPA1	Lewis Lung carcinoma	LLC-2	adhesion	[33]
TRPC1	Breast cancer	MDA-MB-231/MCF-10A	migration proliferation	[34] [35]
	Pancreatic cancer PDAC	BxPc3 Capan-1	migration	[36]
	Non-small cell lung cancer (NSCLC)	A549/H1299	proliferation	[37]
	Nasopharyngeal carcinoma	CNE2	adhesion	[38]
	Glioblastoma	U251	migration	[39]
	Thyroid cancer	ML-1	migration, invasion	[40]
TRPC4	Medulloblastoma	DAOY, ONS76, UW228-1	migration	[41]
TRPC5	Colon cancer	SW620/HT29/tissue	proliferation, migration, invasion	[42]
TRPC6	Glioblastoma	U373MG	tumor growth, invasion, angiogenesis	[43]
	NSCLC	A549	proliferation, invasion	[44]
	Prostate cancer	tissue	expression in metastatic tissues	[45]
	Liver cancer	Huh-7/tissue	proliferation, expression	[46]
TRPM7	Pancreatic cancer PDAC	Panc-1/MiaPaCa2/tissue	proliferation, invasion	[28,47]
	NSCLC	A549	migration	[48]
	Breast cancer	MDA-MB-231/tissue MDA-MB-231 MDA-MB-435 * MDA-MB-468	migration, adhesion, cell tension, lung metastasis migration, expression in invasive ER⁻ ductal carcinoma tissue migration, EMT transition	[49] [50] [51] [52]
	Nasopharyngeal carcinoma	NPC SUNE1/5-8F	migration	[53]
	Ovarian cancer	SKVO-3	migration, adhesion, colony formation	[54]
TRPM8	Oral squamous cell carcinoma	HSC3/4	migration, MMP	[55]
	Breast cancer	MCF-7/MDA-MB-231	migration	[56]
	Lewis Lung cancer	LLC-2	adhesion	[33]
	Glioblastoma	U-87MG/T98G	migration/chemotaxis	[57]
	Pancreatic cancer	Panc-1	migration, invasion	[58]
	Prostate cancer	PC-3 LNCaP	migration cell survival	[59] [60]
TRPV2	Prostate cancer	PC-3	migration	[61]
	Breast cancer	MCF-7/MDA-MB-231	migration	[62]
TRPV4	Breast cancer	MDA-MB-435s *	migration, invasion, metastasis, transendothelial migration	[26,63]
	Gastric cancer	MKN45 and SGC-7901	proliferation, migration	[64]
TRPV6	Breast cancer	MCF-7/MDA-MB-231/tissue	migration/chemotaxis expression in invasive areas	[65]
	Pancreatic cancer	Pancreatic cancer cells/tissue	proliferation, migration, invasion	[66]

* Recently recognized as of melanoma origin [67].

Table 2. TRP channel expression in different cancer types and its correlation with patient prognosis.

Channel	Cancer Type	Expression	Prognosis	Ref.
TRPC1	Breast cancer Basal tumors/lymph nodes	high	poor	[25]
TRPC5	Colon cancer	high	poor	[42]
TRPC6	Glioblastoma	high	no information	[43]
	Prostate cancer	high	no information	[45]
	Esophageal squamous cell carcinoma	high	poor	[68]
TRPM2	Breast cancer	low	poor	[27]
TRPM7	Pancreatic cancer PDAC/lymph nodes	high	poor	[28,47,69]
	Breast cancer Negative (ER(-)) invasive ductal carcinoma/lymph nodes	high high	poor poor	[49] [50,51]
TRPM8	Urothelial carcinoma of bladder	high	poor	[29]
	Osteosarcoma	high	poor	[30]
TRPV2	Prostate cancer	high	poor	[61]
	Breast cancer	high	better	[31]
	Esophageal squamous cell carcinoma	high	poor	[32]
TRPV4	Breast cancer	high	poor	[26,63]
	Gastric cancer	high	poor	[63]
	Ovarian cancer	high	poor	[63]
TRPV6	Breast cancer	high	poor	[65]
	Pancreatic cancer	high	no information	[66]

2. TRP Channels in Cancer Cell Migration and Invasion

Cell migration involves a large variety of temporally and spatially coordinated processes ranging from cell polarization, adhesion/de-adhesion to/from the surrounding matrix and/or neighboring cells, as well as extensive cytoskeletal and membrane dynamics [70–72]. Many components of the migration machinery are Ca^{2+}-sensitive, including myosin-II [73], focal adhesions [74] or Ca^{2+}-sensitive ion channels [72]. Hence, the intracellular Ca^{2+} concentration of migrating tumor (stroma) cells is tightly regulated, both spatially and temporally [75]. In fact, it is widely accepted that ion transport across the plasma membrane via numerous Na^+, Ca^{2+} and K^+ channels and transporters is crucial for cell migration [7,72,76]. Additionally, ion and H_2O fluxes strongly depend on an appropriate plasma membrane potential (V_m). V_m as a key biophysical signal thereby regulates e.g., cell volume and migration and provides the driving force for Ca^{2+} influx. Hyperpolarization and depolarization can directly affect normal cell as well as cancer cell function. A depolarized V_m in many cancer types could be linked to e.g., cancer cell proliferation (reviewed in [77]). The following chapter will focus on the role of TRP channels in cancer cell migration and invasion.

Before summarizing recent findings in the field, we would like to critically discuss the experimental approaches. The gold standard is intravital microscopy because cells are migrating in their complex physiological environment. But it is not trivial to control and manipulate individual components of the tumor microenvironment such as pH or mechanical properties. Controlling the ambient conditions is more easily achieved in an in vitro setting, yet in a reductionist fashion. Boyden chambers for example are popular for in vitro assays of tumor cell invasion. A frequently used protocol is to coat the filter membranes with matrix proteins and induce "invasion" by applying a chemotactic gradient. However, under such experimental conditions it is impossible to distinguish "invasion" from chemotaxis. Inhibiting chemotaxis will lead to the same readout as inhibiting "invasion" since the steering mechanisms can be affected without impairing the migration motor [78,79]. Inhibiting either mechanism will lead to a reduced number of cells reaching the lower compartment of the Boyden chamber. Unfortunately, the proper control experiments, i.e., the use of Boyden chambers in the absence of chemotactic gradients are not always performed. Wound healing assays are also often used for migration analysis and can be a suitable approach to evaluate directionality of cell movement. Migration analysis within a 3D matrix as well can be a useful tool to analyze the matrix invasion of tumor cells; here, translocation as well as matrix digestion via e.g., MMP secretion should be taken into account. The papers cited below are mainly limited to studies considering the above-mentioned criteria.

2.1. TRPM7

TRPM7 is involved in several aspects of cell motility such as polarization [80], adhesion [81,82] and migration [83]. It is a Ca^{2+}- and Mg^{2+}-permeable channel with an α-kinase domain [84]. TRPM7 is essential for PDAC progression and invasion. TRPM7 expression in primary tumors is associated with PDAC lymph node metastasis [28]. Its over-expression correlates with increased tumor size and advanced tumor stages of pancreatic cancer and hence, inversely with patient prognosis [47,85]. Silencing of TRPM7 in PDAC cell lines leads to a reduction of cancer cell invasion [28]. TRPM7 function in PDAC invasion can be partly explained by TRMP7-mediated Mg^{2+} influx and subsequent kinase activation and heat shock protein secretion. Activation of TRPM7 and Hsp90a secretion could be linked to MMP-2 secretion which is an important step to degrade surrounding ECM and initiate cancer cell invasion [28]. In the non-small cell lung cancer (NSCLC) cell line A549 TRPM7 is upregulated after epidermal growth factor (EGF) stimulation and contributes to EGF-mediated increase in cell migration. Accordingly, shRNA-based silencing of TRPM7 attenuates the stimulation by EGF [48]. In breast cancer, myosin-II-based cell tensions and de-adhesion of cell-matrix contacts are TRPM7-dependent and TRPM7 is necessary for breast cancer metastasis into the lung in a murine model [49] (see also below). Silencing of TRPM7 in MDA-MB-435 breast cancer cells leads to a reduced migration. This can be accounted for a TRPM7-dependent regulation of Src and MAPK kinase pathways [51]. However, it should be noted that the origin of MDA-MB-435 cells has recently been questioned [65]. These findings suggest that at least part of the role of TRPM7 is calcium-independent. It rather involves its α-kinase domain which is needed for phosphorylation of myosin-IIA heavy chain [50,51,86]. A similar role of TRPM7 in cancer cell migration was found in a number of other tumors such as nasopharyngeal carcinoma and ovarian cancer [53,54]. In addition, TRPM7 is also known for its role in tumor cell proliferation [65,87,88].

2.2. TRPM8

There are numerous reports describing a role for TRPM8 in cancer cell migration and invasion. However, depending on the type of cancer its impact may be pro- or anti-migratory. In oral squamous cell carcinoma, activation of TRPM8 leads to an increase of MMP-9 activity and cell migration [55]. In breast cancer, TRPM8 promotes the aggressiveness of breast cancer cells by regulating epithelial-mesenchymal transition (EMT) via the activation of the AKT/GSK-3β pathway [56]. Silencing of TRPM8 decreases and over-expression increases the motility of MDA-MB-231 or MCF-7 breast cancer cells. Activation of TRPM8 in combination with TRPA1 leads to enhanced motility also in lung cancer cells, whereas knockdown shows the opposite effect [33]. In glioblastoma cells, TRPM8 inhibition reduces the migration and chemotaxis [57]. In contrast, in PDAC cells and in prostate cancer cells TRPM8 function and expression reduces cell motility [58,59,89]. TRPM8 function is also linked to cell survival in prostate cancer and TRMP8 suppression lead to oxidative stress and apoptosis [60]. TRPM8 channels are also regulated by intracellular proteins, so called TRP channel-associated factors (TCAFs). E.g.,TCAF1 leads to a reduction of prostate cancer cell velocity and migration directionality [90]. A modification of TRPM8 channels can also be mediated via N-glycosylation in HEK293 cells, but not in PDAC cell lines Panc-1, MiaPaCa2 or

BxPc3, which express non-glycosylated channel isoforms [91]. Independently of its conductive function, TRPM8 acts as a Rap1 GTPase inhibitor, inhibiting endothelial cell migration [92].

2.3. TRPV2

Some TRPV channels have been found to be involved in cell proliferation, apoptosis, angiogenesis, migration, invasion, and generally in cancer progression [93]. The elevated expression of TRPV2 in metastatic prostate cancer points to a role of this channel in the metastatic cascade [61]. TRPV2 promotes cell migration and the invasive cancer cell phenotype [94]. Antimicrobial peptide LL-37, which is released from infiltrating immune cells, is able to activate TRPV2 and the Ca^{2+}-activated K^+ channel ($K_{Ca}1.1$) in different breast cancer cell lines leading to increased migration [62]. High TRPV2 expression is also correlated with a poor prognosis of esophageal squamous cell carcinoma (ESCC) [32].

2.4. TRPV4

TRPV4 is upregulated in breast cancer patients. TRPV4-mediated activation of protein kinase B leads to enhanced Akt and focal adhesion kinase (FAK) phosphorylation, which are both associated with cell migration. Pharmacological activation of TRPV4 in a breast cancer cell line causes downregulation of adhesion molecules like E-cadherin and β-catenin [26]. Upregulation of TRPV4 is accompanied by changes of the cytoskeletal network, enhanced blebability and reduced cell stiffness, facilitating cancer metastasis through neighboring tissues. It was suggested that TRPV4 activation thereby regulates breast cancer cell extravasation [63]. In gastric cancer, TRPV4 can be activated by co-localized calcium-sensing receptors, leading to Ca^{2+}-induced proliferation, migration and invasion [64]. TRPV4 channels are also important players in tumor vascularization by regulating endothelial cell migration [95] (see chapter "TRP channels in tumor vascularization"). Moreover, they modulate the endothelial barrier permeability (see chapter "Extravasation of tumor cells" below).

2.5. TRPV6

TRPV6 is associated with both pancreatic and breast cancer. TRPV6 is upregulated in human pancreatic cancer specimens and silencing of TRPV6 significantly inhibits invasion, proliferation and migration of pancreatic cancer cells [66]. In breast cancer, TRPV6 expression is higher in invasive areas of breast cancer tissues in comparison to the corresponding non-invasive areas. Moreover, TRPV6 silencing inhibits MDA-MB-231 and MCF-7 breast cancer cell migration. Therefore, TRPV6 is suggested to be involved in the metastatic process of breast cancer [65].

2.6. TRPC1

TRPC1 is required for PDGF- and EGF-mediated directional migration in glioma cells [39,96] by cooperating with chloride channels that are activated by TRPC1-mediated Ca^{2+} influx [97]. TRPC1 channels are also necessary for VEGF signaling and thyroid cancer migration and invasion [40]. TRPC1-mediated Ca^{2+} influx is needed for NSCLC proliferation in response to EGF signaling [37]. Transforming growth factor β1 (TGF-β1) induces Ca^{2+} entry likely via TRPC1 and NCX1 that raise cytosolic Ca^{2+} in pancreatic cancer cells so that knockdown of TRPC1 reverses TGF-β1-induced pancreatic cancer cell motility [36]. Silencing of TRPC1 or its activator STIM1 reduce TGF-β1 mediated calpain activation and subsequent cell migration, as well as expression of EMT markers such as N-cadherin and vimentin [34]. TRPC1 together with STIM1/Orai1 is also needed for colon cancer cell line (HCT-116) migration [98].

2.7. TRPC4

TRPC4 contributes to enhanced invasion and metastasis of granule precursor-derived human medulloblastoma [41]. Here, the authors use OGR1 to induce the expression of TRPC4 which promotes the migration of medulloblastoma cells.

2.8. TRPC5

It has been shown that overexpression of TRPC5 correlates with a poor prognosis in colon cancer by promoting tumor metastasis via the hypoxia-induced factor 1α (HIF-1α) -Twist signaling pathway [42].

2.9. TRPC6

TRPC6 is linked to several cancer types such as prostate, lung and colon cancer as well as glioblastoma. In prostate cancer, TRPC6 is suggested to be involved in cancer cell invasion into a "matrigel-based" matrix [99]. TRPC6 is detected in benign and malignant human prostate tumor tissues as well as in prostate cancer cell lines and its expression levels are associated with the histological grade [45]. Expression profiles of some TRP channels including TRPC6 are changing during the progression of prostate cancer towards the more aggressive and hormone-refractory stages [100]. TRPC6 also has been linked to lung cancer [44]: inhibition of TRPC6 channels lowers the intracellular Ca^{2+} concentration in A549 cells and strongly reduces the invasion of A549 cells. In human glioblastoma cells, TRPC6 expression is augmented by hypoxia and increases proliferation and cell invasion [43]. Here, TRPC6 is suggested to be a key mediator of Notch-driven glioblastoma invasiveness and angiogenesis. TRPC6 was also found to be upregulated in esophageal squamous cell carcinoma in which it negatively correlates with patients survival [68].

2.10. Other TRP Channels

The TRPA1 channel is involved in cellular invasion. It has been shown with transwell-invasion-assays that methyl syringate, a TRPA1 agonist inhibits induction of COX-2 and cell invasion of the NSCLC cell line A549 and of the fibrosarcoma cell line HT-1080 under hypoxic conditions [101].

To the best knowledge of the authors, there is no direct evidence linking TRPML channels to cancer invasiveness and metastasis, although the channel has an altered expression in glioblastoma and breast cancer [102]. This might be due to the subcellular localization of TRPML channels, as they are primarily expressed in endosomes and lysosomes, and they are not as easily investigated as channels residing in the plasma membrane. Moreover, the literature focuses on the effect of TRPML on autophagy and autophagy-related signaling that is independent of the calcium permeability of the channel [102]. However, these channels are key regulators of lysosomal calcium release, and moreover, their expression is linked to ERK1/2 and Akt signaling which plays a role in cell migration.

3. Influence of the Tumor Microenvironment on TRP Channels

The initial step of cancer cell invasion and migration out of the primary tumor is strongly regulated by a variety of tumor microenvironmental factors like pH, hypoxia, matrix stiffness, cytokines and the infiltrating cellular components such as fibroblasts and immune cells. The following chapter will link these factors to TRP channel function in tumor progression and invasion.

3.1. pH

Due to insufficient vascularization, limited supply of metabolic substrates, metabolic reprogramming towards the so-called aerobic glycolysis (Warburg effect) and-at least in later stages–tumor anemia, primary tumors and cancer cells export increased amounts of H^+ and the tumor microenvironment (TME) becomes acidified [103–106]. In PDAC the extracellular pH landscape is superimposed by an intermittent postprandial acidification of the interstitium which is a consequence of the massive HCO_3^- secretion into the pancreatic ducts [107,108]. Similarly, the pH landscapes of stomach, bone or skin tumors are superimposed by the respective characteristic acid-base homeostasis of these organs. Several TRP channels are regulated by an extra-/intracellular acidosis [19,109]. They can either be activated, e.g., TRPV1/3 [20], TRPC5 [110] or inhibited by an acidosis such as TRPM2 [111] and TRPM8 [112], or their selectivity is regulated by pH (e.g., TRPM7; [113]). There is a close interrelation between the regulation of TRPM7 by protons and the divalent cations Ca^{2+} and

Mg^{2+}. On the one hand, the effect of the extracellular pH on TRPM7 activity depends on the presence of extracellular Ca^{2+} and Mg^{2+} [114]. On the other hand, the selectivity of TRPM7 channels for mono- or divalent cations is regulated by the extracellular pH. An acidification (e.g., pH 6) increases the permeability for monovalent cations [113]. For tumor cells, the impact of an intracellular alkalization (pH >7.2) is more relevant because tumor cells are frequently characterized by an alkaline intracellular pH [105]. TRMP7 channels are activated by an alkaline pH in these cells [115].

TRPV1 is a nonselective cation channel that is not only regulated by protons but also permeable for protons [20,116]. Low extracellular pH in lymphatic endothelial cells induces lymph-angiogenesis in a TRPV1-dependent manner [117]. This pH-dependent activation of TRPV1 also induces cytokine production (IL8) by endothelial cells.

The effect of pH on TRPV4 cells is controversially. Heterologously expressed TRPV4 channels can be activated by a drop of extracellular pH in CHO cells [118]. However, in esophageal epithelial cells TRPV4 activity is suppressed by an acidic pH [119].

TRPC4 and TRPC5 channels are already activated by a modest decrease of the extracellular pH (e.g., pH 7.0) when expressed in HEK293 cells [110].

TRPM2 channels are inhibited by extracellular acidification (pH 6.5) as protons compete with other cations like Ca^{2+} or Na^+ for channel permeation and act as competitive TRPM2 antagonists [111]. Another possible mechanism for proton-dependent regulation of TRP channel activity was shown for TRPM8; the channel activity is reduced by extracellular divalent cations as well as by protons. The authors showed that this is due to a change in the membrane surface charge caused by an increased proton concentration [112].

3.2. Hypoxia

The high metabolic demand of the tumor cells and the insufficient blood and oxygen supply due the compression and inadequate number of vessels frequently cause hypoxia of the tumor stroma [120–122]. Hypoxia can be sensed by several TRP channels such as TRPM7 and TRPA1 [123], TRPC1 [25,40], TRPC6 [43,124–126], both in cancer cells and in stromal cells [126,127]. Hypoxia is commonly associated with increased production of reactive oxygen species (ROS) that can elicit both protumorigenic and antitumor effects [128]. TRPC6, TRPV1, TRPM2/4/7, TRPA1 are activated by ROS [19], and they are regulators of relevant steps of the metastatic cascade.

TRPM2 channels can be activated by hypoxia. They are expressed in several cancer types, for instance in breast cancer [129], neuroblastoma [130] and malignant melanoma [131]. In neuroblastoma cells, TRPM2 depletion leads to a suppressed HIF-1α signaling. Inhibiting TRPM2 function by mutating its pore region increases mitochondrial ROS production [132]. Accordingly, TRPM2 activation by oxidative stress in ischemic hearts prevents ROS production in the hypoxic heart [133]. A protective role of TRPM2 under hypoxia can also be found in neuroblastoma cells, in which activated TRPM2 channels lead to increased expression of superoxide dismutase 2 (SOD2) and reduced ROS levels [130,132].

TRPM7 as well as TRPA1 can be activated by hypoxia and increased ROS levels [123,134,135]. The prominent role of TRPM7 channels in cancer progression and cancer cell migration has already been discussed (see "TRP channels in cancer cell migration and invasion").

TPRV1 and TRPV4 channels are activated under hypoxic conditions in pulmonary artery smooth muscle cells and induce migration [136].

In the follicular thyroid cancer cell line ML-1, knockdown of TRPC1 channels leads to decreased HIF-1α levels [40]. Corresponding results were found in breast cancer cells, in which hypoxia increases TRPC1 expression and TRPC1 regulates hypoxia-induced signaling [25].

In glioma cells, TRPC6 is upregulated and required for the hypoxia-mediated increase in proliferation and cell invasion [43]. Activated TRPC6 stabilizes HIF-1α in hypoxic glioma cells and supports hypoxic glucose metabolism of cancer cells via the GLUT1 transporter [124]. TRPC6 channels are also activated in a hypoxic environment in pancreatic stellate cells, which are the main producers of extracellular matrix proteins in PDAC [126,137]. Similar results were found in hepatic stellate cells, in which TRPC6 expression increases under hypoxic conditions [127].

3.3. Cytokines

The tumor microenvironment is a rich source of cytokines and growth factors secreted by tumor cells, stromal cells and infiltrating immune cells. Cytokine and growth factor receptors frequently trigger TRP channel-dependent signaling cascades [137]. In addition, TRP channels can also modify cytokine secretion of cancer and stroma cells and thereby modify the composition of the tumor microenvironment. However, it must be stated at this point that many of the studies investigating the role of TRP channels in cytokine secretion were not made with tumor cells. Nonetheless, they can be taken as proof-of-principle and studies made with immune cells are highly relevant because of the consistent immune cell infiltration of the tumor stroma.

TRPM2 is important for secretion of IL-2, IFN$_Y$ and IL-17 in T-lymphocytes [138] as well as for IL-8 secretion in monocytes [139]. Stimulation of TRPM3 channels leads to activation of extracellular signal-regulated protein kinase (ERK1/2) and transcription of IL-8, a proinflammatory CXC chemokine important for proliferation, survival and migration of cancer cells in lung cancer and PDAC [140–143]. TRPM8 inhibition in murine peritoneal macrophages leads to a pro-inflammatory cytokine profile with increased TNFα and decreased IL-6 secretion [144]. TRPM8 activators like eucalyptol inhibit secretion of TNFα, IL-1β, IL-6 and IL-8 in monocytes [145]. In lung epithelial cells, TRPM8 activation increases transcription of IL-1α, IL-1β, IL-4, IL-6, IL-8, IL-13 and TNFα [146].

Ca^{2+} entry through TRPV2 was shown to be involved in IL-6 secretion in RAW264 and murine macrophages [147]. IL-8 secretion in human non-melanoma skin cancer can be stimulated by TRPV4, thereby leading to a possibly inhibitory autocrine circuitry, because IL-8 induces the downregulation of TRPV4 channels [148]. In human airway epithelial NCI-H292 cells, TRPV4 activation triggers Ca^{2+} entry and release of IL-8 and prostaglandin E_2 (PGE_2) in vitro and increases KC levels in in vivo murine bronchoalveolar lavage fluids [149].

3.4. Mechanical Properties of Tumor Cells and the Tumor Microenvironment

In addition to the above mentioned chemical stimuli, metastasizing tumor cells and stromal cells are also exposed to mechanical stimuli [150]. Altered mechanics is one of the main characteristics of most cancer types. In fact, the clinical detection of a tumor by palpation relies on the typical mechanical properties of the tumor tissue [150,151]. The elasticity of the tumor stroma [150,152] and the tissue pressure [121,153] are usually higher than those of the normal organs. PDAC and breast cancer may serve as prominent examples [154–157]. Altered mechanical properties not only stimulate the cancer cells. They have an equal impact on stromal cells as illustrated by the response of pancreatic stellate cells to a mechanical load. They are activated by an elevated tissue pressure and substrate rigidity [152,158].

Moreover, circulating tumor cells are exposed to massive shear forces while in the bloodstream and prior to extravasation. Finally, tumor and stroma cell migration itself also generates mechanical signals within the cells that–via TRP channel activation–modulate the migratory behavior [159]. There is ample evidence that TRP channels are involved in mechano-signaling [125]. TRPC1 [158,160], TRPM7 [161], TRPV4 [63], TRPA1 channels [162] are some of the relevant TRP channels that are also required for specific steps of the metastatic cascade.

TRPC1 channels are found at the rear end of polarized U2OS osteosarcoma cells. TRPC1 knockdown leads to disturbed cell polarity, decreased cell stiffness and disorganization of the actin filaments and microtubules [163]. In pancreatic stellate cells TRPC1 is involved in responding to an increase of the ambient pressure and its activation leads to increased migratory activity of pancreatic stellate cells [158]. TRPC1 also contributes to mechano-signaling during migration of MDCK-F cells and fibroblasts. Knockdown or knockout of TRPC1 attenuates calcium transients following mechanical stretch. Moreover, TRPC1 channels are needed for MDCK-F cells to respond to directional mechanical cues [160].

TRPM7 can be activated by mechanical stimuli like membrane stretch as well as through phospholipase C (PLC) signaling [164,165]. TRPM7 channels are involved in calpain signaling and myosin-II activation and modulate actomyosin cytoskeleton contraction [81,86]. In neuroblastoma cells TRPM7 modulates the cytoskeletal organization and affects the malignancy of tumor cells by regulating actomyosin dynamics and cell-matrix interactions [166].

In tumor-derived endothelial cells TRPV4 expression levels are lowered. This leads to decreased mechanosensitivity and increased cell spreading on stiff matrices—an effect that is restored by overexpression of TRPV4. Prostate cancer-derived endothelial cells with low TRPV4 expression showed increased migration and abnormal angiogenesis [167]. TRPV4 is also required for breast cancer cell invasion. In breast cancer, TRPV4 overexpression leads to cancer cell softening, increased cell blebbing and actin reorganization. Altered mechanics were assessed indirectly with a micropipette aspiration technique. This was proposed to point to a role of TRPV4 channels in cancer cell extravasation by reducing cancer cell rigidity and improving the ability of cancer cells to infiltrate through the surrounding tissue [63].

3.5. Stroma Cells

The function of stromal cells such as fibroblast and immune cells, that are recruited and activated by cancer cells, is regulated by different TRP channels as well [137]. Our group has begun a systematic analysis of the (TRP) channels regulating the function of pancreatic stellate cells. These cells play a major role in PDAC progression by underlying the desmoplastic reaction within the tumor stroma and they are also involved in acute and chronic pancreatitis. Their functions rely on intracellular Ca^{2+} signaling [168,169]. Blockade of Ca^{2+}-release-activated Ca^{2+}-channels (CRAC) by GSK-7975A inhibits Ca^{2+} signaling in pancreatic stellate cells and attenuates pancreatitis [169].

Activation and migration of pancreatic stellate cells depend on TRPC1 channel expression. As mentioned in the preceding paragraph, TRPC1 is involved in the mechano-signaling of murine pancreatic stellate cells and needed for pressure-dependent activation [158]. TRPC3 channels are upregulated in the PDAC stroma. By cooperation with $K_{Ca}3.1$ channels they are necessary for pancreatic stellate cell migration and chemotaxis by mediating Ca^{2+} influx necessary for calpain stimulation [170]. TRPC6 channels are required for hypoxia-induced activation and autocrine stimulation of pancreatic stellate cells [126].

In hepatic stellate cells, TRPM7 is in involved in cell activation via the ERK and phosphoinositide 3-kinase (PI3K) pathway [171]. Inhibition or knockdown of TRPM7 lead to reduced proliferation and attenuated expression of activation markers like α-smooth muscle actin and Col1α1 in response to platelet-derived growth factor (PDGF) and TGF-β1 stimulation [171,172]. TRPM7 also underlies Ca^{2+} signaling at the leading edge of migrating lung fibroblasts [173]. In prostate cancer-associated fibroblasts, activation of TRPA1 leads to increased Ca^{2+} levels and elevated hepatocyte growth factor (HGF) and vascular endothelial growth factor (VEGF) secretion. Co-cultured prostate cancer cells are rescued from apoptosis by TRPA1 activation [174].

Infiltrating immune cells like neutrophils are important constituents of the tumor stroma in numerous tumors, including PDAC [175,176]. Neutrophils are recruited to the PDAC stroma via CXCR2 signaling [177] which in turn relies on TRPC6 channel activity [79]. It is discussed controversially whether TRPM2 channels contribute to neutrophil chemotaxis [139,178–180] Other neutrophilic TRP channels that are linked to chemotaxis or tissue infiltration include TRPM7 [139,178–180] and TRPV4 [181]. For a detailed overview of TRP channel function in neutrophil granulocytes we refer to a recent review from our group [23].

Taken together, the tumor microenvironment encompasses a wealth of different stimuli that shape cancer and stromal cell behavior. TRP channels are not only the sensors for these stimuli, they are also involved in transducing these external stimuli to altered cellular behavior and finally modify the tumor microenvironment by inducing e.g., cytokine secretion.

4. TRP Channels in Tumor Vascularization

Tumor cells must have access to blood or lymph vessels in order to spread within the body. They can either enter already existing vessels in the host organ, or they can enter newly formed vessels within the tumor. Thus, tumor angiogenesis is generally a prerequisite for metastasis. Tumor angiogenesis is initiated among others by growth factors secreted by tumor cells into the hypoxic tumor microenvironment such as VEGF, EGF and many others [95]. It strongly relies on intracellular Ca^{2+} signaling which may in part be mediated by TRP channels (reviewed in [95,182,183]). However, there are discrepancies between in vitro and in vivo studies. While the former reveal a participation of TRPC1 and TRPC6 channels in endothelial tube formation [184,185], the respective knockout mice appear to have a normal vasculature [3,186]. On the other hand, modulating TRPV4 channel activity pharmacologically (4α-PDD; [187]) or mechanically [188] elicits concordant effects in vivo and in vitro. It is interesting to note that altered expression of TRP channels is also observed in tumor-derived endothelial cells. This has been well documented for TRPV4 channels in breast cancer and prostate cancer-derived endothelial cells [167,189,190].

5. Extravasation of Tumor Cells

Extravasation of circulating tumor cells may originate from single tumor cells or cell clusters [12]. Prior to crossing the vessel wall, tumor cells have to adhere to endothelial cells. For extravasation of single tumor cells, analogies with immune cells are evident. Accordingly, adhesion molecules expressed by endothelial and tumor cells are crucial. Prominent examples are the family of cadherins, selectins, integrins or the Ig superfamily, including ICAM-1 or VCAM-1. There are several examples showing that the expression of adhesion molecules in endothelial cells is modulated by Ca^{2+}-permeable ion channels. Overexpression of Orai1 potentiates the expression of ICAM-1 and VCAM-1 [191], silencing of TRPC1 attenuates cisplatin-induced ICAM-1 expression and endothelial dysfunction [192] and overexpression of TRPC3 enhances TNFα-induced VCAM-1 expression. Binding of selectins to their ligands is Ca^{2+}-dependent. P-selectin has been identified to mediate adhesion of various leukocytes and certain types of cancer cells [193]. Its expression in endothelial cells is upregulated by TRPV4 agonists [194]. E-selectin with its ligands sialyl-Lewis-a or sialyl-Lewis-x and CD44 is important for the early attachment of cancer cells to endothelial cells [15]. Most studies only investigate the invasion of tumor cells which precedes intravasation and follows extravasation. We have referred to the role of TRP channels therein in one of the earlier sections of this review.

By analogy with the increased adhesion of monocytes to endothelial cells that is indirectly mediated by TRPC3 channels [195], one would expect a similar behavior for tumor cells as well. Channel-mediated upregulation of endothelial vascular cell adhesion molecule (VCAM)-1 should lead to an increase of adhesion of tumor cells to the endothelium. However, so far there are only very few studies investigating this aspect of the metastatic cascade. Using single cell force spectroscopy we recently measured cell-cell adhesion forces between A549 non-small cell lung cancer cells and human microvascular endothelial (HMEC-1) cells. We could show that inhibition or silencing of the Ca^{2+}-activated potassium channel $K_{Ca}3.1$, which, by transporting positive charges to the extracellular space, provides electrical driving force for Ca^{2+} influx via TRP channels [170], increases ICAM-1-dependent adhesion between A549 and HMEC-1 cells [17]. One important conclusion of our study is that the adhesion of tumor cells to endothelial cells is largely regulated by *endothelial* $K_{Ca}3.1$ channels. Since inhibition of $K_{Ca}3.1$ channels leads to a decrease of the intracellular Ca^{2+} concentration [170,196], these channels must regulate ICAM-1 expression in a different manner than Orai1 or TRPC1 which mediate an increase of the intracellular Ca^{2+} concentration [184,185].

The limited knowledge on the role of ion channels in cell-cell adhesion contrasts with that on cell-matrix adhesion. Several studies have shown a role of TRP channels in this process. A few examples are listed in the following: inhibition of TRPC1 decreases adhesiveness of CNE2 nasopharyngeal tumor cells [38], TRPC2 channels regulate adhesion of rat thyroid FRTL-5 cells [197], silencing TRPM7 channels increases the adhesiveness of human umbilical vein endothelial (HUVEC) cells [82] and

TRPM8 activation leads to inhibition of the GTPase Rap1 and impaired ß1 integrin-dependent adhesion and migration of endothelial cell line (HMECs) [92].

Once tumor cells are adherent to endothelial cells they will eventually breach the endothelial barrier and invade the underlying tissue. It is well known that cadherin-mediated cell-cell adhesion of endothelial cells is Ca^{2+}-dependent [198]. The cadherin-mediated barrier integrity also depends on intracellular Ca^{2+} signaling that in turn is regulated, among others, by TRPV4 channels as shown for retinal endothelial cells [199] or for pulmonary vessels [12,200]. Endothelial TRPV4 channels cooperate with $K_{Ca}3.1$ channels in the regulation of the endothelial barrier integrity [201]. The barrier integrity can also be modulated by endothelial TRPM2 channels. When they are activated by oxidants generated by neutrophil granulocytes, endothelial cell junctions open and facilitate transmigration of neutrophils [202]. It remains to be seen whether such a mechanism also applies for tumor cell extravasation. Moreover, endothelial TRPC6 [203] and $K_{2P}2.1$ channels [204] control the transendothelial migration of leukocytes. To the best of our knowledge, a role of TRP channels in transendothelial migration of tumor cells has not been directly shown. Our study showing that inhibition of endothelial $K_{Ca}3.1$ channels also impairs lung cancer cell transmigration [17] may serve as a further proof-of-principle for the role of ion channels in this process.

6. Pharmacologic Targeting of TRP Channels in Cancer

This review emphasizes the therapeutic potential of targeting TRP channels in cancer. TRP channels can already be used as prognostic and predictive clinical markers because TRP channel expression strongly correlates with patient survival (e.g., [205–209]). The pharmacological targeting of TRP channels offers the advantage that tumor, stroma and immune cells can be targeted simultaneously with potentially only one drug. For example, TRPC6 channels are expressed in hepatocellular carcinoma cells [210], in hepatic stellate cells [127], endothelial cells [203] and in neutrophil granulocytes [79]. Moreover, their inhibition is at least partially effective in tumors that are resistantt to chemotherapy [210]. Thus, TRP channel blockade may not only interrupt the mutual activation of tumor and stroma cells. When combined with conventional chemotherapeutics it also offers the opportunity to reduce their dosage and thereby lessen the severity of side effects. The challenge will be to selectively target TRP channel modulators to the tumor in order to avoid systemic side effects. We refer to the review by Gautier and colleagues for an overview of the pharmacological approach of targeting TRP channels in cancer [211].

Some approaches use the fact that TRP channels are upregulated in tumorigenic cells, so that targeted TRP channel activation leads to Ca^{2+} and Na^+ influx, disruption of the ionic homeostasis and subsequent cell death. For the TRPM8 activator D3263, a clinical Phase 1 dose escalation study (NCT00839631) led to disease stabilization in prostate cancer patients. Another TRPM8 activator, WS-12, may be used as a diagnostic marker for prostate cancer by incorporating radiohalogens [212,213]. Another example is the Phase 1 trial of SOR-C13 (NCT01578564), a TRPV6 inhibitor. TRPV6 inhibition aims to suppress Ca^{2+}-mediated cancer proliferation and metastasis e.g., in SCLC, prostate or pancreas cancer [66,214,215].

For ion channel inhibitors, the possible target is typically located in plasma membrane. The drug must only diffuse through the capillaries and the tissue to reach its target. Disease- and drug-derived factors (e.g., interstitial pH) significantly contribute to the differential distribution in the tissues. Therefore, relying solely on total drug concentration has the potential to introduce significant errors into the interpretation of drug delivery mechanisms. To assess the pharmacokinetic properties of potential drugs, it is crucial to also assess the free, unbound drug concentration, which refers to compounds that are for example not bound to plasma proteins [216]. In case of TRP channel inhibitors, it is still necessary to assess the amount of unbound drug concentration in the vicinity of the migrating cancer cells.

However, most of the cancer-associated TRP channels are far away from being targeted in clinical trials and developing suitable TRP channel modulators in combination with cancer-specific applications is urgently needed.

7. Conclusions and Open Questions

Recapitulating our knowledge on TRP channel regulation and function, it becomes obvious, that they play an important role in the dissemination of cancer cells and in disease progression (see Figure 1). In our view their contribution to cancer progression can be attributed at least in part to the fact that they are multimodal sensors and transducers/effectors of microenvironmental cues encountered by cancer cells during the metastatic cascade. They respond to many of the chemico-physical stimuli that are relevant for the metastatic spread of cancer cells. In light of the prognostic relevance of metastases, it is not surprising that there are strong correlations between TRP channel expression in tumors and the overall survival of the diseased patients. This review also shows that TRP channel functions in metastasis and cancer in general are still far from being fully understood. Many studies do not provide a detailed look on the mechanistic steps and signaling cascades regulated by TRP channels. Moreover, there is an almost complete lack of knowledge concerning the role of TRP channels in the processes of intra- and extravasation. It is equally unknown whether they play a role in circulating tumor cells. Circulating tumor cells are exposed to a massive mechanical stress so that one can expect a strong activation of mechanosensitive TRP and PIEZO channels potentially leading to a Ca^{2+} overload. While the overexpression of many TRP channels involved in mechano-signaling promotes aggressive tumor cell behavior, this may not be the case for the "success" of circulating tumor cells.

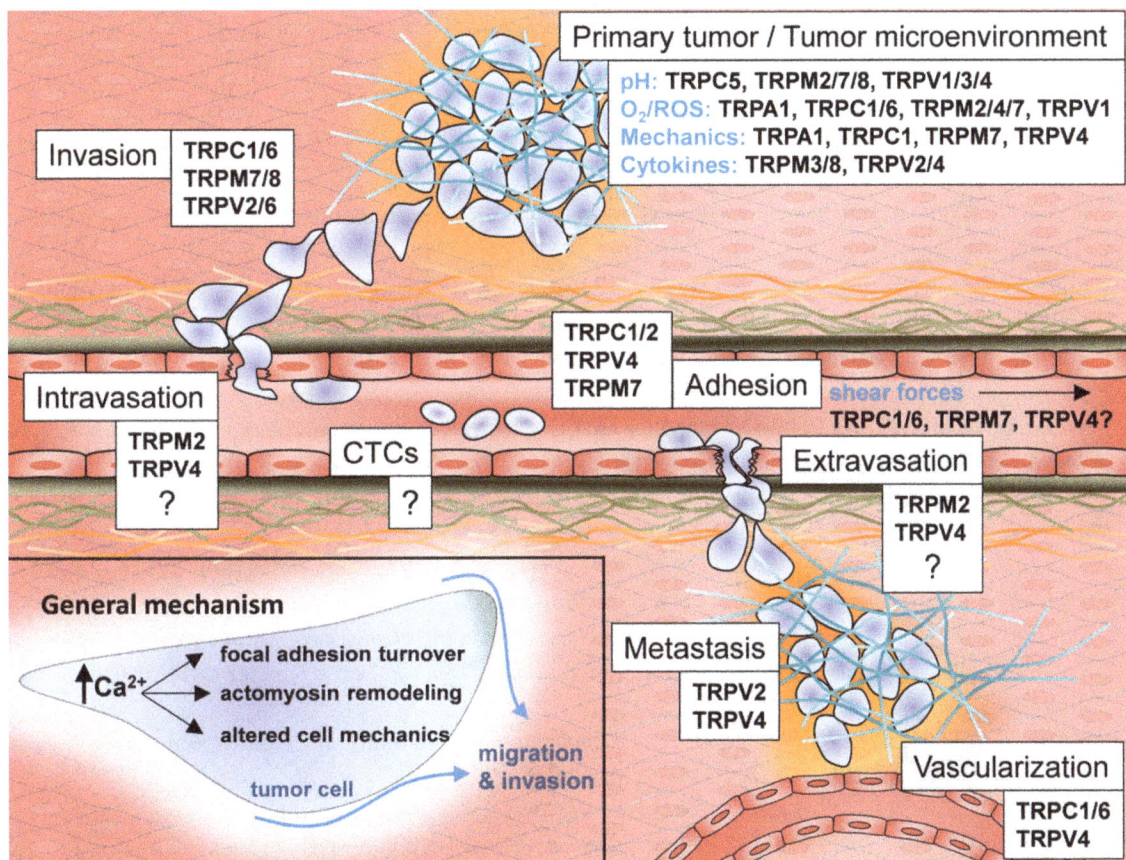

Figure 1. TRP channels in the metastatic cascade.

During the metastatic cascade, cancer cells have to respond to various chemico-physical stimuli such as changes in pH, hypoxia, ROS, mechanical cues and growth factor and cytokine gradients. Cancer cells use TRP channels to sense, modify and regulate these stimuli during the different steps of the metastatic cascade/during tumor progression. This figure highlights important TRP channels within the metastatic cascade. Open questions are stressed with question marks.

There are clearly two major quests for the field of TRP channels in cancer. One is to delineate in more detail the contribution of TRP channels to the metastatic cascade. A molecular understanding of the role of TRP channels therein is a prerequisite for developing new (TRP channel-targeting) therapeutic concepts. Novel microfluidic techniques as well as biophysical techniques such as atomic force microscopy will be valuable approaches for deciphering the role of TRP channels in intra- and extravasation of tumor cells and also in circulating tumor cells. The second challenge is to continue the development of new and specific TRP channel modulators so that the therapeutic potential of aberrant TRP channel function in the metastatic cascade can be evaluated pharmacologically and eventually be translated clinically. In our view, the responsiveness of TRP channels to cues from the tumor microenvironment makes them very attractive targets. Their attractiveness is reinforced by the fact that they allow simultaneous targeting of both tumor and stromal cells. Moreover, there is growing evidence that TRP channel modulation constitutes a new approach to overcome resistance to "conventional" cancer therapeutics (e.g., [210,217]). Thereby, the vicious cycle of mutual activation of tumor and stromal cells can potentially be interrupted.

Acknowledgments: The authors wish to thank past and present members of their laboratory whose enthusiastic work contributed largely to developing the concepts described in this review. A.S. acknowledges support from the Deutsche Forschungsgemeinschaft (DFG; SCHW 407/17-1), Cells-in-Motion Cluster of Excellence (EXC 1003-CiM), University of Münster, Germany and IZKF Münster (Schw2/020/18). B.F. received support from Cells-in-Motion Cluster of Excellence (EXC 1003-CiM; PP 2016-12).

References

1. Riggi, N.; Aguet, M.; Stamenkovic, I. Cancer Metastasis: A Reappraisal of Its Underlying Mechanisms and Their Relevance to Treatment. *Annu. Rev. Pathol.* **2018**, *13*, 117–140. [CrossRef] [PubMed]

2. Carrato, A.; Falcone, A.; Ducreux, M.; Valle, J.W.; Parnaby, A.; Djazouli, K.; Alnwick-Allu, K.; Hutchings, A.; Palaska, C.; Parthenaki, I. A Systematic Review of the Burden of Pancreatic Cancer in Europe: Real-World Impact on Survival, Quality of Life and Costs. *J. Gastrointest. Cancer* **2015**, *46*, 201–211. [CrossRef] [PubMed]

3. De Angelis, R.; Sant, M.; Coleman, M.P.; Francisci, S.; Baili, P.; Pierannunzio, D.; Trama, A.; Visser, O.; Brenner, H.; Ardanaz, E.; et al. EUROCARE-5 Working Group Cancer survival in Europe 1999–2007 by country and age: Results of EUROCARE–5-a population-based study. *Lancet Oncol.* **2014**, *15*, 23–34. [CrossRef]

4. Hanahan, D.; Weinberg, R.A. Hallmarks of cancer: The next generation. *Cell* **2011**, *144*, 646–674. [CrossRef] [PubMed]

5. Djamgoz, M.B.A.; Coombes, R.C.; Schwab, A. Ion transport and cancer: From initiation to metastasis. *Philos. Trans. R. Soc. Lond. B. Biol. Sci.* **2014**, *369*, 20130092. [CrossRef] [PubMed]

6. Andersen, A.P.; Moreira, J.M.A.; Pedersen, S.F. Interactions of ion transporters and channels with cancer cell metabolism and the tumour microenvironment. *Philos. Trans. R. Soc. B Biol. Sci.* **2014**, *369*. [CrossRef] [PubMed]

7. Schwab, A.; Stock, C. Ion channels and transporters in tumour cell migration and invasion. *Philos. Trans. R. Soc. Lond. B. Biol. Sci.* **2014**, *369*, 20130102. [CrossRef] [PubMed]

8. Urrego, D.; Tomczak, A.P.; Zahed, F.; Stühmer, W.; Pardo, L.A. Potassium channels in cell cycle and cell proliferation. *Philos. Trans. R. Soc. B Biol. Sci.* **2014**, *369*. [CrossRef] [PubMed]

9. Wanitchakool, P.; Wolf, L.; Koehl, G.E.; Sirianant, L.; Schreiber, R.; Kulkarni, S.; Duvvuri, U.; Kunzelmann, K. Role of anoctamins in cancer and apoptosis. *Philos. Trans. R. Soc. Lond. B. Biol. Sci.* **2014**, *369*, 20130096. [CrossRef] [PubMed]

10. Bernardini, M.; Fiorio Pla, A.; Prevarskaya, N.; Gkika, D. Human transient receptor potential (TRP) channel expression profiling in carcinogenesis. *Int. J. Dev. Biol.* **2015**, *59*, 399–406. [CrossRef] [PubMed]

11. Prevarskaya, N.; Skryma, R.; Shuba, Y. Ion Channels in Cancer: Are Cancer Hallmarks Oncochannelopathies? *Physiol. Rev.* **2018**, *98*, 559–621. [CrossRef] [PubMed]

12. Micalizzi, D.S.; Maheswaran, S.; Haber, D.A. A conduit to metastasis: Circulating tumor cell biology. *Genes Dev.* **2017**, *31*, 1827–1840. [CrossRef] [PubMed]

13. Franco, A.T.; Corken, A.; Ware, J. Platelets at the interface of thrombosis, inflammation, and cancer. *Blood* **2015**, *126*, 582–588. [CrossRef] [PubMed]

14. Velez, J.; Enciso, L.J.; Suarez, M.; Fiegl, M.; Grismaldo, A.; López, C.; Barreto, A.; Cardozo, C.; Palacios, P.; Morales, L.; et al. Platelets promote mitochondrial uncoupling and resistance to apoptosis in leukemia cells: A novel paradigm for the bone marrow microenvironment. *Cancer Microenviron.* **2014**, *7*, 79–90. [CrossRef] [PubMed]

15. Reymond, N.; d'Água, B.B.; Ridley, A.J. Crossing the endothelial barrier during metastasis. *Nat. Rev. Cancer* **2013**, *13*, 858–870. [CrossRef] [PubMed]

16. Pick, R.; Brechtefeld, D.; Walzog, B. Intraluminal crawling versus interstitial neutrophil migration during inflammation. *Mol. Immunol.* **2013**, *55*, 70–75. [CrossRef] [PubMed]

17. Bulk, E.; Kramko, N.; Liashkovich, I.; Glaser, F.; Schillers, H.; Schnittler, H.-J.; Oberleithner, H.; Schwab, A. KCa3.1 channel inhibition leads to an ICAM-1 dependent increase of cell-cell adhesion between A549 lung cancer and HMEC-1 endothelial cells. *Oncotarget* **2017**, *8*, 112268–112282. [CrossRef] [PubMed]

18. Soto, M.S.; O'Brien, E.R.; Andreou, K.; Scrace, S.F.; Zakaria, R.; Jenkinson, M.D.; O'Neill, E.; Sibson, N.R. Disruption of tumour-host communication by downregulation of LFA-1 reduces COX-2 and e-NOS expression and inhibits brain metastasis growth. *Oncotarget* **2016**, *7*, 52375–52391. [CrossRef] [PubMed]

19. Nilius, B.; Szallasi, A. Transient receptor potential channels as drug targets: From the science of basic research to the art of medicine. *Pharmacol. Rev.* **2014**, *66*, 676–814. [CrossRef] [PubMed]

20. Szolcsányi, J.; Sándor, Z. Multisteric TRPV1 nocisensor: A target for analgesics. *Trends Pharmacol. Sci.* **2012**, *33*, 646–655. [CrossRef] [PubMed]

21. Khalil, M.; Alliger, K.; Weidinger, C.; Yerinde, C.; Wirtz, S.; Becker, C.; Engel, M.A. Functional Role of Transient Receptor Potential Channels in Immune Cells and Epithelia. *Front. Immunol.* **2018**, *9*, 174. [CrossRef] [PubMed]

22. van Goor, M.K.C.; Hoenderop, J.G.J.; van der Wijst, J. TRP channels in calcium homeostasis: From hormonal control to structure-function relationship of TRPV5 and TRPV6. *Biochim. Biophys. Acta* **2017**, *1864*, 883–893. [CrossRef] [PubMed]

23. Najder, K.; Musset, B.; Lindemann, O.; Bulk, E.; Schwab, A.; Fels, B. The function of TRP channels in neutrophil granulocytes. *Pflüg. Arch.* **2018**. [CrossRef] [PubMed]

24. Vrenken, K.S.; Jalink, K.; van Leeuwen, F.N.; Middelbeek, J. Beyond ion-conduction: Channel-dependent and -independent roles of TRP channels during development and tissue homeostasis. *Biochim. Biophys. Acta* **2016**, *1863*, 1436–1446. [CrossRef] [PubMed]

25. Azimi, I.; Milevskiy, M.J.G.; Kaemmerer, E.; Turner, D.; Yapa, K.T.D.S.; Brown, M.A.; Thompson, E.W.; Roberts-Thomson, S.J.; Monteith, G.R. TRPC1 is a differential regulator of hypoxia-mediated events and Akt signalling in PTEN-deficient breast cancer cells. *J. Cell Sci.* **2017**, *130*, 2292–2305. [CrossRef] [PubMed]

26. Lee, W.H.; Choong, L.Y.; Jin, T.H.; Mon, N.N.; Chong, S.; Liew, C.S.; Putti, T.; Lu, S.Y.; Harteneck, C.; Lim, Y.P. TRPV4 plays a role in breast cancer cell migration via Ca^{2+}-dependent activation of AKT and downregulation of E-cadherin cell cortex protein. *Oncogenesis* **2017**, *6*, e338. [CrossRef] [PubMed]

27. Sumoza-Toledo, A.; Espinoza-Gabriel, M.I.; Montiel-Condado, D. Evaluation of the TRPM2 channel as a biomarker in breast cancer using public databases analysis. *Bol. Méd. Hosp. Infant. México* **2016**, *73*, 397–404. [CrossRef] [PubMed]

28. Rybarczyk, P.; Vanlaeys, A.; Brassart, B.; Dhennin-Duthille, I.; Chatelain, D.; Sevestre, H.; Ouadid-Ahidouch, H.; Gautier, M. The Transient Receptor Potential Melastatin 7 Channel Regulates Pancreatic Cancer Cell Invasion through the Hsp90α/uPA/MMP2 pathway. *Neoplasia* **2017**, *19*, 288–300. [CrossRef] [PubMed]

29. Xiao, N.; Jiang, L.M.; Ge, B.; Zhang, T.Y.; Zhao, X.K.; Zhou, X. Over-expression of TRPM8 is associated with poor prognosis in urothelial carcinoma of bladder. *Tumour Biol.* **2014**, *35*, 11499–11504. [CrossRef] [PubMed]

30. Zhao, W.; Xu, H. High expression of TRPM8 predicts poor prognosis in patients with osteosarcoma. *Oncol. Lett.* **2016**, *12*, 1373–1379. [CrossRef] [PubMed]

31. Elbaz, M.; Ahirwar, D.; Xiaoli, Z.; Zhou, X.; Lustberg, M.; Nasser, M.W.; Shilo, K.; Ganju, R.K. TRPV2 is a novel biomarker and therapeutic target in triple negative breast cancer. *Oncotarget* **2016**, *5*. [CrossRef]

32. Zhou, K.; Zhang, S.-S.; Yan, Y.; Zhao, S. Overexpression of transient receptor potential vanilloid 2 is associated

with poor prognosis in patients with esophageal squamous cell carcinoma. *Med. Oncol.* **2014**, *31*, 17. [CrossRef] [PubMed]

33. Du, G.-J.; Li, J.-H.; Liu, W.-J.; Liu, Y.-H.; Zhao, B.; Li, H.-R.; Hou, X.-D.; Li, H.; Qi, X.-X.; Duan, Y.-J. The combination of TRPM8 and TRPA1 expression causes an invasive phenotype in lung cancer. *Tumour Biol.* **2014**, *35*, 1251–1261. [CrossRef] [PubMed]

34. Schaar, A.; Sukumaran, P.; Sun, Y.; Dhasarathy, A.; Singh, B.B. TRPC1-STIM1 activation modulates transforming growth factor β-induced epithelial-to-mesenchymal transition. *Oncotarget* **2016**, *7*, 80554–80567. [CrossRef] [PubMed]

35. Faouzi, M.; Hague, F.; Geerts, D.; Ay, A.-S.; Potier-Cartereau, M.; Ahidouch, A.; Ouadid-Ahidouch, H. Functional cooperation between KCa3.1 and TRPC1 channels in human breast cancer: Role in cell proliferation and patient prognosis. *Oncotarget* **2016**, *7*, 36419–36435. [CrossRef] [PubMed]

36. Dong, H.; Shim, K.-N.; Li, J.M.J.; Estrema, C.; Ornelas, T.A.; Nguyen, F.; Liu, S.; Ramamoorthy, S.L.; Ho, S.; Carethers, J.M.; et al. Molecular mechanisms underlying Ca^{2+}-mediated motility of human pancreatic duct cells. *Am. J. Physiol. Cell Physiol.* **2010**, *299*, C1493–1503. [CrossRef] [PubMed]

37. Tajeddine, N.; Gailly, P. TRPC1 protein channel is major regulator of epidermal growth factor receptor signaling. *J. Biol. Chem.* **2012**, *287*, 16146–16157. [CrossRef] [PubMed]

38. He, B.; Liu, F.; Ruan, J.; Li, A.; Chen, J.; Li, R.; Shen, J.; Zheng, D.; Luo, R. Silencing TRPC1 expression inhibits invasion of CNE2 nasopharyngeal tumor cells. *Oncol. Rep.* **2012**, *27*, 1548–1554. [CrossRef] [PubMed]

39. Lepannetier, S.; Zanou, N.; Yerna, X.; Emeriau, N.; Dufour, I.; Masquelier, J.; Muccioli, G.; Tajeddine, N.; Gailly, P. Sphingosine-1-phosphate-activated TRPC1 channel controls chemotaxis of glioblastoma cells. *Cell Calcium* **2016**, *60*, 373–383. [CrossRef] [PubMed]

40. Asghar, M.Y.; Magnusson, M.; Kemppainen, K.; Sukumaran, P.; Löf, C.; Pulli, I.; Kalhori, V.; Törnquist, K. Transient Receptor Potential Canonical 1 (TRPC1) Channels as Regulators of Sphingolipid and VEGF Receptor Expression: Implications for thyroid cancer cell migration and proliferation. *J. Biol. Chem.* **2015**, *290*, 16116–16131. [CrossRef] [PubMed]

41. Wei, W.-C.; Huang, W.-C.; Lin, Y.-P.; Becker, E.B.E.; Ansorge, O.; Flockerzi, V.; Conti, D.; Cenacchi, G.; Glitsch, M.D. Functional expression of calcium-permeable canonical transient receptor potential 4-containing channels promotes migration of medulloblastoma cells. *J. Physiol.* **2017**, *595*, 5525–5544. [CrossRef] [PubMed]

42. Chen, Z.; Zhu, Y.; Dong, Y.; Zhang, P.; Han, X.; Jin, J.; Ma, X. Overexpression of TrpC5 promotes tumor metastasis via the HIF-1α-Twist signaling pathway in colon cancer. *Clin. Sci. Lond. Engl. 1979* **2017**, *131*, 2439–2450. [CrossRef] [PubMed]

43. Chigurupati, S.; Venkataraman, R.; Barrera, D.; Naganathan, A.; Madan, M.; Paul, L.; Pattisapu, J.V.; Kyriazis, G.A.; Sugaya, K.; Bushnev, S.; et al. Receptor channel TRPC6 is a key mediator of Notch-driven glioblastoma growth and invasiveness. *Cancer Res.* **2010**, *70*, 418–427. [CrossRef] [PubMed]

44. Yang, L.-L.; Liu, B.-C.; Lu, X.-Y.; Yan, Y.; Zhai, Y.-J.; Bao, Q.; Doetsch, P.W.; Deng, X.; Thai, T.L.; Alli, A.A.; et al. Inhibition of TRPC6 reduces non-small cell lung cancer cell proliferation and invasion. *Oncotarget* **2017**, *8*, 5123–5134. [CrossRef] [PubMed]

45. Yue, D.; Wang, Y.; Xiao, J.-Y.; Wang, P.; Ren, C.-S. Expression of TRPC6 in benign and malignant human prostate tissues. *Asian J. Androl.* **2009**, *11*, 541–547. [CrossRef] [PubMed]

46. El Boustany, C.; Bidaux, G.; Enfissi, A.; Delcourt, P.; Prevarskaya, N.; Capiod, T. Capacitative calcium entry and transient receptor potential canonical 6 expression control human hepatoma cell proliferation. *Hepatology* **2008**, *47*, 2068–2077. [CrossRef] [PubMed]

47. Yee, N.S.; Kazi, A.A.; Li, Q.; Yang, Z.; Berg, A.; Yee, R.K. Aberrant over-expression of TRPM7 ion channels in pancreatic cancer: Required for cancer cell invasion and implicated in tumor growth and metastasis. *Biol. Open* **2015**, *4*, 507–514. [CrossRef] [PubMed]

48. Gao, H.; Chen, X.; Du, X.; Guan, B.; Liu, Y.; Zhang, H. EGF enhances the migration of cancer cells by up-regulation of TRPM7. *Cell Calcium* **2011**, *50*, 559–568. [CrossRef] [PubMed]

49. Middelbeek, J.; Kuipers, A.J.; Henneman, L.; Visser, D.; Eidhof, I.; van Horssen, R.; Wieringa, B.; Canisius, S.V.; Zwart, W.; Wessels, L.F.; et al. TRPM7 is required for breast tumor cell metastasis. *Cancer Res.* **2012**, *72*, 4250–4261. [CrossRef] [PubMed]

50. Guilbert, A.; Gautier, M.; Dhennin-Duthille, I.; Rybarczyk, P.; Sahni, J.; Sevestre, H.; Scharenberg, A.M.;

Ouadid-Ahidouch, H. Transient receptor potential melastatin 7 is involved in oestrogen receptor-negative metastatic breast cancer cells migration through its kinase domain. *Eur. J. Cancer* **2013**, *49*, 3694–3707. [CrossRef] [PubMed]

51. Meng, X.; Cai, C.; Wu, J.; Cai, S.; Ye, C.; Chen, H.; Yang, Z.; Zeng, H.; Shen, Q.; Zou, F. TRPM7 mediates breast cancer cell migration and invasion through the MAPK pathway. *Cancer Lett.* **2013**, *333*, 96–102. [CrossRef] [PubMed]

52. Davis, F.M.; Azimi, I.; Faville, R.A.; Peters, A.A.; Jalink, K.; Putney, J.W.; Goodhill, G.J.; Thompson, E.W.; Roberts-Thomson, S.J.; Monteith, G.R. Induction of epithelial-mesenchymal transition (EMT) in breast cancer cells is calcium signal dependent. *Oncogene* **2014**, *33*, 2307–2316. [CrossRef] [PubMed]

53. Chen, J.-P.; Luan, Y.; You, C.-X.; Chen, X.-H.; Luo, R.-C.; Li, R. TRPM7 regulates the migration of human nasopharyngeal carcinoma cell by mediating Ca^{2+} influx. *Cell Calcium* **2010**, *47*, 425–432. [CrossRef] [PubMed]

54. Wang, J.; Liao, Q.-J.; Zhang, Y.; Zhou, H.; Luo, C.-H.; Tang, J.; Wang, Y.; Tang, Y.; Zhao, M.; Zhao, X.-H.; et al. TRPM7 is required for ovarian cancer cell growth, migration and invasion. *Biochem. Biophys. Res. Commun.* **2014**, *454*, 547–553. [CrossRef] [PubMed]

55. Okamoto, Y.; Ohkubo, T.; Ikebe, T.; Yamazaki, J. Blockade of TRPM8 activity reduces the invasion potential of oral squamous carcinoma cell lines. *Int. J. Oncol.* **2012**, *40*, 1431–1440. [CrossRef] [PubMed]

56. Liu, J.; Chen, Y.; Shuai, S.; Ding, D.; Li, R.; Luo, R. TRPM8 promotes aggressiveness of breast cancer cells by regulating EMT via activating AKT/GSK-3β pathway. *Tumour Biol.* **2014**, *35*, 8969–8977. [CrossRef] [PubMed]

57. Klumpp, D.; Frank, S.C.; Klumpp, L.; Sezgin, E.C.; Eckert, M.; Edalat, L.; Bastmeyer, M.; Zips, D.; Ruth, P.; Huber, S.M. TRPM8 is required for survival and radioresistance of glioblastoma cells. *Oncotarget* **2017**, *8*, 95896–95913. [CrossRef] [PubMed]

58. Cucu, D.; Chiritoiu, G.; Petrescu, S.; Babes, A.; Stanica, L.; Duda, D.G.; Horii, A.; Dima, S.O.; Popescu, I. Characterization of functional transient receptor potential melastatin 8 channels in human pancreatic ductal adenocarcinoma cells. *Pancreas* **2014**, *43*, 795–800. [CrossRef] [PubMed]

59. Yang, Z.-H.; Wang, X.-H.; Wang, H.-P.; Hu, L.-Q. Effects of TRPM8 on the proliferation and motility of prostate cancer PC-3 cells. *Asian J. Androl.* **2009**, *11*, 157–165. [CrossRef] [PubMed]

60. Bidaux, G.; Borowiec, A.-S.; Dubois, C.; Delcourt, P.; Schulz, C.; Vanden Abeele, F.; Lepage, G.; Desruelles, E.; Bokhobza, A.; Dewailly, E.; et al. Targeting of short TRPM8 isoforms induces 4TM-TRPM8-dependent apoptosis in prostate cancer cells. *Oncotarget* **2016**, *7*, 29063–29080. [CrossRef] [PubMed]

61. Monet, M.; Lehen'kyi, V. 'yacheslav; Gackiere, F.; Firlej, V.; Vandenberghe, M.; Roudbaraki, M.; Gkika, D.; Pourtier, A.; Bidaux, G.; Slomianny, C.; Delcourt, P.; et al. Role of cationic channel TRPV2 in promoting prostate cancer migration and progression to androgen resistance. *Cancer Res.* **2010**, *70*, 1225–1235. [CrossRef] [PubMed]

62. Gambade, A.; Zreika, S.; Guéguinou, M.; Chourpa, I.; Fromont, G.; Bouchet, A.M.; Burlaud-Gaillard, J.; Potier-Cartereau, M.; Roger, S.; Aucagne, V.; et al. Activation of TRPV2 and BKCa channels by the LL-37 enantiomers stimulates calcium entry and migration of cancer cells. *Oncotarget* **2016**, *7*, 23785–23800. [CrossRef] [PubMed]

63. Lee, W.H.; Choong, L.Y.; Mon, N.N.; Lu, S.; Lin, Q.; Pang, B.; Yan, B.; Krishna, V.S.R.; Singh, H.; Tan, T.Z.; et al. TRPV4 Regulates Breast Cancer Cell Extravasation, Stiffness and Actin Cortex. *Sci. Rep.* **2016**, *6*, 27903. [CrossRef] [PubMed]

64. Xie, R.; Xu, J.; Xiao, Y.; Wu, J.; Wan, H.; Tang, B.; Liu, J.; Fan, Y.; Wang, S.; Wu, Y.; et al. Calcium Promotes Human Gastric Cancer via a Novel Coupling of Calcium-Sensing Receptor and TRPV4 Channel. *Cancer Res.* **2017**, *77*, 6499–6512. [CrossRef] [PubMed]

65. Dhennin-Duthille, I.; Gautier, M.; Faouzi, M.; Guilbert, A.; Brevet, M.; Vaudry, D.; Ahidouch, A.; Sevestre, H.; Ouadid-Ahidouch, H. High expression of transient receptor potential channels in human breast cancer epithelial cells and tissues: Correlation with pathological parameters. *Cell. Physiol. Biochem.* **2011**, *28*, 813–822. [CrossRef] [PubMed]

66. Song, H.; Dong, M.; Zhou, J.; Sheng, W.; Li, X.; Gao, W. Expression and prognostic significance of TRPV6 in the development and progression of pancreatic cancer. *Oncol. Rep.* **2018**, *39*, 1432–1440. [CrossRef] [PubMed]

67. Rae, J.M.; Creighton, C.J.; Meck, J.M.; Haddad, B.R.; Johnson, M.D. MDA-MB-435 cells are derived from M14

Melanoma cells—a loss for breast cancer, but a boon for melanoma research. *Breast Cancer Res. Treat.* **2007**, *104*, 13–19. [CrossRef] [PubMed]

68. Zhang, S.-S.; Wen, J.; Yang, F.; Cai, X.-L.; Yang, H.; Luo, K.-J.; Liu, Q.W.; Hu, R.-G.; Xie, X.; Huang, Q.-Y.; et al. High expression of transient potential receptor C6 correlated with poor prognosis in patients with esophageal squamous cell carcinoma. *Med. Oncol.* **2013**, *30*, 607. [CrossRef] [PubMed]

69. Rybarczyk, P.; Gautier, M.; Hague, F.; Dhennin-Duthille, I.; Chatelain, D.; Kerr-Conte, J.; Pattou, F.; Regimbeau, J.-M.; Sevestre, H.; Ouadid-Ahidouch, H. Transient receptor potential melastatin-related 7 channel is overexpressed in human pancreatic ductal adenocarcinomas and regulates human pancreatic cancer cell migration. *Int. J. Cancer* **2012**, *131*, E851–E861. [CrossRef] [PubMed]

70. Fife, C.M.; McCarroll, J.A.; Kavallaris, M. Movers and shakers: Cell cytoskeleton in cancer metastasis. *Br. J. Pharmacol.* **2014**, *171*, 5507–5523. [CrossRef] [PubMed]

71. Friedl, P.; Mayor, R. Tuning Collective Cell Migration by Cell-Cell Junction Regulation. *Cold Spring Harb. Perspect. Biol.* **2017**, *9*. [CrossRef] [PubMed]

72. Schwab, A.; Fabian, A.; Hanley, P.J.; Stock, C. Role of ion channels and transporters in cell migration. *Physiol. Rev.* **2012**, *92*, 1865–1913. [CrossRef] [PubMed]

73. Betapudi, V.; Rai, V.; Beach, J.R.; Egelhoff, T. Novel regulation and dynamics of myosin II activation during epidermal wound responses. *Exp. Cell Res.* **2010**, *316*, 980–991. [CrossRef] [PubMed]

74. Giannone, G.; Rondé, P.; Gaire, M.; Beaudouin, J.; Haiech, J.; Ellenberg, J.; Takeda, K. Calcium rises locally trigger focal adhesion disassembly and enhance residency of focal adhesion kinase at focal adhesions. *J. Biol. Chem.* **2004**, *279*, 28715–28723. [CrossRef] [PubMed]

75. Iamshanova, O.; Fiorio Pla, A.; Prevarskaya, N. Molecular mechanisms of tumour invasion: Regulation by calcium signals. *J. Physiol.* **2017**, *595*, 3063–3075. [CrossRef] [PubMed]

76. Stock, C.; Ludwig, F.T.; Hanley, P.J.; Schwab, A. Roles of ion transport in control of cell motility. *Compr. Physiol.* **2013**, *3*, 59–119. [CrossRef] [PubMed]

77. Yang, M.; Brackenbury, W.J. Membrane potential and cancer progression. *Front. Physiol.* **2013**, *4*. [CrossRef] [PubMed]

78. Kronlage, M.; Song, J.; Sorokin, L.; Isfort, K.; Schwerdtle, T.; Leipziger, J.; Robaye, B.; Conley, P.B.; Kim, H.-C.; Sargin, S.; et al. Autocrine Purinergic Receptor Signaling Is Essential for Macrophage Chemotaxis. *Sci. Signal* **2010**, *3*, ra55. [CrossRef] [PubMed]

79. Lindemann, O.; Umlauf, D.; Frank, S.; Schimmelpfennig, S.; Bertrand, J.; Pap, T.; Hanley, P.J.; Fabian, A.; Dietrich, A.; Schwab, A. TRPC6 regulates CXCR2-mediated chemotaxis of murine neutrophils. *J. Immunol.* **2013**, *190*, 5496–5505. [CrossRef] [PubMed]

80. Schilling, T.; Miralles, F.; Eder, C. TRPM7 regulates proliferation and polarisation of macrophages. *J. Cell Sci.* **2014**, *127*, 4561–4566. [CrossRef] [PubMed]

81. Clark, K.; Langeslag, M.; van Leeuwen, B.; Ran, L.; Ryazanov, A.G.; Figdor, C.G.; Moolenaar, W.H.; Jalink, K.; van Leeuwen, F.N. TRPM7, a novel regulator of actomyosin contractility and cell adhesion. *EMBO J.* **2006**, *25*, 290–301. [CrossRef] [PubMed]

82. Nishitani, W.S.; Alencar, A.M.; Wang, Y. Rapid and Localized Mechanical Stimulation and Adhesion Assay: TRPM7 Involvement in Calcium Signaling and Cell Adhesion. *PLoS ONE* **2015**, *10*, e0126440. [CrossRef]

83. Gao, S.-L.; Kong, C.-Z.; Zhang, Z.; Li, Z.-L.; Bi, J.-B.; Liu, X.-K. TRPM7 is overexpressed in bladder cancer and promotes proliferation, migration, invasion and tumor growth. *Oncol. Rep.* **2017**, *38*, 1967–1976. [CrossRef] [PubMed]

84. Chubanov, V.; Mittermeier, L.; Gudermann, T. Role of kinase-coupled TRP channels in mineral homeostasis. *Pharmacol. Ther.* **2018**, *184*, 159–176. [CrossRef] [PubMed]

85. Yee, N.S.; Chan, A.S.; Yee, J.D.; Yee, R.K. TRPM7 and TRPM8 Ion Channels in Pancreatic Adenocarcinoma: Potential Roles as Cancer Biomarkers and Targets. *Scientifica* **2012**, *2012*, 415158. [CrossRef] [PubMed]

86. Clark, K.; Middelbeek, J.; Lasonder, E.; Dulyaninova, N.G.; Morrice, N.A.; Ryazanov, A.G.; Bresnick, A.R.; Figdor, C.G.; van Leeuwen, F.N. TRPM7 regulates myosin IIA filament stability and protein localization by heavy chain phosphorylation. *J. Mol. Biol.* **2008**, *378*, 790–803. [CrossRef] [PubMed]

87. Jiang, J.; Li, M.-H.; Inoue, K.; Chu, X.-P.; Seeds, J.; Xiong, Z.-G. Transient Receptor Potential Melastatin 7–like

Current in Human Head and Neck Carcinoma Cells: Role in Cell Proliferation. *Cancer Res.* **2007**, *67*, 10929–10938. [CrossRef] [PubMed]

88. Yee, N.S.; Zhou, W.; Liang, I.-C. Transient receptor potential ion channel Trpm7 regulates exocrine pancreatic epithelial proliferation by Mg^{2+}-sensitive Socs3a signaling in development and cancer. *Dis. Model. Mech.* **2011**, *4*, 240–254. [CrossRef] [PubMed]

89. Gkika, D.; Flourakis, M.; Lemonnier, L.; Prevarskaya, N. PSA reduces prostate cancer cell motility by stimulating TRPM8 activity and plasma membrane expression. *Oncogene* **2010**, *29*, 4611–4616. [CrossRef] [PubMed]

90. Gkika, D.; Lemonnier, L.; Shapovalov, G.; Gordienko, D.; Poux, C.; Bernardini, M.; Bokhobza, A.; Bidaux, G.; Degerny, C.; Verreman, K.; et al. TRP channel-associated factors are a novel protein family that regulates TRPM8 trafficking and activity. *J. Cell Biol.* **2015**, *208*, 89–107. [CrossRef] [PubMed]

91. Ulăreanu, R.; Chirițoiu, G.; Cojocaru, F.; Deftu, A.; Ristoiu, V.; Stănică, L.; Mihăilescu, D.F.; Cucu, D. N-glycosylation of the transient receptor potential melastatin 8 channel is altered in pancreatic cancer cells. *Tumour Biol.* **2017**, *39*. [CrossRef] [PubMed]

92. Genova, T.; Grolez, G.P.; Camillo, C.; Bernardini, M.; Bokhobza, A.; Richard, E.; Scianna, M.; Lemonnier, L.; Valdembri, D.; Munaron, L.; et al. TRPM8 inhibits endothelial cell migration via a non-channel function by trapping the small GTPase Rap1. *J. Cell Biol.* **2017**, *216*, 2107–2130. [CrossRef] [PubMed]

93. Santoni, G.; Farfariello, V.; Amantini, C. TRPV channels in tumor growth and progression. *Adv. Exp. Med. Biol.* **2011**, *704*, 947–967. [CrossRef] [PubMed]

94. Oulidi, A.; Bokhobza, A.; Gkika, D.; Vanden Abeele, F.; Lehen'kyi, V.; Ouafik, L.H.; Mauroy, B.; Prevarskaya, N. TRPV2 mediates adrenomedullin stimulation of prostate and urothelial cancer cell adhesion, migration and invasion. *PLoS ONE* **2013**, *8*, e64885. [CrossRef] [PubMed]

95. Moccia, F. Endothelial Ca^{2+} Signaling and the Resistance to Anticancer Treatments: Partners in Crime. *Int. J. Mol. Sci.* **2018**, *19*, 217. [CrossRef] [PubMed]

96. Bomben, V.C.; Turner, K.L.; Barclay, T.-T.C.; Sontheimer, H. Transient receptor potential canonical channels are essential for chemotactic migration of human malignant gliomas. *J. Cell. Physiol.* **2011**, *226*, 1879–1888. [CrossRef] [PubMed]

97. Cuddapah, V.A.; Turner, K.L.; Sontheimer, H. Calcium entry via TRPC1 channels activates chloride currents in human glioma cells. *Cell Calcium* **2013**, *53*, 187–194. [CrossRef] [PubMed]

98. Guéguinou, M.; Harnois, T.; Crottes, D.; Uguen, A.; Deliot, N.; Gambade, A.; Chantôme, A.; Haelters, J.P.; Jaffrès, P.A.; Jourdan, M.L.; et al. SK3/TRPC1/Orai1 complex regulates SOCE-dependent colon cancer cell migration: A novel opportunity to modulate anti-EGFR mAb action by the alkyl-lipid Ohmline. *Oncotarget* **2016**, *7*, 36168–36184. [CrossRef] [PubMed]

99. Wang, D.; Li, X.; Liu, J.; Li, J.; Li, L.-J.; Qiu, M.-X. Effects of TRPC6 on invasibility of low-differentiated prostate cancer cells. *Asian Pac. J. Trop. Med.* **2014**, *7*, 44–47. [CrossRef]

100. Gkika, D.; Prevarskaya, N. TRP channels in prostate cancer: The good, the bad and the ugly? *Asian J. Androl.* **2011**, *13*, 673–676. [CrossRef] [PubMed]

101. Park, J.; Shim, M.K.; Jin, M.; Rhyu, M.-R.; Lee, Y. Methyl syringate, a TRPA1 agonist represses hypoxia-induced cyclooxygenase-2 in lung cancer cells. *Phytomedicine* **2016**, *23*, 324–329. [CrossRef] [PubMed]

102. Morelli, M.B.; Nabissi, M.; Amantini, C.; Tomassoni, D.; Rossi, F.; Cardinali, C.; Santoni, M.; Arcella, A.; Oliva, M.A.; Santoni, A.; et al. Overexpression of transient receptor potential mucolipin-2 ion channels in gliomas: Role in tumor growth and progression. *Oncotarget* **2016**, *7*, 43654–43668. [CrossRef] [PubMed]

103. Estrella, V.; Chen, T.; Lloyd, M.; Wojtkowiak, J.; Cornnell, H.H.; Ibrahim-Hashim, A.; Bailey, K.; Balagurunathan, Y.; Rothberg, J.M.; Sloane, B.F.; et al. Acidity generated by the tumor microenvironment drives local invasion. *Cancer Res.* **2013**, *73*, 1524–1535. [CrossRef] [PubMed]

104. Helmlinger, G.; Yuan, F.; Dellian, M.; Jain, R.K. Interstitial pH and pO2 gradients in solid tumors in vivo: High-resolution measurements reveal a lack of correlation. *Nat. Med.* **1997**, *3*, 177–182. [CrossRef] [PubMed]

105. Reshkin, S.J.; Cardone, R.A.; Harguindey, S. Na^+-H^+ exchanger, pH regulation and cancer. *Recent Pat. Anticancer Drug Discov.* **2013**, *8*, 85–99. [CrossRef] [PubMed]

106. Vaupel, P.; Kallinowski, F.; Okunieff, P. Blood flow, oxygen and nutrient supply, and metabolic microenvironment of human tumors: A review. *Cancer Res.* **1989**, *49*, 6449–6465. [PubMed]

107. Novak, I.; Haanes, K.A.; Wang, J. Acid-base transport in pancreas—New challenges. *Front. Physiol.* **2013**, *4*. [CrossRef] [PubMed]

108. Pedersen, S.F.; Novak, I.; Alves, F.; Schwab, A.; Pardo, L.A. Alternating pH landscapes shape epithelial cancer initiation and progression: Focus on pancreatic cancer. *Bioessays* **2017**. [CrossRef] [PubMed]

109. Holzer, P. Acid-Sensitive Ion Channels and Receptors. In *Sensory Nerves*; Canning, B.J., Spina, D., Eds.; Springer: Berlin/Heidelberg, Germany, 2009; Volume 194, pp. 283–332. ISBN 978-3-540-79089-1.

110. Semtner, M.; Schaefer, M.; Pinkenburg, O.; Plant, T.D. Potentiation of TRPC5 by Protons. *J. Biol. Chem.* **2007**, *282*, 33868–33878. [CrossRef] [PubMed]

111. Starkus, J.G.; Fleig, A.; Penner, R. The calcium-permeable non-selective cation channel TRPM2 is modulated by cellular acidification. *J. Physiol.* **2010**, *588*, 1227–1240. [CrossRef] [PubMed]

112. Mahieu, F.; Janssens, A.; Gees, M.; Talavera, K.; Nilius, B.; Voets, T. Modulation of the cold-activated cation channel TRPM8 by surface charge screening. *J. Physiol.* **2010**, *588*, 315–324. [CrossRef] [PubMed]

113. Jiang, J.; Li, M.; Yue, L. Potentiation of TRPM7 inward currents by protons. *J. Gen. Physiol.* **2005**, *126*, 137–150. [CrossRef] [PubMed]

114. Mačianskienė, R.; Almanaitytė, M.; Jekabsone, A.; Mubagwa, K. Modulation of Human Cardiac TRPM7 Current by Extracellular Acidic pH Depends upon Extracellular Concentrations of Divalent Cations. *PLoS ONE* **2017**, *12*, e0170923. [CrossRef] [PubMed]

115. Chokshi, R.; Matsushita, M.; Kozak, J.A. Detailed examination of Mg2+ and pH sensitivity of human TRPM7 channels. *Am. J. Physiol. Cell Physiol.* **2012**, *302*, C1004–C1011. [CrossRef] [PubMed]

116. Hellwig, N.; Plant, T.D.; Janson, W.; Schäfer, M.; Schultz, G.; Schaefer, M. TRPV1 acts as proton channel to induce acidification in nociceptive neurons. *J. Biol. Chem.* **2004**, *279*, 34553–34561. [CrossRef] [PubMed]

117. Nakanishi, M.; Morita, Y.; Hata, K.; Muragaki, Y. Acidic microenvironments induce lymphangiogenesis and IL-8 production via TRPV1 activation in human lymphatic endothelial cells. *Exp. Cell Res.* **2016**, *345*, 180–189. [CrossRef] [PubMed]

118. Suzuki, M.; Mizuno, A.; Kodaira, K.; Imai, M. Impaired pressure sensation in mice lacking TRPV4. *J. Biol. Chem.* **2003**, *278*, 22664–22668. [CrossRef] [PubMed]

119. Shikano, M.; Ueda, T.; Kamiya, T.; Ishida, Y.; Yamada, T.; Mizushima, T.; Shimura, T.; Mizoshita, T.; Tanida, S.; Kataoka, H.; et al. Acid inhibits TRPV4-mediated Ca^{2+} influx in mouse esophageal epithelial cells. *Neurogastroenterol. Motil.* **2011**, *23*, 1020–1028. [CrossRef] [PubMed]

120. Muz, B.; de la Puente, P.; Azab, F.; Azab, A.K. The role of hypoxia in cancer progression, angiogenesis, metastasis, and resistance to therapy. *Hypoxia* **2015**, *3*, 83–92. [CrossRef] [PubMed]

121. Provenzano, P.P.; Cuevas, C.; Chang, A.E.; Goel, V.K.; Von Hoff, D.D.; Hingorani, S.R. Enzymatic targeting of the stroma ablates physical barriers to treatment of pancreatic ductal adenocarcinoma. *Cancer Cell* **2012**, *21*, 418–429. [CrossRef] [PubMed]

122. Semenza, G.L. The hypoxic tumor microenvironment: A driving force for breast cancer progression. *Biochim. Biophys. Acta* **2016**, *1863*, 382–391. [CrossRef] [PubMed]

123. Mori, Y.; Takahashi, N.; Polat, O.K.; Kurokawa, T.; Takeda, N.; Inoue, M. Redox-sensitive transient receptor potential channels in oxygen sensing and adaptation. *Pflüg. Arch.* **2016**, *468*, 85–97. [CrossRef] [PubMed]

124. Li, S.; Wang, J.; Wei, Y.; Liu, Y.; Ding, X.; Dong, B.; Xu, Y.; Wang, Y. Crucial role of TRPC6 in maintaining the stability of HIF-1α in glioma cells under hypoxia. *J. Cell Sci.* **2015**, *128*, 3317–3329. [CrossRef] [PubMed]

125. Liu, C.; Montell, C. Forcing open TRP channels: Mechanical gating as a unifying activation mechanism. *Biochem. Biophys. Res. Commun.* **2015**, *460*, 22–25. [CrossRef] [PubMed]

126. Nielsen, M.F.B.; Mortensen, M.B.; Detlefsen, S. Identification of markers for quiescent pancreatic stellate cells in the normal human pancreas. *Histochem. Cell Biol.* **2017**. [CrossRef] [PubMed]

127. Iyer, S.C.; Kannan, A.; Devaraj, N.; Halagowder, D. Receptor channel TRPC6 orchestrate the activation of human hepatic stellate cell under hypoxia condition. *Exp. Cell Res.* **2015**. [CrossRef] [PubMed]

128. Yang, Y.; Karakhanova, S.; Werner, J.; Bazhin, A.V. Reactive oxygen species in cancer biology and anticancer therapy. *Curr. Med. Chem.* **2013**, *20*, 3677–3692. [CrossRef] [PubMed]

129. Miller, B.A.; Cheung, J.Y. TRPM2 protects against tissue damage following oxidative stress and ischaemia-reperfusion. *J. Physiol.* **2016**, *594*, 4181–4191. [CrossRef] [PubMed]

130. Chen, S.; Hoffman, N.E.; Shanmughapriya, S.; Bao, L.; Keefer, K.; Conrad, K.; Merali, S.; Takahashi, Y.; Abraham, T.; Hirschler-Laszkiewicz, I.; et al. A splice variant of the human ion channel TRPM2 modulates neuroblastoma tumor growth through hypoxia-inducible factor (HIF)-1/2α. *J. Biol. Chem.* **2014**, *289*, 36284–36302. [CrossRef] [PubMed]

131. Orfanelli, U.; Wenke, A.-K.; Doglioni, C.; Russo, V.; Bosserhoff, A.K.; Lavorgna, G. Identification of novel sense and antisense transcription at the TRPM2 locus in cancer. *Cell Res.* **2008**, *18*, 1128–1140. [CrossRef] [PubMed]

132. Bao, L.; Chen, S.-J.; Conrad, K.; Keefer, K.; Abraham, T.; Lee, J.P.; Wang, J.; Zhang, X.-Q.; Hirschler-Laszkiewicz, I.; Wang, H.-G.; et al. Depletion of the Human Ion Channel TRPM2 in Neuroblastoma Demonstrates Its Key Role in Cell Survival through Modulation of Mitochondrial Reactive Oxygen Species and Bioenergetics. *J. Biol. Chem.* **2016**, *291*, 24449–24464. [CrossRef] [PubMed]

133. Miller, B.A.; Hoffman, N.E.; Merali, S.; Zhang, X.-Q.; Wang, J.; Rajan, S.; Shanmughapriya, S.; Gao, E.; Barrero, C.A.; Mallilankaraman, K.; et al. TRPM2 channels protect against cardiac ischemia-reperfusion injury: Role of mitochondria. *J. Biol. Chem.* **2014**, *289*, 7615–7629. [CrossRef] [PubMed]

134. Aarts, M.; Iihara, K.; Wei, W.-L.; Xiong, Z.-G.; Arundine, M.; Cerwinski, W.; MacDonald, J.F.; Tymianski, M. A key role for TRPM7 channels in anoxic neuronal death. *Cell* **2003**, *115*, 863–877. [CrossRef]

135. Takahashi, N.; Kuwaki, T.; Kiyonaka, S.; Numata, T.; Kozai, D.; Mizuno, Y.; Yamamoto, S.; Naito, S.; Knevels, E.; Carmeliet, P.; et al. TRPA1 underlies a sensing mechanism for O$_2$. *Nat. Chem. Biol.* **2011**, *7*, 701–711. [CrossRef] [PubMed]

136. Parpaite, T.; Cardouat, G.; Mauroux, M.; Gillibert-Duplantier, J.; Robillard, P.; Quignard, J.-F.; Marthan, R.; Savineau, J.-P.; Ducret, T. Effect of hypoxia on TRPV1 and TRPV4 channels in rat pulmonary arterial smooth muscle cells. *Pflüg. Arch.* **2016**, *468*, 111–130. [CrossRef] [PubMed]

137. Nielsen, N.; Lindemann, O.; Schwab, A. TRP channels and STIM/ORAI proteins: Sensors and effectors of cancer and stroma cell migration. *Br. J. Pharmacol.* **2014**, *171*, 5524–5540. [CrossRef] [PubMed]

138. Melzer, N.; Hicking, G.; Göbel, K.; Wiendl, H. TRPM2 cation channels modulate T cell effector functions and contribute to autoimmune CNS inflammation. *PLoS ONE* **2012**, *7*, e47617. [CrossRef] [PubMed]

139. Yamamoto, S.; Shimizu, S.; Kiyonaka, S.; Takahashi, N.; Wajima, T.; Hara, Y.; Negoro, T.; Hiroi, T.; Kiuchi, Y.; Okada, T.; et al. TRPM2-mediated Ca^{2+} influx induces chemokine production in monocytes that aggravates inflammatory neutrophil infiltration. *Nat. Med.* **2008**, *14*, 738–747. [CrossRef] [PubMed]

140. Luppi, F.; Longo, A.M.; de Boer, W.I.; Rabe, K.F.; Hiemstra, P.S. Interleukin-8 stimulates cell proliferation in non-small cell lung cancer through epidermal growth factor receptor transactivation. *Lung Cancer* **2007**, *56*, 25–33. [CrossRef] [PubMed]

141. Rubil, S.; Lesch, A.; Mukaida, N.; Thiel, G. Stimulation of transient receptor potential M3 (TRPM3) channels increases interleukin-8 gene promoter activity involving AP-1 and extracellular signal-regulated protein kinase. *Cytokine* **2018**, *103*, 133–141. [CrossRef] [PubMed]

142. Takamori, H.; Oades, Z.G.; Hoch, O.C.; Burger, M.; Schraufstatter, I.U. Autocrine growth effect of IL-8 and GROalpha on a human pancreatic cancer cell line, Capan-1. *Pancreas* **2000**, *21*, 52–56. [CrossRef] [PubMed]

143. Waugh, D.J.J.; Wilson, C. The interleukin-8 pathway in cancer. *Clin. Cancer Res.* **2008**, *14*, 6735–6741. [CrossRef] [PubMed]

144. Khalil, M.; Babes, A.; Lakra, R.; Försch, S.; Reeh, P.W.; Wirtz, S.; Becker, C.; Neurath, M.F.; Engel, M.A. Transient receptor potential melastatin 8 ion channel in macrophages modulates colitis through a balance-shift in TNF-alpha and interleukin-10 production. *Mucosal Immunol.* **2016**, *9*, 1500–1513. [CrossRef] [PubMed]

145. Juergens, U.R.; Engelen, T.; Racké, K.; Stöber, M.; Gillissen, A.; Vetter, H. Inhibitory activity of 1,8-cineol (eucalyptol) on cytokine production in cultured human lymphocytes and monocytes. *Pulm. Pharmacol. Ther.* **2004**, *17*, 281–287. [CrossRef] [PubMed]

146. Sabnis, A.S.; Reilly, C.A.; Veranth, J.M.; Yost, G.S. Increased transcription of cytokine genes in human lung epithelial cells through activation of a TRPM8 variant by cold temperatures. *Am. J. Physiol. Lung Cell. Mol. Physiol.* **2008**, *295*, L194–200. [CrossRef] [PubMed]

147. Yamashiro, K.; Sasano, T.; Tojo, K.; Namekata, I.; Kurokawa, J.; Sawada, N.; Suganami, T.; Kamei, Y.; Tanaka, H.; Tajima, N.; et al. Role of transient receptor potential vanilloid 2 in LPS-induced cytokine production in macrophages. *Biochem. Biophys. Res. Commun.* **2010**, *398*, 284–289. [CrossRef] [PubMed]

148. Fusi, C.; Materazzi, S.; Minocci, D.; Maio, V.; Oranges, T.; Massi, D.; Nassini, R. Transient receptor potential vanilloid 4 (TRPV4) is downregulated in keratinocytes in human non-melanoma skin cancer. *J. Investig. Dermatol.* **2014**, *134*, 2408–2417. [CrossRef] [PubMed]

149. Henry, C.O.; Dalloneau, E.; Pérez-Berezo, M.-T.; Plata, C.; Wu, Y.; Guillon, A.; Morello, E.; Aimar, R.-F.; Potier-Cartereau, M.; Esnard, F.; et al. In vitro and in vivo evidence for an inflammatory role of the calcium channel TRPV4 in lung epithelium: Potential involvement in cystic fibrosis. *Am. J. Physiol. Lung Cell. Mol. Physiol.* **2016**, *311*, L664–675. [CrossRef] [PubMed]

150. Northey, J.J.; Przybyla, L.; Weaver, V.M. Tissue Force Programs Cell Fate and Tumor Aggression. *Cancer Discov.* **2017**, *7*, 1224–1237. [CrossRef] [PubMed]

151. Pickup, M.W.; Mouw, J.K.; Weaver, V.M. The extracellular matrix modulates the hallmarks of cancer. *EMBO Rep.* **2014**, *15*, 1243–1253. [CrossRef] [PubMed]

152. Lachowski, D.; Cortes, E.; Pink, D.; Chronopoulos, A.; Karim, S.A.; Morton, J.; del Río Hernández, A.E. Substrate Rigidity Controls Activation and Durotaxis in Pancreatic Stellate Cells. *Sci. Rep.* **2017**, *7*, 2506. [CrossRef] [PubMed]

153. Stylianopoulos, T.; Martin, J.D.; Chauhan, V.P.; Jain, S.R.; Diop-Frimpong, B.; Bardeesy, N.; Smith, B.L.; Ferrone, C.R.; Hornicek, F.J.; Boucher, Y.; et al. Causes, consequences, and remedies for growth-induced solid stress in murine and human tumors. *Proc. Natl. Acad. Sci. USA* **2012**, *109*, 15101–15108. [CrossRef] [PubMed]

154. Acerbi, I.; Cassereau, L.; Dean, I.; Shi, Q.; Au, A.; Park, C.; Chen, Y.Y.; Liphardt, J.; Hwang, E.S.; Weaver, V.M. Human breast cancer invasion and aggression correlates with ECM stiffening and immune cell infiltration. *Integr. Biol.* **2015**, *7*, 1120–1134. [CrossRef] [PubMed]

155. Paszek, M.J.; Zahir, N.; Johnson, K.R.; Lakins, J.N.; Rozenberg, G.I.; Gefen, A.; Reinhart-King, C.A.; Margulies, S.S.; Dembo, M.; Boettiger, D.; et al. Tensional homeostasis and the malignant phenotype. *Cancer Cell* **2005**, *8*, 241–254. [CrossRef] [PubMed]

156. Reid, S.E.; Kay, E.J.; Neilson, L.J.; Henze, A.; Serneels, J.; McGhee, E.J.; Dhayade, S.; Nixon, C.; Mackey, J.B.; Santi, A.; et al. Tumor matrix stiffness promotes metastatic cancer cell interaction with the endothelium. *EMBO J.* **2017**, *36*, 2373–2389. [CrossRef] [PubMed]

157. Rice, A.J.; Cortes, E.; Lachowski, D.; Cheung, B.C.H.; Karim, S.A.; Morton, J.P.; del Río Hernández, A. Matrix stiffness induces epithelial–mesenchymal transition and promotes chemoresistance in pancreatic cancer cells. *Oncogenesis* **2017**, *6*, e352. [CrossRef] [PubMed]

158. Fels, B.; Nielsen, N.; Schwab, A. Role of TRPC1 channels in pressure-mediated activation of murine pancreatic stellate cells. *Eur. Biophys. J.* **2016**, 1–14. [CrossRef] [PubMed]

159. Mrkonjić, S.; Garcia-Elias, A.; Pardo-Pastor, C.; Bazellières, E.; Trepat, X.; Vriens, J.; Ghosh, D.; Voets, T.; Vicente, R.; Valverde, M.A. TRPV4 participates in the establishment of trailing adhesions and directional persistence of migrating cells. *Pflüg. Arch.* **2015**, *467*, 2107–2119. [CrossRef] [PubMed]

160. Fabian, A.; Bertrand, J.; Lindemann, O.; Pap, T.; Schwab, A. Transient receptor potential canonical channel 1 impacts on mechanosignaling during cell migration. *Pflüg. Arch.* **2012**, *464*, 623–630. [CrossRef] [PubMed]

161. Liu, Y.-S.; Liu, Y.-A.; Huang, C.-J.; Yen, M.-H.; Tseng, C.-T.; Chien, S.; Lee, O.K. Mechanosensitive TRPM7 mediates shear stress and modulates osteogenic differentiation of mesenchymal stromal cells through Osterix pathway. *Sci. Rep.* **2015**, *5*, 16522. [CrossRef] [PubMed]

162. Lennertz, R.C.; Kossyreva, E.A.; Smith, A.K.; Stucky, C.L. TRPA1 Mediates Mechanical Sensitization in Nociceptors during Inflammation. *PLoS ONE* **2012**, *7*, e43597. [CrossRef] [PubMed]

163. Huang, Y.-W.; Chang, S.-J.; Harn, H.I.-C.; Huang, H.-T.; Lin, H.-H.; Shen, M.-R.; Tang, M.-J.; Chiu, W.-T. Mechanosensitive store-operated calcium entry regulates the formation of cell polarity. *J. Cell. Physiol.* **2015**, *230*, 2086–2097. [CrossRef] [PubMed]

164. Kim, J.M.; Choi, S.; Park, K. TRPM7 Is Involved in Volume Regulation in Salivary Glands. *J. Dent. Res.* **2017**, *96*, 1044–1050. [CrossRef] [PubMed]

165. Won, J.; Vang, H.; Kim, J.H.; Lee, P.R.; Kang, Y.; Oh, S.B. TRPM7 Mediates Mechanosensitivity in Adult Rat Odontoblasts. *J. Dent. Res.* **2018**, 22034518759947. [CrossRef] [PubMed]

166. Middelbeek, J.; Vrenken, K.; Visser, D.; Lasonder, E.; Koster, J.; Jalink, K.; Clark, K.; van Leeuwen, F.N. The TRPM7 interactome defines a cytoskeletal complex linked to neuroblastoma progression. *Eur. J. Cell Biol.* **2016**, *95*, 465–474. [CrossRef] [PubMed]

167. Adapala, R.K.; Thoppil, R.J.; Ghosh, K.; Cappelli, H.C.; Dudley, A.C.; Paruchuri, S.; Keshamouni, V.; Klagsbrun, M.; Meszaros, J.G.; Chilian, W.M.; et al. Activation of mechanosensitive ion channel TRPV4 normalizes tumor vasculature and improves cancer therapy. *Oncogene* **2015**. [CrossRef] [PubMed]

168. Ferdek, P.E.; Jakubowska, M.A. Biology of pancreatic stellate cells-more than just pancreatic cancer. *Pflüg. Arch.* **2017**. [CrossRef]

169. Gryshchenko, O.; Gerasimenko, J.V.; Gerasimenko, O.V.; Petersen, O.H. Ca(2+) signals mediated by bradykinin type 2 receptors in normal pancreatic stellate cells can be inhibited by specific Ca(2+) channel blockade. *J. Physiol.* **2015**. [CrossRef]

170. Storck, H.; Hild, B.; Schimmelpfennig, S.; Sargin, S.; Nielsen, N.; Zaccagnino, A.; Budde, T.; Novak, I.; Kalthoff, H.; Schwab, A. Ion channels in control of pancreatic stellate cell migration. *Oncotarget* **2017**. [CrossRef] [PubMed]

171. Fang, L.; Zhan, S.; Huang, C.; Cheng, X.; Lv, X.; Si, H.; Li, J. TRPM7 channel regulates PDGF-BB-induced proliferation of hepatic stellate cells via PI3K and ERK pathways. *Toxicol. Appl. Pharmacol.* **2013**, *272*, 713–725. [CrossRef] [PubMed]

172. Fang, L.; Huang, C.; Meng, X.; Wu, B.; Ma, T.; Liu, X.; Zhu, Q.; Zhan, S.; Li, J. TGF-β1-elevated TRPM7 channel regulates collagen expression in hepatic stellate cells via TGF-β1/Smad pathway. *Toxicol. Appl. Pharmacol.* **2014**, *280*, 335–344. [CrossRef] [PubMed]

173. Wei, C.; Wang, X.; Chen, M.; Ouyang, K.; Song, L.-S.; Cheng, H. Calcium flickers steer cell migration. *Nature* **2009**, *457*, 901–905. [CrossRef] [PubMed]

174. Vancauwenberghe, E.; Noyer, L.; Derouiche, S.; Lemonnier, L.; Gosset, P.; Sadofsky, L.R.; Mariot, P.; Warnier, M.; Bokhobza, A.; Slomianny, C.; et al. Activation of mutated TRPA1 ion channel by resveratrol in human prostate cancer associated fibroblasts (CAF). *Mol. Carcinog.* **2017**, *56*, 1851–1867. [CrossRef] [PubMed]

175. Mayer, P.; Dinkic, C.; Jesenofsky, R.; Klauss, M.; Schirmacher, P.; Dapunt, U.; Hackert, T.; Uhle, F.; Hänsch, G.M.; Gaida, M.M. Changes in the microarchitecture of the pancreatic cancer stroma are linked to neutrophil-dependent reprogramming of stellate cells and reflected by diffusion-weighted magnetic resonance imaging. *Theranostics* **2018**, *8*, 13–30. [CrossRef] [PubMed]

176. Powell, D.R.; Huttenlocher, A. Neutrophils in the Tumor Microenvironment. *Trends Immunol.* **2016**, *37*, 41–52. [CrossRef] [PubMed]

177. Nywening, T.M.; Belt, B.A.; Cullinan, D.R.; Panni, R.Z.; Han, B.J.; Sanford, D.E.; Jacobs, R.C.; Ye, J.; Patel, A.A.; Gillanders, W.E.; et al. Targeting both tumour-associated CXCR2+neutrophils and CCR2+macrophages disrupts myeloid recruitment and improves chemotherapeutic responses in pancreatic ductal adenocarcinoma. *Gut* **2017**. [CrossRef] [PubMed]

178. Di, A.; Gao, X.-P.; Qian, F.; Kawamura, T.; Han, J.; Hecquet, C.; Ye, R.D.; Vogel, S.M.; Malik, A.B. The redox-sensitive cation channel TRPM2 modulates phagocyte ROS production and inflammation. *Nat. Immunol.* **2011**, *13*, 29–34. [CrossRef] [PubMed]

179. Haraguchi, K.; Kawamoto, A.; Isami, K.; Maeda, S.; Kusano, A.; Asakura, K.; Shirakawa, H.; Mori, Y.; Nakagawa, T.; Kaneko, S. TRPM2 contributes to inflammatory and neuropathic pain through the aggravation of pronociceptive inflammatory responses in mice. *J. Neurosci.* **2012**, *32*, 3931–3941. [CrossRef] [PubMed]

180. Wang, C.-H.; Rong, M.-Y.; Wang, L.; Ren, Z.; Chen, L.-N.; Jia, J.-F.; Li, X.-Y.; Wu, Z.-B.; Chen, Z.-N.; Zhu, P. CD147 up-regulates calcium-induced chemotaxis, adhesion ability and invasiveness of human neutrophils via a TRPM-7-mediated mechanism. *Rheumatology* **2014**, *53*, 2288–2296. [CrossRef] [PubMed]

181. Yin, J.; Michalick, L.; Tang, C.; Tabuchi, A.; Goldenberg, N.; Dan, Q.; Awwad, K.; Wang, L.; Erfinanda, L.; Nouailles, G.; et al. Role of Transient Receptor Potential Vanilloid 4 in Neutrophil Activation and Acute Lung Injury. *Am. J. Respir. Cell Mol. Biol.* **2016**, *54*, 370–383. [CrossRef] [PubMed]

182. Earley, S.; Brayden, J.E. Transient receptor potential channels in the vasculature. *Physiol. Rev.* **2015**, *95*, 645–690. [CrossRef] [PubMed]

183. Fiorio Pla, A.; Gkika, D. Emerging role of TRP channels in cell migration: From tumor vascularization to metastasis. *Front. Physiol.* **2013**, *4*. [CrossRef] [PubMed]

184. Hamdollah Zadeh, M.A.; Glass, C.A.; Magnussen, A.; Hancox, J.C.; Bates, D.O. VEGF-mediated elevated intracellular calcium and angiogenesis in human microvascular endothelial cells in vitro are inhibited by dominant negative TRPC6. *Microcirculation* **2008**, *15*, 605–614. [CrossRef] [PubMed]

185. Kini, V.; Chavez, A.; Mehta, D. A new role for PTEN in regulating transient receptor potential canonical channel 6-mediated Ca^{2+} entry, endothelial permeability, and angiogenesis. *J. Biol. Chem.* **2010**, *285*, 33082–33091. [CrossRef] [PubMed]

186. Schmidt, K.; Dubrovska, G.; Nielsen, G.; Fesüs, G.; Uhrenholt, T.R.; Hansen, P.B.; Gudermann, T.; Dietrich, A.; Gollasch, M.; de Wit, C.; Köhler, R. Amplification of EDHF-type vasodilatations in TRPC1-deficient mice. *Br. J. Pharmacol.* **2010**, *161*, 1722–1733. [CrossRef] [PubMed]

187. Chen, C.-K.; Hsu, P.-Y.; Wang, T.-M.; Miao, Z.-F.; Lin, R.-T.; Juo, S.-H.H. TRPV4 Activation Contributes Functional Recovery from Ischemic Stroke via Angiogenesis and Neurogenesis. *Mol. Neurobiol.* **2017**. [CrossRef] [PubMed]

188. Thodeti, C.K.; Matthews, B.; Ravi, A.; Mammoto, A.; Ghosh, K.; Bracha, A.L.; Ingber, D.E. TRPV4 channels mediate cyclic strain-induced endothelial cell reorientation through integrin-to-integrin signaling. *Circ. Res.* **2009**, *104*, 1123–1130. [CrossRef] [PubMed]

189. Fiorio Pla, A.; Ong, H.L.; Cheng, K.T.; Brossa, A.; Bussolati, B.; Lockwich, T.; Paria, B.; Munaron, L.; Ambudkar, I.S. TRPV4 mediates tumor-derived endothelial cell migration via arachidonic acid-activated actin remodeling. *Oncogene* **2012**, *31*, 200–212. [CrossRef] [PubMed]

190. Thoppil, R.J.; Cappelli, H.C.; Adapala, R.K.; Kanugula, A.K.; Paruchuri, S.; Thodeti, C.K. TRPV4 channels regulate tumor angiogenesis via modulation of Rho/Rho kinase pathway. *Oncotarget* **2016**, *7*, 25849–25861. [CrossRef] [PubMed]

191. Yu, B.-X.; Yuan, J.-N.; Zhang, F.-R.; Liu, Y.-Y.; Zhang, T.-T.; Li, K.; Lv, X.-F.; Zhou, J.-G.; Huang, L.-Y.; Shang, J.-Y.; et al. Inhibition of Orai1-mediated Ca^{2+} entry limits endothelial cell inflammation by suppressing calcineurin-NFATc4 signaling pathway. *Biochem. Biophys. Res. Commun.* **2018**, *495*, 1864–1870. [CrossRef] [PubMed]

192. Bodiga, V.L.; Kudle, M.R.; Bodiga, S. Silencing of PKC-α, TRPC1 or NF-κB expression attenuates cisplatin-induced ICAM-1 expression and endothelial dysfunction. *Biochem. Pharmacol.* **2015**, *98*, 78–91. [CrossRef] [PubMed]

193. Kaytes, P.S.; Geng, J.G. P-selectin mediates adhesion of the human melanoma cell line NKI-4: Identification of glycoprotein ligands. *Biochemistry* **1998**, *37*, 10514–10521. [CrossRef] [PubMed]

194. Bihari, S.; Dixon, D.-L.; Lawrence, M.D.; De Bellis, D.; Bonder, C.S.; Dimasi, D.P.; Bersten, A.D. Fluid-induced lung injury-role of TRPV4 channels. *Pflüg. Arch.* **2017**, *469*, 1121–1134. [CrossRef] [PubMed]

195. Smedlund, K.; Tano, J.-Y.; Vazquez, G. The constitutive function of native TRPC3 channels modulates vascular cell adhesion molecule-1 expression in coronary endothelial cells through nuclear factor kappaB signaling. *Circ. Res.* **2010**, *106*, 1479–1488. [CrossRef] [PubMed]

196. Bulk, E.; Ay, A.-S.; Hammadi, M.; Ouadid-Ahidouch, H.; Schelhaas, S.; Hascher, A.; Rohde, C.; Thoennissen, N.H.; Wiewrodt, R.; Schmidt, E.; et al. Epigentic dysregulation of KCa 3.1 channels induces poor prognosis in lung cancer. *Int. J. Cancer J. Int. Cancer* **2015**. [CrossRef] [PubMed]

197. Sukumaran, P.; Löf, C.; Pulli, I.; Kemppainen, K.; Viitanen, T.; Törnquist, K. Significance of the transient receptor potential canonical 2 (TRPC2) channel in the regulation of rat thyroid FRTL-5 cell proliferation, migration, adhesion and invasion. *Mol. Cell. Endocrinol.* **2013**, *374*, 10–21. [CrossRef] [PubMed]

198. Nagafuchi, A.; Takeichi, M. Cell binding function of E-cadherin is regulated by the cytoplasmic domain. *EMBO J.* **1988**, *7*, 3679–3684. [PubMed]

199. Phuong, T.T.T.; Redmon, S.N.; Yarishkin, O.; Winter, J.M.; Li, D.Y.; Križaj, D. Calcium influx through TRPV4 channels modulates the adherens contacts between retinal microvascular endothelial cells. *J. Physiol.* **2017**, *595*, 6869–6885. [CrossRef] [PubMed]

200. Simonsen, U.; Wandall-Frostholm, C.; Oliván-Viguera, A.; Köhler, R. Emerging roles of calcium-activated K channels and TRPV4 channels in lung oedema and pulmonary circulatory collapse. *Acta Physiol. Oxf. Engl.* **2017**, *219*, 176–187. [CrossRef] [PubMed]

201. Wandall-Frostholm, C.; Dalsgaard, T.; Bajoriūnas, V.; Oliván-Viguera, A.; Sadda, V.; Beck, L.; Mogensen, S.; Stankevicius, E.; Simonsen, U.; Köhler, R. Genetic deficit of KCa 3.1 channels protects against pulmonary circulatory collapse induced by TRPV4 channel activation. *Br. J. Pharmacol.* **2015**. [CrossRef] [PubMed]

202. Mittal, M.; Nepal, S.; Tsukasaki, Y.; Hecquet, C.M.; Soni, D.; Rehman, J.; Tiruppathi, C.; Malik, A.B. Neutrophil Activation of Endothelial Cell-Expressed TRPM2 Mediates Transendothelial Neutrophil Migration and Vascular Injury. *Circ. Res.* **2017**, *121*, 1081–1091. [CrossRef] [PubMed]

203. Weber, E.W.; Han, F.; Tauseef, M.; Birnbaumer, L.; Mehta, D.; Muller, W.A. TRPC6 is the endothelial calcium channel that regulates leukocyte transendothelial migration during the inflammatory response. *J. Exp. Med.* **2015**, *212*, 1883–1899. [CrossRef] [PubMed]

204. Bittner, S.; Ruck, T.; Schuhmann, M.K.; Herrmann, A.M.; Maati, H.M.; ou Bobak, N.; Göbel, K.; Langhauser, F.; Stegner, D.; Ehling, P.; Borsotto, M.; et al. Endothelial TWIK-related potassium channel-1 (TREK1) regulates immune-cell trafficking into the CNS. *Nat. Med.* **2013**, *19*, 1161–1165. [CrossRef] [PubMed]

205. Cui, C.; Merritt, R.; Fu, L.; Pan, Z. Targeting calcium signaling in cancer therapy. *Acta Pharm. Sin. B* **2017**, *7*, 3–17. [CrossRef] [PubMed]

206. Zhang, L.; Barritt, G.J. TRPM8 in prostate cancer cells: A potential diagnostic and prognostic marker with a secretory function? *Endocr. Relat. Cancer* **2006**, *13*, 27–38. [CrossRef] [PubMed]

207. Ouadid-Ahidouch, H.; Dhennin-Duthille, I.; Gautier, M.; Sevestre, H.; Ahidouch, A. TRP channels: Diagnostic markers and therapeutic targets for breast cancer? *Trends Mol. Med.* **2013**, *19*, 117–124. [CrossRef] [PubMed]

208. Peters, A.A.; Simpson, P.T.; Bassett, J.J.; Lee, J.M.; Da Silva, L.; Reid, L.E.; Song, S.; Parat, M.-O.; Lakhani, S.R.; Kenny, P.A.; et al. Calcium channel TRPV6 as a potential therapeutic target in estrogen receptor-negative breast cancer. *Mol. Cancer Ther.* **2012**, *11*, 2158–2168. [CrossRef] [PubMed]

209. Alptekin, M.; Eroglu, S.; Tutar, E.; Sencan, S.; Geyik, M.A.; Ulasli, M.; Demiryurek, A.T.; Camci, C. Gene expressions of TRP channels in glioblastoma multiforme and relation with survival. *Tumour Biol.* **2015**, *36*, 9209–9213. [CrossRef] [PubMed]

210. Wen, L.; Liang, C.; Chen, E.; Chen, W.; Liang, F.; Zhi, X.; Wei, T.; Xue, F.; Li, G.; Yang, Q.; et al. Regulation of Multi-drug Resistance in hepatocellular carcinoma cells is TRPC6/Calcium Dependent. *Sci. Rep.* **2016**, *6*, 23269. [CrossRef] [PubMed]

211. Gautier, M.; Dhennin-Duthille, I.; Ay, A.S.; Rybarczyk, P.; Korichneva, I.; Ouadid-Ahidouch, H. New insights into pharmacological tools to TR(i)P cancer up. *Br. J. Pharmacol.* **2014**, *171*, 2582–2592. [CrossRef] [PubMed]

212. Beck, B.; Bidaux, G.; Bavencoffe, A.; Lemonnier, L.; Thebault, S.; Shuba, Y.; Barrit, G.; Skryma, R.; Prevarskaya, N. Prospects for prostate cancer imaging and therapy using high-affinity TRPM8 activators. *Cell Calcium* **2007**, *41*, 285–294. [CrossRef] [PubMed]

213. Boonstra, M.C.; de Geus, S.W.L.; Prevoo, H.A.J.M.; Hawinkels, L.J.A.C.; van de Velde, C.J.H.; Kuppen, P.J.K.; Vahrmeijer, A.L.; Sier, C.F.M. Selecting Targets for Tumor Imaging: An Overview of Cancer-Associated Membrane Proteins. *Biomark. Cancer* **2016**, *8*, 119–133. [CrossRef] [PubMed]

214. Lehen'Kyi, V.; Flourakis, M.; Skryma, R.; Prevarskaya, N. TRPV6 channel controls prostate cancer cell proliferation via Ca(2+)/NFAT-dependent pathways. *Oncogene* **2007**, *26*, 7380–7385. [CrossRef] [PubMed]

215. Lau, J.K.; Brown, K.C.; Dom, A.M.; Witte, T.R.; Thornhill, B.A.; Crabtree, C.M.; Perry, H.E.; Brown, J.M.; Ball, J.G.; Creel, R.G.; et al. Capsaicin induces apoptosis in human small cell lung cancer via the TRPV6 receptor and the calpain pathway. *Apoptosis* **2014**, *19*, 1190–1201. [CrossRef] [PubMed]

216. Stern, S.T.; Martinez, M.N.; Stevens, D.M. When Is It Important to Measure Unbound Drug in Evaluating Nanomedicine Pharmacokinetics? *Drug Metab. Dispos.* **2016**, *44*, 1934–1939. [CrossRef] [PubMed]

217. Nabissi, M.; Morelli, M.B.; Santoni, M.; Santoni, G. Triggering of the TRPV2 channel by cannabidiol sensitizes glioblastoma cells to cytotoxic chemotherapeutic agents. *Carcinogenesis* **2013**, *34*, 48–57. [CrossRef] [PubMed]

5

Multidirectional Efficacy of Biologically Active Nitro Compounds Included in Medicines

Dorota Olender, Justyna Żwawiak *⬤ and Lucjusz Zaprutko ⬤

Department of Organic Chemistry, Pharmaceutical Faculty, Poznan University of Medical Sciences, Grunwaldzka 6, 60-780 Poznan, Poland; dolender@ump.edu.pl (D.O.); zaprutko@ump.edu.pl (L.Z.)
* Correspondence: jzwawiak@ump.edu.pl

Abstract: The current concept in searching for new bioactive products, including mainly original active substances with potential application in pharmacy and medicine, is based on compounds with a previously determined structure, well-known properties, and biological activity profile. Nowadays, many commonly used drugs originated from natural sources. Moreover, some natural materials have become the source of leading structures for processing further chemical modifications. Many organic compounds with great therapeutic significance have the nitro group in their structure. Very often, nitro compounds are active substances in many well-known preparations belonging to different groups of medicines that are classified according to their pharmacological potencies. Moreover, the nitro group is part of the chemical structure of veterinary drugs. In this review, we describe many bioactive substances with the nitro group, divided into ten categories, including substances with exciting activity and that are currently undergoing clinical trials.

Keywords: nitro group; nitro compounds; drugs with the nitro group; veterinary medicines with the nitro group

---

1. Introduction

Drugs exert a local action, or, after being absorbed into the body, a general effect. The chemical structure of the active substance is fundamental because of its therapeutic effect on the body. As a result of its connection with specific structures (multiparticulates—receptor), various types of transformations occur, which consequently leads to particular pharmacological effects. Medicines containing the nitro group in their structure constitute a huge family, which is diverse in terms of pharmacology and chemical structure. The nitro group is a chemical functional group containing two oxygen atoms that are bound to a nitrogen atom, which connects the group to the rest of the molecule. With regard to the chemical structure, it should be noted that the nitrogen atom is characterized by a large deficit of negative charge. Therefore, on an aromatic ring, it has a strong electron withdrawing effect that deactivates the ring, because the resonance effect causes the "pull" of electrons from the cyclic aromatic structure. Sometimes the presence of the nitro group may be responsible for the toxicity of certain drugs.

In biological systems, the nitro group undergoes enzymatic reduction, which can take place by both a one- or two- electron mechanism. Sequential two-electron reduction of the NO_2 group gives amines via nitroso and hydroxylamine intermediates. The nitroaromatics and amines remains unchanging, but sometimes the nitroso and hydroxylamine intermediates can react with biomolecules to produce compounds having undesired effects. A one-electron reduction of the nitro group produces a nitro radical anion, which is unstable. Under aerobic conditions, it is reoxidized back to the nitro group by molecular oxygen, which is in turn reduced to form a reactive superoxide anion. This process is named the "futile cycle." In many cases, it is connected with the toxicity of compounds having

NO_2 group. Also, these reactive species are connected with the acting of nitroso compounds as a pro-drug. The wide range of applications suggests, therefore, that nitro drugs are an essential part of chemotherapy.

2. Drugs Used in Cardiovascular Diseases

Nitro compounds are used in the treatment of many diseases, including hypertension, coronary artery disease, and heart failure, and in the prevention of stroke in atrial fibrillation and thromboembolism. Drugs that are used in cardiovascular diseases include organic nitrates that are characterized by $C-ONO_2$, β-blockers, calcium channel blockers, anticoagulants, fibrinolytics, omega 3-fatty acids, and free radical scavengers [1,2].

2.1. Organic Nitrates

Preparations of nitroglycerin (trinitrate glycerol) from the group of organic nitrates are mainly used. These are characterized by very high membrane permeability and very low stability [3]. This group also includes such substances, as: clonitrate, trinitrotriethanolamine diphosphate, pentrinitrol (Petrin) and nitropentaerythritol. To avoid the accidental explosion, nitropentaerythritol is combined with lactose and D-glucitol derivatives. Isosorbide dinitrate is used in the treatment and the prophylaxis of angina pectoris and is partially metabolized to weaker but much longer acting 5-isosorbide mononitrate. 5-Isosorbide mononitrate is also known as a separate formulation [2,3] (Figure 1).

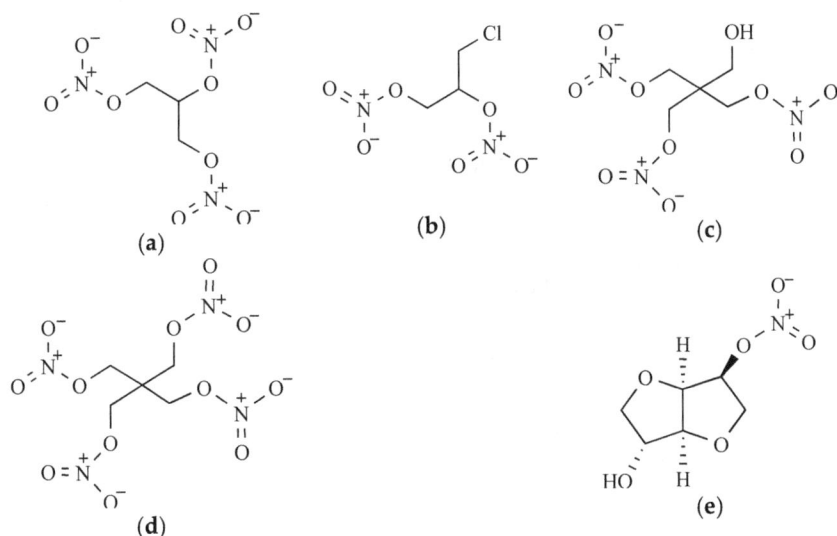

Figure 1. The chemical structure of some organic nitrates: (a) Nitroglicerinum; (b) Clonitrate; (c) Pentrinitrol; (d) Nitropentaerythritol; and (e) 5-Isosorbide mononitrate.

Organic Nitrates' Mechanism of Action

Organic nitrates act as prodrugs for nitric oxide and are used to treat or prevent acute attacks of angina pectoris. These agents have been in full-scale use for many decades and have not been implicated in causing serum enzyme elevations or clinically apparent liver injury. Organic nitrates do not release NO in a simple way. Very often, nitrate groups react with enzymes and intracellular -SH groups cause a reduction in the nitrate groups to NO or to S-nitrosothiol, which then undergoes reduction producing NO. Nitric oxide activates smooth muscle soluble guanylyl cyclase (GC) to form cGMP. Increased intracellular cGMP inhibits calcium entry into the cell, thereby decreasing intracellular Ca concentrations and causing smooth muscle relaxation. NO also influences K^+ channels, which leads to hyperpolarization and relaxation. Finally, when acting through cGMP, NO can stimulate a cGMP-dependent protein kinase that activates myosin light chain phosphatase, which is the enzyme that dephosphorylates myosin light chains, which leads to relaxation [4].

The pharmacological action of nitrate involves the vasodilation of venous and arterial vessels (including coronary arteries), thereby reducing pre- and afterload of the left ventricle, as well as improving coronary blood flow. Smooth muscle is probably due to the activation of guanylate cyclase and increasing cyclic GMP levels that are responsible for NO formed from an organic nitrate. For stable coronary heart disease, myocardial infarction acute heart failure or hypertensive crisis, preparations of nitroglycerin can be used. Nitrates are typically given sublingually and have a rapid onset of action and a somewhat short duration of action. Frequently appeared side effects of nitrates are a headache (caused by cerebral vasodilation) and cutaneous flushing. Other side effects include hypotension and reflex tachycardia. Excessive hypotension and tachycardia can worsen angina by increasing the oxygen demand.

2.2. β-Blockers Others Cardiovascular Drugs

In the long-term treatment of angina, nicorandil, which is a derivative of nicotinic acid amide, and nipradilol is one of the β-blockers from the benzopyran group are also helpful [3].

2.3. Calcium Channel Blockers

The nitro drugs class also includes nifedipine derivatives, which in chemical terms are derivatives of 1,4-dihydropyridine (Table 1). The presence of the nitro group in their structure sensitizes nifedipines to light [1]. It has been found that the best therapeutic properties belong to compounds containing a hydrogen atom on the nitrogen atom in the dihydropyridine ring and where methyl or cyano groups are present in positions 2 and 6. Moreover, the ester group should be attached to the C-3 and C-5 position, and an aromatic substituent should be on the C-4 atom of this ring.

Table 1. Nifedipine derivatives.

General Structure	Derivative	Nitro Group Position	R^1	R^2	R^3
	Aranidipine	ortho	-CH$_3$		
	Barnidipine	meta	-CH$_3$		
	Benidipine	meta	-CH$_3$		
	Cylnidipine	meta	-CH$_3$		
	Efonidipine	meta	-CH$_3$		
	Nifedipine	ortho	-CH$_3$		-CH$_3$
	Nicardipine	meta	-CH$_3$		

Table 1. *Cont.*

General Structure	Derivative	Nitro Group Position	R¹	R²	R³
	Nilvadipine	*meta*	-CN	H₃C–O–C(=O)–	–CH(CH₃)CH₃
	Nisoldipine	*ortho*	-CH₃	H₃C–O–C(=O)–	–CH₂CH(CH₃)CH₃
	Nitrendipine	*meta*	-CH₃	H₃C–O–C(=O)–	-CH₂CH₃
	Pranidipine	*meta*	-CH₃	H₃C–O–C(=O)–	–CH₂CH=CH–Ph
	Nimodipine	*meta*	-CH₃	(H₃C)₂CH–O–C(=O)–	–CH₂CH₂–O–CH₃
	Manidipine	*ortho*	-CH₃	H₃C–O–C(=O)–	–CH₂CH₂–N(piperazine)N–CH(Ph)(Ph)
	Falnidipine	*ortho*	-CH₃	H₃C–O–C(=O)–	–CH₂–(tetrahydrofuran)

Nifedipine Derivatives' Mechanism of Action

The pharmacological activity mechanism of nifedipine derivatives categorizes this class of compounds as selective calcium channel blockers which can affect different aspects of the body to serve specific purposes based on a person's unique health conditions. Calcium has several effects on the body, one of which is triggering heart muscle contraction by blocking calcium channels in vascular smooth muscle, nifedipine prevents them from opening during stimulation [5]. Even in small doses, it inhibits the penetration of calcium ions into smooth muscle cells throughout the vascular system, including renal and cerebral vessels. This reduces the concentration of Ca^{2+} in the cytosol, thereby decreasing the strength of the muscle contraction [6]. Nifedipine inhibits voltage-dependent L-type calcium channels, which leads to vascular (and other) smooth muscle relaxation, and it has an anti-anginal and antihypertensive effect.

Vasodilation, followed by a baroreceptor-mediated increase in sympathetic tone then results in reflex tachycardia [7].

2.4. Treatment of Thromboembolic Disease

In the prevention and treatment of thromboembolic disease acenocoumarol, a 4-hydroxycoumarin derivative is applied (Figure 2) [8]. Acenocoumarol is a mono-coumarin derivative with a racemic mixture of R (+) and S (−) enantiomers.

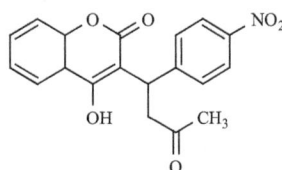

Figure 2. The chemical structure of acenocoumarol.

This drug is a vitamin K reductase antagonist. It inhibits the biosynthesis of clotting factors, including prothrombin. Acenocoumarol is one of the more frequently used oral anticoagulant therapies. Oral anticoagulant therapy is indicated for many diseases, including the prevention of stroke in atrial fibrillation, mechanical heart valve prosthesis and some valvular diseases, deep vein thrombosis, and pulmonary embolism. Acenocoumarol is effective and safe for all age groups [9].

3. Anxiolytics

Benzodiazepines are the most frequently represented pharmacologically active substances with anxiolytic activity with the nitro group. They are mostly a series of derivatives of 1,4-benzodiazepin-2-one. The presence of specific substituents is important for the scope of their activity. The nitro group or halogen (Cl, Br) at the 7-position, enhances the therapeutic action of the drug, and it is relatively strongly hypnotic. Similarly, the presence of the methyl group at the 1-position increases its activity, while an ethyl substituent reduces this effect. An increase in pharmacological effect also occurs in the event of hydroxyl moiety at the 3-position and the halogen atom in the ortho position of the phenyl substituent at C-5.

Benzodiazepines that are used in therapy include the following compounds with the nitro group (Figure 3):

- Nitrazepam is used in short-term insomnia, and as adjunctive therapy in the treatment of epilepsy and preparation for surgery (a day before surgery overnight) [10].
- Flunitrazepam is a fluorine-benzodiazepine derivative with a strong sedative and hypnotic activity being applied for the treatment of sleep disorders, including premedication as an agent in anesthesia and intensive care [11].
- Clonazepam is a chloro derivative of nitrazepam, which is characterized by anti-convulsant activity. Clonazepam, more than other benzodiazepines, is of benefit in the treatment of some types of myoclonus. Its mechanism of action is to facilitate GABAergic transmission in the brain directly on benzodiazepine receptors [12]. It is one of the most effective antiepileptic drugs.
- Nimetazepam is the N-methyl derivative of nitrazepam with a sedative and hypnotic effect. This drug is not registered in Poland.
- Loprazolam is a tricyclic derivative of imidazo-1,4-benzodiazepine, and it mainly exhibits hypnotics, anxiolytics, sedatives, anticonvulsants, and muscle relaxants effects [13].

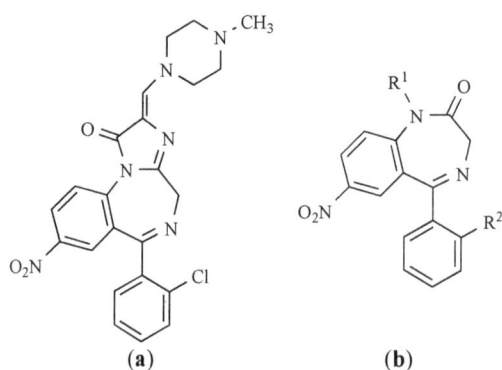

Figure 3. The chemical structure of benzodiazepine derivatives: (**a**) Loprazolam; (**b**) Nitrazepam: R^1, $R^2 = H$, Clonazepam: $R^1 = H$, $R^2 = Cl$, Flunitrazepam: $R^1 = CH_3$, $R^2 = F$, Nimetazepam: $R^1 = CH_3$, $R^2 = H$.

In addition to anxiolytic activity, these compounds also have sedative, anticonvulsant, and muscle relaxant effects. They cause polysynaptic reflexes by inhibiting the spinal cord, but long-term use can lead to a state of drug dependency. All of these actions are the results of potentiating neuronal inhibition mediated by specific receptors. Benzodiazepine forms an integral part of the $GABA_A$-ionophore (channel) chloride complex.

4. Drugs Used in Parkinson's Disease

Parkinson's disease treatment works to restore the neurohormonal balance in the extrapyramidal system, which can be achieved by increasing the dopamine concentration using levodopa (dopamine precursor) agents that inhibit the metabolism of dopamine or drugs, which increase the release of dopamine from the synaptic granules. Pharmaceuticals with the nitro group, which increase the concentration of dopamine, including entacapone and tolcapone [1] withdrawn from the treatment due to the large hepatotoxicity. In these compounds, nitro group is connected with the benzene ring (Figure 4).

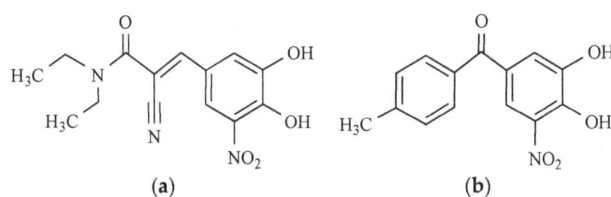

Figure 4. Parkinson's disease drugs: (**a**) Entacapone; and (**b**) Tolcapone.

Entacapone is structurally and pharmacologically similar to tolcapone, but unlike tolcapone, it is not associated with hepatotoxicity. Entacapone is used in the treatment of Parkinson's disease as an adjunct to levodopa/carbidopa therapy [14]. These two drugs are selective and potent catechol-O-methyltransferase (COMT) inhibitors that slow down the metabolism of levodopa, thus prolonging its effects. Entacapone represents one of the cornerstones of therapy for Parkinsons' disease, and which is particularly useful in motor fluctuations. The main side effects usually consist of dyskinesia and gastrointestinal symptoms, and although adverse cardiovascular effects have been identified, the drug has so far demonstrated an acceptable safety profile.

However, adjunctive therapy with tolcapone can significantly reduce the dose of levodopa that is required for illness treatment. Moreover, the use of tolcapone significantly reduces wearing off and on-off periods in fluctuating patients and improves "on" time in patients with stable disease. Tolcapone produces the expected dopaminergic side effects, such as a headache, nausea, insomnia, and diarrhea. Fortunately, these undesirable effects are mild and as a rule do not result in the discontinuation of therapy [15,16].

5. Drugs Used in Peptic Ulcer

Antiulcer drugs containing the nitro group in their structure, in terms of the mechanism through which they act in the organism, are H_2 receptor antagonists. They are characterized by their possessing the aromatic ring in their structure with basic heteroatoms (e.g., imidazole) or the neutral aromatic ring, but containing the basic substituent, polar group, and alkyl chain. Replacing imidazole moiety with the furan ring, weakens the strength of the drug. Introducing the furan cyclic structure with a dimethylaminomethyl substituent as a side chain, yields a highly potent compound named ranitidine. A similar effect in activity was achieved as a result of introducing a plane thiazole ring, which is substituted with the same dimethylaminomethyl group, which contributed to a drug called nizatidine (Figure 5).

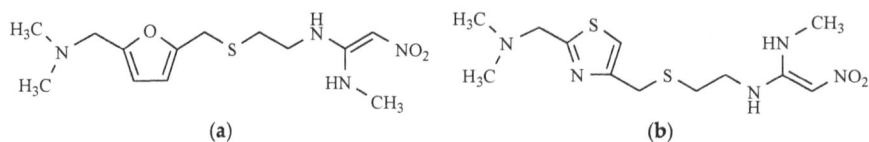

Figure 5. Antiulcerative drugs: (a) Ranitidine; and (b) Nizatidine.

In both of these substances, the polar nitro group decreased the lipophilicity of the compounds. Ranitidine is an H_2 histamine receptor antagonist. It inhibits gastric acid secretion that is stimulated by histamine H_2, pentagastrin, insulin, caffeine, and food, which explains its use with active peptic ulcers of the stomach and duodenum, and inflammation of the esophagus, which is the consequence of gastroesophageal reflux disease [17,18]. This drug is also used as an agent for preventing the recurrence of duodenal ulcer and stress ulcer formation. By inhibiting the excessive secretion of hydrochloric acid by the parietal cells of the gastric mucosa, nizatidine reduces both the volume of gastric acid secretion and pepsin content thereof. It can also be used in the treatment of dyspepsia [19].

6. Anticancer Agents

Advances in the field of oncology have led to the development of many anticancer agents for the treatment of cancer.

6.1. Flutamide and Nilutamide

The antiandrogenic drugs containing the nitro group, flutamide, and nilutamide are widely used in the treatment of carcinoma of the prostate. They are used in combination with agonists of luliberine, resulting in a total androgen blockade [20]. Flutamide and nilutamide contain the nitro group in the benzene ring (Figure 6).

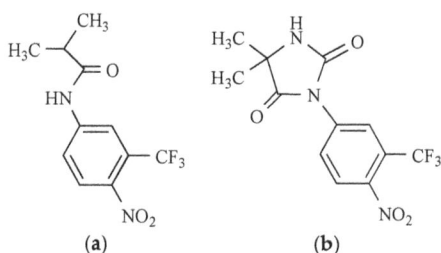

Figure 6. Anticancer drugs: (a) Flutamide; and (b) Nilutamide.

Phenylpropanamide androgen antagonists are among the anticancer active compounds with the nitro substituent. They inhibit transportation to the cell and the binding of dihydrotestosterone in the cell nucleus, which in turn inhibits prostate cell growth and division [13].

Different studies show the principal role of CYP1A2 in the metabolism of flutamide to 2-hydroxyflutamide. The mechanism of flutamide is to block the action of both endogenous and exogenous testosterone, and moreover, it is a potent inhibitor of testosterone-stimulated prostatic DNA synthesis. It is also capable of inhibiting the prostatic nuclear uptake of androgen [21].

The therapeutic effects of nilutamide are overshadowed by the occurrence of adverse reactions, mediated by mechanisms that remain elusive. Studies demonstrate that nilutamide is reduced to its hydroxylamine and amino derivatives and this reduction is oxygen-sensitive [22].

6.2. Azathioprine

Active anti-immune suppressants bearing the nitro group include a pro-drug azathioprine. Azathioprine is a thiopurine that is linked to a second heterocycle (an imidazole derivative) via a thioether (Figure 7).

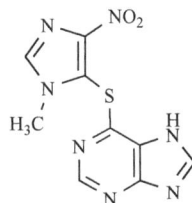

Figure 7. Anti-immunosuppressants: Azathioprine.

Azathioprine is converted into 6-mercaptopurine in the body where it blocks purine metabolism and DNA synthesis. The inclusion of thioanalogs of purines in the DNA chain causes DNA helix damage. Azathioprine is used to prevent allograft rejection, severe rheumatoid arthritis, dermatomyositis-muscular, autoimmune chronic active hepatitis, and multiple sclerosis, and also in dermatology [23]. The most recognized uses of azathioprine in dermatology are for immunobullous diseases, photodermatoses, and generalized eczematous disorders [24]. Azathioprine is commonly administered with other drugs, mainly with corticosteroids.

6.3. Nitracrine and Rubitecan

Furthermore, nitracrine and rubitecan are anticancer drugs. Nitracrine is an acridine derivative. While rubitecan is a derivative of camptothecin (Figure 8).

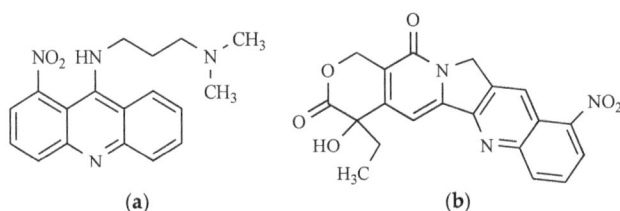

Figure 8. Anticancer drugs: (a) Nitracrine; and (b) Rubitecan.

It is approved for the treatment of patients with breast and ovarian cancer because it inhibits the synthesis of RNA. Reducing the nitro group seems to be one of the steps leading to the formation of nitracrine metabolites. It has been found that a lack of the nitro group or its replacement by methyl or halogen at different positions of the acridine ring reduces the activity of the compound obtained. Similarly, the translocation of the nitro group to another position of the benzene ring results in a decrease in activity.

Rubitecan is a derivative of camptothecin, an alkaloid that is extracted from *Camptotheca acuminata* (*Nyssaceae*). Camptothecin has a broad range of anticancer activity, especially against colon cancer and other solid tumors and leukemias. It is not used in therapy due to its high toxicity, which is particularly manifested in hemorrhagic cystitis, gastrointestinal toxicity, and myelosuppression [25]. Rubitecan exists in a 1:1 ratio as 9-nitro-camptothecin and 9-amino-camptothecin. Both of the compounds contain a lactone ring that is required for optimal activity with the carboxylic acid (open ring) forms being significantly less active or inactive. Preclinically, rubitecan has shown activity against a broad spectrum of tumor types in in vitro and in vivo human tumor xenograft models. Unfortunately, the level of activity of an agent in preclinical models has not always translated into similar activity against human tumors in clinical trials. To date, with the exception of pancreatic and possibly ovarian cancer, rubitecan has exhibited disappointing activity against some other solid tumors in relatively small Phase I/II trials; however, it has shown sufficient activity against pancreatic cancer, which is a malignancy [26].

Rubitecan was withdrawn in 2006 because of the existence of serious adverse events in patients that were treated with this substance.

7. Antibacterial Drugs

The class of antibacterial nitro drugs includes numerous derivatives of 5-nitrofuran, 2-nitro- and 5-nitroimidazole, 5-nitrothiazole, 5-nitroquinoline, and chloramphenicol.

7.1. Derivatives of 5-Nitrofuran

The furan ring system is the basic skeleton of many compounds with biological activities. These moieties are found widely in antibacterial, antiviral, anti-inflammatory, antifungal, anticancer, antihyperglycemic analgesic, anticonvulsant, and other agents. Slight changes in substitution patterns in the furan nucleus cause distinguishable differences in their biological activities. The presence of the nitro group at the C-5 position in the furan ring is essential for antibacterial activity (Tables 2 and 3). These drugs act as bacteriostatic and antiseptics, and they also show an antifungal and antiprotozoal effect. Nitrofurans act even in small doses, and they do not cause the formation of resistant strains. They have antibacterial potency against pathogenic both Gram-positive and Gram-negative, such as *Escherichia, Klebsiella, Enterobacter, Salmonella, Shigella*, and *Vibrio* genus. On the other hand, they are not effective against infections that are caused by *Proteus sp.* and *Pseudomonas aeruginosa*.

Table 2. 5-Nitrofuran analogues with antibacterial activity.

Compound	R	Compound	R
Nitrofurantoin		Furazidine	
Furazolidone		Nifurzide	
Nifuroxime	-OH	Nitrovin	
Nifurtoinol		Nifurmazole	
Nifuratel		Nifurizone	
Nifuradene		Nifurvidine	

Table 2. *Cont.*

Compound	R	Compound	R
Nifurimide		Nifuralide	
Nifurtimox		Nifurpirinol	
Furaltadone		Nifurprazine	
Nifurfoline			

Table 3. 5-Nitrofuran analogues with antibacterial activity.

Compound	R^1	R^2	Compound	R
Nifuroxazide	-H		Nifurthiazole	
Nifurpipone	-H		Nifuratrone	
Nifuraldezone	-H		Furazolium	
Nifurethazone	-(CH$_2$)$_2$N(CH$_3$)$_2$	-NH$_2$	Nifuroquine	
Nitrofural	-H	-NH$_2$		
Nidroxyzone	-(CH$_2$)$_2$OH	-NH$_2$		
Nihydrazone	-H	-CH$_3$		

The most widely used drugs from this class are nitrofurantoin, furazidin, nifuroxazide, furazolidone or nifurtoinol, nitrofural, nifurzide, and nifuratel. Nitrofurantoin is a substance that is active against the majority of microorganisms causing urinary tract infections, especially with *E. coli*. Furazidin is a nitrofurantoin analog that has the stronger effect than its parent compound on Gram-positive and Gram-negative bacteria, and also against sulfonamide and some antibiotic-resistant pathogenic strains. Furazidin activity increases in acidic urine. The higher the pH value, the more its effectiveness decreases. Furazidin is used in both acute and chronic urinary tract infections (e.g., suppurative inflammation of renal pelvis, inflammation of prostate and bladder). Moreover, it can be useful in the long-term prevention of infections [27–29], and locally for irrigation of wounds, burns and abscesses [2]. Effective therapeutics in bacterial and protozoal diseases of the gastrointestinal tract are nifuroxazide and furazolidone as they are active against *Escherichia, Shigella, Salmonella,* and *Klebsiella*.

These drugs are used in acute and chronic bacterial diarrhoea (also in infants), and during inflammation of the colon and small intestine. Furthermore, nifuroxazide exhibits antiseptic potency. On the other hand, furazolidone is an active agent in trichomonas infection and vaginal thrush [30]. Nihydrazone, nifuroxime, and nifuratel show both antibacterial and antiprotozoal activity. Nifuratel is considered as the alternative to metronidazole, as it has a similar effect on protozoa (*Trichomonas* and *Giardia lamblia*) and *Gardnerella*, with no effect on lactobacilli. Nifuratel is provided with an inhibitory effect on the growth of strains of *Atopobium*, which are strongly associated with bacterial vaginosis, but are resistant to metronidazole [31]. Nifuratel is also effective against *Candida albicans* infections because it damages the structures of enzymes Hwp 1 (Hyphal wall protein 1) and also the cytoplasmic membrane of fungi. By combining methylmercadone with nystatin, a full antibacterial effect is achieved, which determines the broad spectrum of activity, including *Chlamydia, Trichomonas vaginalis*, anaerobes, and aerobic Gram-positive and Gram-negative bacteria.

The group of drugs with a 5-nitrofuran moiety also includes nitrovin, which in addition to antimicrobial properties, is also used in veterinary medicine as a growth promoter [32].

Among the derivatives of 5-nitrofuran, other preparations with antibacterial activity should also be emphasised, namely: nifurthiazole, nifurvidine, nifuralide, and nifuratrone, which are used for controlling *Salmonella choleraesuis* in swine, nifurethazone, nifurimide, nifurizone, and nifurmazole. Nifurpipone, nifurtoinol, nifuraldezone, and nifuradene are used in the treatment of urinary tract infections.

5-Nitrofuran Derivatives' Mechanism of Action

The mode of action of 5-nitrofuran analogues is based on red-ox biotransformation. The active moiety is 5-nitro-2-furyl, which can be activated by a biological reduction of the nitro to the hydroxylamino group. These compounds must undergo activation before mediating its cytotoxic effects [33]. These are reactions are catalyzed by nitroreductase (NTR) enzymes. Based on their cofactors, oxygen sensitivities, and product profiles, NTRs can be broadly divided into two groups (reaction 1 and 2, Scheme 1). The ubiquitous oxygen-sensitive type II NTRs are flavin (flavin mononucleotide [FMN] or flavin adenine dinucleotide [FAD]) binding NAD(P)H-dependent enzymes that mediate the $1e^-$ reduction of the nitro substrate to form a nitro radical anion (reaction 1, Scheme 1). In an aerobic environment, this radical undergoes futile cycling, resulting in the formation of superoxide anions and the regeneration of the parent nitro compound (reaction 2, Scheme 1). Free radicals can readily react with cellular macromolecules, and they are directly responsible for antibacterial action. As a result, lipids oxidation, cell membrane damages, enzyme inactivation, and, finally fragmentation of the DNA sequence is observed.

reaction 1: $R\text{-}NO_2$ + $\overline{e}$ $\longrightarrow$ $R\text{-}NO_2^{\bullet\,-}$

reaction 2: $R\text{-}NO_2^{\bullet\,-}$ + O_2 $\longrightarrow$ $R\text{-}NO_2$ + $O_2^{\bullet\,-}$ $R = furyl$

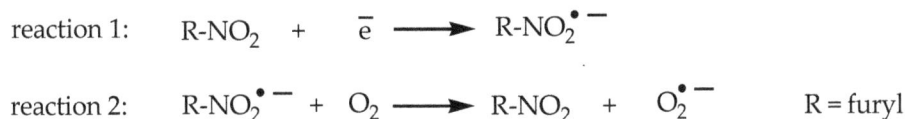

Scheme 1. The red-ox reactions of 5-nitrofurans.

7.2. Derivatives of 2-Nitro-, 5-Nitroimidazole and 5-Nitrothiazole

The discovery of azomycine (2-nitroimidazole) and the confirmation of its biological activity directed against both Gram-positive and Gram-negative and anaerobic microorganisms resulted in increased interest in this group of chemicals. 2-Nitroimidazoles were the first class of nitroimidazoles with reported anti-tubercular activity. A vast array of compounds belonging to this class substituted at 1- and 5-positions was screened against Gram-positive and Gram-negative bacteria, as well as fungi. Taking into account the structure-activity relationship, it should be stated that an increase in lipophilicity at the 5-position of the 2-nitroimidazoles increased the antimicrobial activity of Gram-positive bacteria, including Mycobacterium tuberculosis (Figure 9) [34].

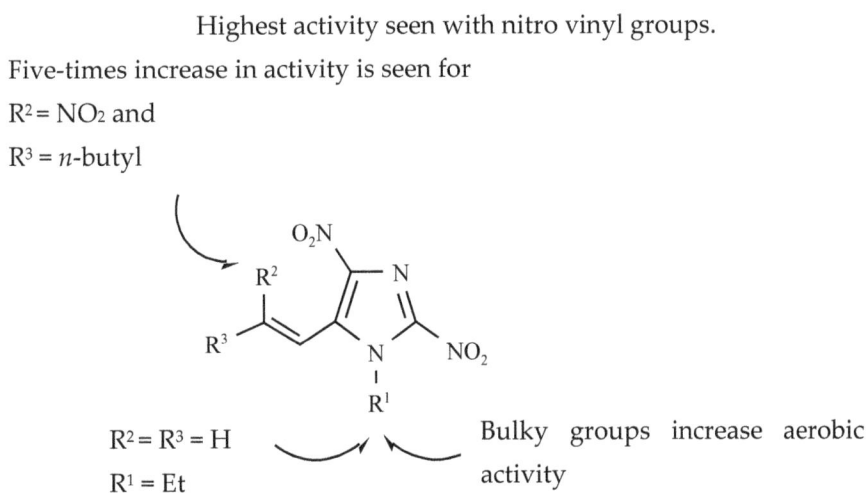

Highest activity seen with nitro vinyl groups.

Five-times increase in activity is seen for

$R^2 = NO_2$ and

$R^3 = n$-butyl

$R^2 = R^3 = H$ Bulky groups increase aerobic

$R^1 = Et$ activity

Figure 9. Structure-activity relationships of 2-nitroimidazoles [34].

Derivatives of 5-nitroimidazole (azanidazole, ipronidazole, metronidazole, tinidazole, nimorazole, ornidazole, and many others) (Table 4) and 5-nitrothiazole (e.g., niridazole and nitazoxanide) have two-way activity [35]. This strictly concerns anaerobic bacteria and protozoa. In some countries, azanidazole is also approved for the treatment of trichomoniasis. Ipronidazole is mainly used for the veterinary purposes of combating histomoniasis in turkeys and dysentery in pigs. Derivatives of azomycine damage DNA by forming complexes or terminating the thread. Under such anaerobic conditions, the transformation of the reactive metabolites attacking the DNA results in bactericidal activity.

Table 4. Antibacterial 5-nitroimidazole derivatives.

General Structure	Derivative	R^1	R^2
	Metronidazole	(OH)	$-CH_3$
	Nimorazole	(morpholine)	-H
	Ornidazole	(Cl, OH)	$-CH_3$
	Secnidazole	(CH₃, OH)	$-CH_3$
	Tinidazole	(sulfonyl ethyl)	$-CH_3$
	Ipronidazole	$-CH_3$	(isopropyl)
	Azanidazole	$-CH_3$	(aminopyrimidine vinyl)
	Megazole	$-CH_3$	(amino-thiadiazole)
	Propenidazole	$-CH_3$	(acetyl acrylate ester)

Nitroimidazoles are weakly basic compounds, moderately lipophilic with a low molecular weight, making it easy to penetrate cell membranes and allowing for almost complete absorption into the blood circulation system. In the gastrointestinal tract, they are absorbed quickly, but at different rates. 5-Nitroimidazoles are readily oxidized in the liver (at the C-2 position of the imidazole ring) to hydroxy, acetyl, and carboxylic derivatives, and then they are subjected to conjugation with glucuronic acid and sulphuric acid. Metronidazole shows bactericidal activity against the most important anaerobic microorganisms, from the clinical point of view, including types of *Bacteroides*, *Fusobacterium*, *Megasphaera*, and *Clostridium*, sometimes *Peptococcus*, *Peptostreptococcus* and *Veillonella*, as well as some of the spirochetes. In contrast, the bacteria of the genus *Propionibacterium* and *Actinomyces* are usually resistant to metronidazole. These are used to treat many bacterial infections, especially in gynecology [36], and dentistry, as well as gastric ulcers and duodenal ulcers caused by *Helicobacter pylori*. It was found that metronidazole and tinidazole exhibit a high degree of activity in the treatment of bacterial infections in combination with clarithromycin. Tinidazole is a drug acting against the bacteria of *Gardnerella*, *Propionibacterium*, *Eubacterium*, *Campylobacter*, *Actinomyces*, and *Spirochetes*. Nimorazole, however, is used in acute necrotizing ulcerative stomatitis, and non-specific inflammation of the vagina (Vincent inflammation) [2] and in the control of amebiasis [37]. Ornidazole is applied in the treatment of infections that are caused by susceptible anaerobic bacteria and preventing the disease in the perioperative period. Moreover, it is used in the treatment of rheumatism [38].

7.3. Antituberculotic Activity of Nitroimidazole Derivatives

In 1990, it was discovered that some derivatives of bicyclic nitroazoles, named nitroimidazo[2,1-b]dihydrooxazole, might have antituberculotic activity [39]. The leading substance from this series was 2-ethyl-5-nitroimidazo[2,1-b]-2,3-dihydrooxazole, designated as CGI-17341 (Figure 10). The results of biological testing showed that the tuberculostatic activity of the compound CGI-17341 was comparable to that of isoniazid (INH) and rifampicin (RIF), which are first-line drugs, and was higher than the activity of antibiotics, such as streptomycin and ciprofloxacin [35]. Furthermore, CGI-17341 showed no cross-resistance with INH and RIF. In a further study, some observations were made regarding the relationship between biological activity and the presence of structural elements in the molecule. It was found that the introduction of a halogen atom in position 2 of the imidazolyl-oxazole system resulted in a 16-fold increase in in vitro activity. The presence of the phenyl ring, as a substituent on the same carbon atom, induced a two-fold increase in tuberculostatic activity, while the long alkyl chain at C-2 decreased potency in vitro. It was also observed that the derivatives with the nitro group in the 5-position of the imidazole ring are two to two thousand times less active (depending on the nature of the substituent at C-2) than isomers of 4-nitroimidazole [40]. The tuberculostatic action mechanisms of compound OPC-67683 (Delamanid) (Figure 10) and isoniazid are very similar and they involve inhibition of mycolic acid synthesis—the main components of the cell wall of *M. tuberculosis*. The difference in behavior between nitroimidazodihydrooxazole and INH is that OPC-67683 is an inhibitor of methoxy- and ketomycolic acids, whereas isoniazid inhibits the formation of all types of these particular fatty acids [41]. OPC-67683 is a prodrug. It is activated by one of the *M. tuberculosis* enzymes, Rv3547, which reduces the nitro group. It is active against strains resistant to rifampicin (RIF), ethambutol (ETH), pyrazinamide (PZA), isoniazid (INH), and streptomycin (SM). OPC-67683 is not mutagenic, and the duration of the therapy can be reduced to two months. It was approved for the European market in 2014 [42]. Only *R* enantiomer is active against mycobacteria. Another extremely promising potential tuberculostatic drug from the group of bicyclic derivatives of nitroimidazoles is a compound signed as PA-824. Interestingly, only *S* enantiomer has tuberculostatic activity. What is more, both chiral forms of PA-824 are active against *Leishmania donovani*, which is the causative agent of visceral leishmaniasis. In leishmania-infected macrophages, (*R*)-PA-824 is even six-fold more active than (*S*)-PA-824 [43]. Chemically, it is a substance with the structure of condensed nitroimidazooxazine (Figure 10) [44].

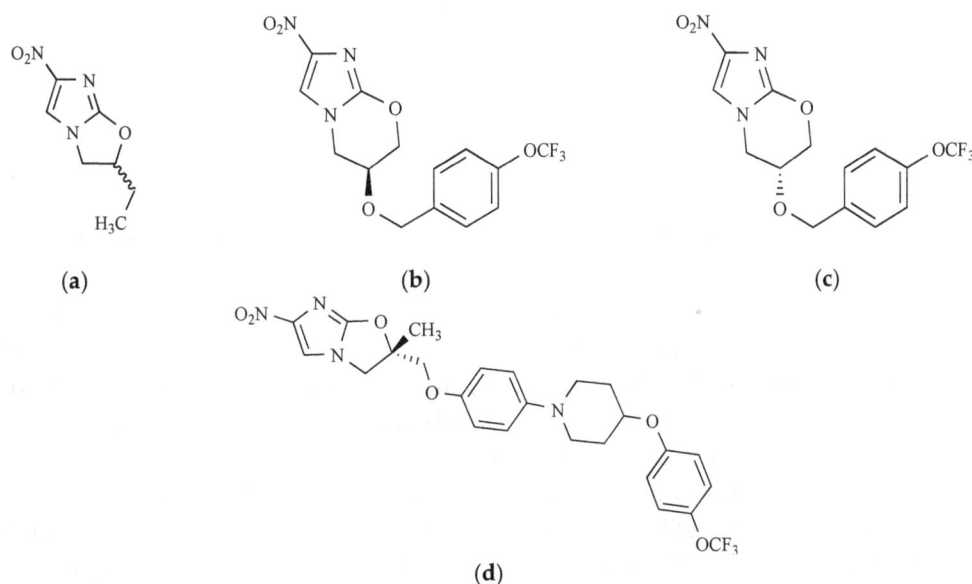

Figure 10. The chemical structure of antitubertulostatic nitroimidazoles: (**a**) CGI-17341; (**b**) (S)-PA-824; (**c**) (R)-PA-824; and (**d**) (S)-OPC-67683.

Tests in vitro confirmed its high activity against tuberculosis bacteria, even against strains that are resistant to other drugs. An essential advantage of this compound is also found not to be cross-resistant to other tuberculostatic drugs [45]. Tests in vivo confirm its activity against non-replicated bacteria. The mechanism of action of PA-824 is not fully compprehended, but presumably, it might rely on the creation of radicals that can damage the DNA of *M. tuberculosis*. It has also been noted that, like OPC-67683, PA-824 inhibits the synthesis of mycolic acids and protein biosynthesis [45]. This compound is a prodrug that is activated inside the cell. The mechanism of antitubercular activity is complex and it depends on the enzyme nitroreductase Ddn (Rv3547) [46]. This enzyme produces a biochemical reduction in three directions, which provides three different products. One of the metabolites is des-nitroimidazole. Its formation is closely related to the simultaneous evolution of reactive nitrogen compounds. PA-824 activity in anaerobic conditions is associated with a large number of released nitric oxide (NO) molecules during reduction, which are toxic to bacteria (Scheme 2).

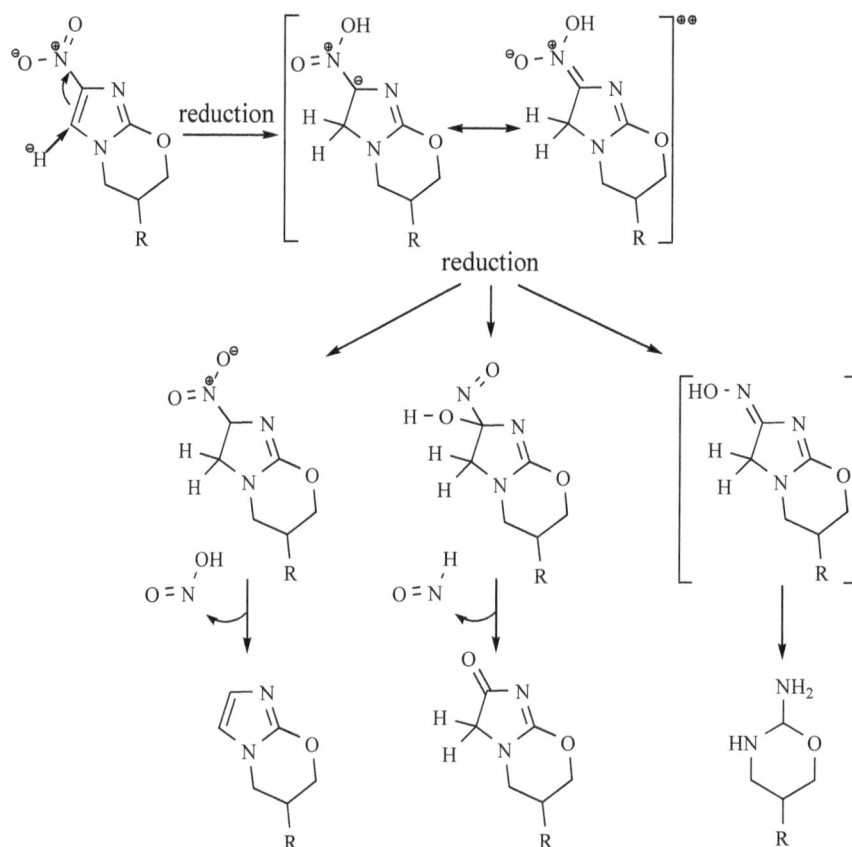

Scheme 2. The proposed mechanism for the anticubercular activity of PA-824 [46].

The success of animal studies paved the way for it to be tested in humans. Pharmacokinetic studies of PA-824 in healthy organisms in single as well as multiple-dose studies have shown that the drug is easily absorbed, has good oral bioavailability, and it is safe and well tolerated, with no serious adverse effects [34]. In the coming years, PA-824 could become the primary drug that is used to treat tuberculosis. Currently, it is in late-stage clinical trials.

Initial structure–activity relationship (SAR) studies have revealed that the replacement of the oxygen atom at the C(9) position of PA-824 with a methylene group results in the loss of antitubercular aerobic and anaerobic activities [47]. However, the 9-position oxygen of the oxazine ring of PA-824 can be replaced by either nitrogen or sulphur, with no significant reduction in MIC value in aerobic conditions, in comparison with the MIC of the parent nitroimidazooxazine [48].

7.4. Quinoline Derivatives

Those drugs containing nitro antibacterial substances also include compounds that are derived from quinoline. Among these drugs with a broad range of antibacterial activity are nitroxoline [49] (Figure 11) and nifuroquine (see: Table 2), which contains the 5-nitrofuran ring.

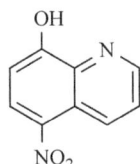

Figure 11. The chemical structure of nitroxoline.

They show substantial antibacterial activity towards microorganisms forming a film layer, Gram-negative, Gram-positive bacteria, and additionally against *Candida albicans*. It is used in both acute and chronic urinary tract infections [2]. The established urinary antibiotic nitroxoline has recently enjoyed considerable attention, due to its potent activities in inhibiting angiogenesis, inducing apoptosis and blocking cancer cell invasion. These features make nitroxoline an excellent candidate for anticancer drug repurposing [50]. The addition of a 2-(ethylamino)acetonitrile group to nitroxoline at position 7 significantly improves its pharmacological characteristics and its potential for use as an anti-cancer drug [51].

7.5. Chloramphenicol and Its Derivatives

The structure of chloramphenicol and its derivative, azidamphenicol (Leukomycin, Posifenicol, Thilocanfol), is presented in Figure 12.

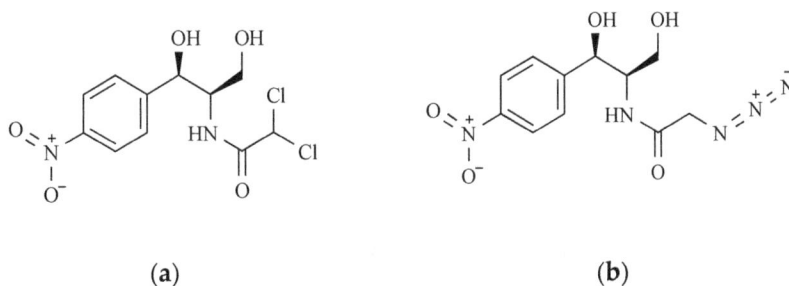

(a)   (b)

Figure 12. The chemical structure of chloramphenicol (**a**) and its derivative—azidamphenicol (**b**).

The Mechanism of the Antibacterial Action of Chloramphenicol

It was originally isolated from the bacterium *Streptomyces venezuelae*, by David Gottlieb. It appeared in clinical practice in 1949, under the trade name Chloromycetin. Azidamfenicol has a similar profile to chloramphenicol. Both drugs have been useful in treating ocular infections that were caused by some bacteria, including *Staphylococcus aureus*, *Streptococcus pneumoniae*, and *Escherichia coli*. They are not effective against *Pseudomonas aeruginosa*. Currently, these drugs are obtained only synthetically [52,53]. The mechanism of the antibacterial action of chloramphenicol is based on blocking protein synthesis in ribosome (Scheme 3).

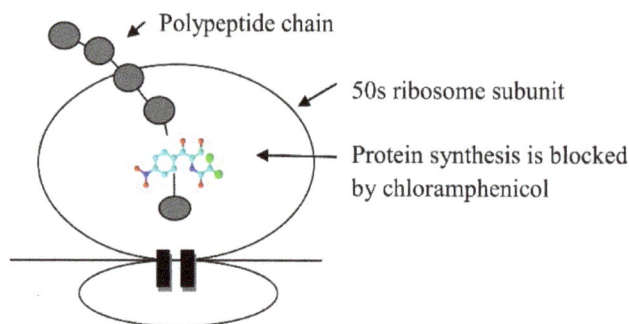

Scheme 3. The mechanism of the antibacterial action of chloramphenicol.

Chloramphenicol has a bacteriostatic effect against *Staphylococcus* and Gram-negative bacteria of the family *Enterobacteriaceae*, and bactericidal against *Haemophilus influenzae*, *Streptococcus pneumoniae*, and *Neisseria meningitidis*.   Because of the risk of severe side effects, this drug is used in exceptional disease states, as an antibiotic alternative for the treatment of life-threatening infections with *Pseudomonas* and *Haemophilus influenzae* (meningitis), brain abscesses, anaerobic infections (destructive lung infections, brain abscess, pelvic abscess), typhoid fever, brucellosis, rickettsiosis, and tularemia.

7.6. Others Antibacterial Nitro Drugs

Among preparations containing a derivative of 5-nitrothiazole as the active ingredient, antibacterial and particularly antiprotozoal properties are exhibited by niridazole, which is an active chemotherapeutic agent in the treatment of schistosomiasis (Figure 11). The group of antibacterial drugs also includes an amide of benzoic acid with two nitro groups, e.g., nitromide (Figure 13). This drug has only found application in veterinary therapy as coccidiostatic [3].

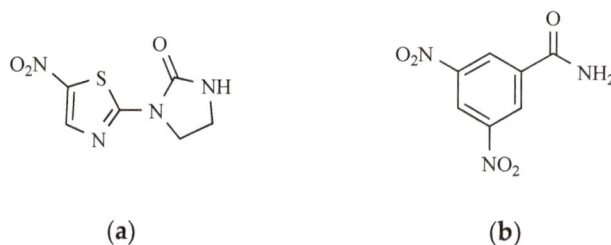

(a)   (b)

Figure 13. The chemical structures of 5-nitrothiazole: (**a**) Niridazole, and (**b**) Nitromide.

8. Anthelmintics

The parasites that cause infections of the gastrointestinal tract in our latitude come from the two families: roundworms (*Nemathelminthes*) and tapeworms (*Plathelminthes*), which include tapeworms (*Cestoda*) and flukes (*Trematoda*) [30]. Drugs used for the control of parasitic diseases belong to different chemical groups, and their mechanism of action also varies. The drug of choice for the treatment of taeniasis, and which contains the nitro group in their structure, is niclosamide (Figure 14). It is used in the taeniasis of the gastrointestinal system that is caused by *Taenia solium*, *Taenia saginata*, *Diphyllobothrium latum*, *Hymenolepis nana*, *Dipylidum caninum*, and *Fasciolopsis buski* [54]. Sometimes niclosamide is used for the treatment of the mollusc *Bulinus* in water reservoirs in the prevention of schistosomiasis endemics [1]. The beneficial effects of the therapy with niclosamide caused the use of other pharmacological agents, such as nitroxynil, which has a strong effect, especially in the mature form of *Fasciola hepatica* and niclofolan (Figure 14). Drugs containing the nitrobenzene ring and exhibiting activity against flatworms are mainly used as veterinary drugs, include netobimin, which belongs to probenzimidazole, nitrodan, and disophenol (Figure 14). Disophenol, for instance, is a nitrophenolic antiparasitic compound that is very useful in controlling several helminth-induced infections in dogs, cats, birds, sheep, and bovines, among other animals. Probenzimidazole is converted in the digestive tract of the host into an active compound belonging to benzimidazole. Netobimin is converted into albendazole.

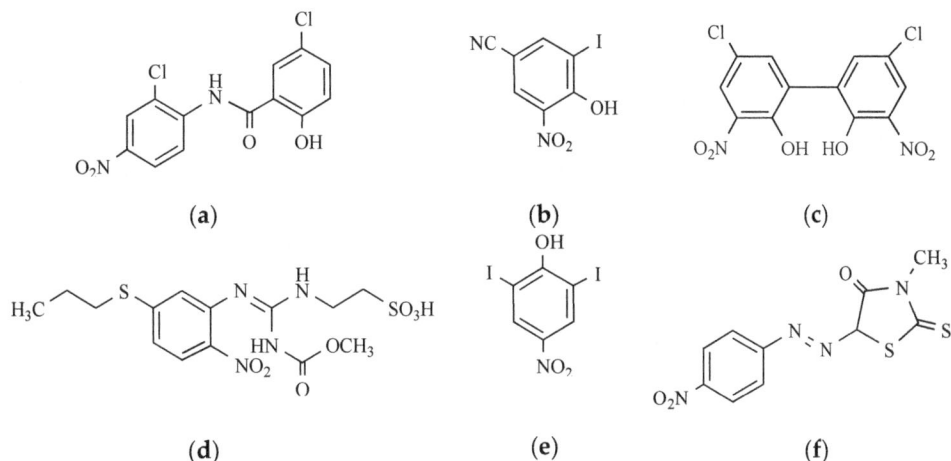

Figure 14. The chemical structure of anthelmintics: (**a**) Niclosamide; (**b**) Nitroxynil; (**c**) Niclofolan; (**d**) Netobimin; (**e**) Disophenol; and (**f**) Nitrodan.

The group of aromatic nitroisothiocyanates includes nitroscanate and a compound with the INN name Amoscanate, which were used in combating flukes and duodenum hookworms. Unfortunately, widespread use of Amoscanate in veterinary medicine is limited because of its high hepatotoxicity.

Oxamniquine is a drug that is used to treat infections of fluke causing a disease called schistosomiasis. (Figure 15).

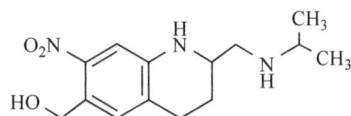

Figure 15. The chemical structure of oxamniquine.

This compound is useful in the treatment of acute and chronic schistosomiasis, which are induced in particular by various forms of *Schistosoma mansoni* and *Schistosoma intercalatum*. Perhaps one of the mechanisms of their action is to cause worms to shift from the mesenteric veins to the liver where the male worms are retained and are subsequently destracted. Females remaining in the mesenteric veins are unable to release eggs [2]. Because of the broad activity against schistosomiasis, niridazole (see Figure 13) is also used, which is characterized by the antibacterial and antiprotozoal potencies, as discussed previously [55]. In contrast to oxamniquine, niridazole has a pharmacological effect on *Schistosoma haematobium* flukes, and also a lesser effect on *Schistosoma mansoni* and *Schistosoma japonicum*. This drug is also effective against *Dracunculus medinensis* nematodes, and in the treatment of amebiasis invasion in cases of resistance developed to other treatment, or the inability to use it. It also shows beneficial effects in the treatment of *Onchocerciasis*, cutaneous leishmaniasis, and infections that are caused by fleas *Tunga penetraus* [2].

Veterinary medicine uses a halogenated derivative pyridine, called nitenpyram (Figure 16), which is intended for controlling external parasites of dogs and cats, such as fleas. Nitenpyram is neonicotinoid (new nicotine-like insecticides) that binds particularly well in the central nervous system of insects, causing their rapid death.

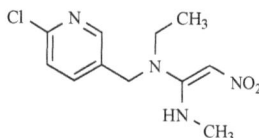

Figure 16. The chemical structure of nitenpyram.

The Mechanisms of Action of Anthelmintic Drugs

One of the mechanisms for the action of anthelmintic drugs is the inhibition of energy processes in the parasite's body. Drugs acting as anthelmintics interfere with the metabolism of carbohydrates, causing the incomplete oxidation of substrates in worms. The primary source of energy production in worms is the process of glycolysis, catalysed by phosphofructokinase. This enzyme facilitates phosphorylation of fructose 6-phosphate to fructose-1,6-diphosphate. The sensitivity of the fructokinase, e.g., in Schistosoma to inhibitors is much greater than the corresponding enzyme in mammals. Blocking the fructokinase that is involved in glycolysis causes an accumulation of the substrate, which is fructose-6-P (Scheme 4).

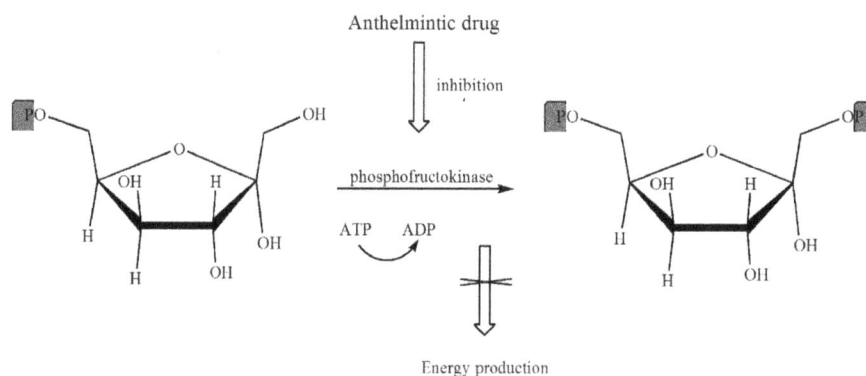

Scheme 4. The mechanism of action of anthelmintic drugs.

9. Antiprotozoal Drugs

Pathogenic protozoa belong to many groups of unicellular organisms, among which the following stand out: dinoflagellates, rugrats, and trypanosomes. In many parts of the world, protozoal infections are the most common causes of diseases. In Poland, however, the most frequently occurring ones are trichomoniasis that are caused by *Trichomonas vaginitis* (*Trichomonas vaginalis*), giardiasis caused by *Lamblia intestinalis* and toxoplasmosis caused by protozoa *Toxoplasma gondii*. A rarer case is amebiasis (amoebic dysentery), which is caused by the amoeba *Entamoeba histolytica* occurring in the gastrointestinal tract [30].

9.1. Nitroimidazole Derivatives

Megazol, which is a 5-nitroimidazole derivative containing the thiadiazole ring (Figure 17), is hugely effective against *Trypanosoma brucei* and *Trypanosoma cruzi*. Another 5-nitroimidazole derivative is fexinidazole (Figure 17), demonstrating potent in vitro and in vivo activity against trichomonas, *Entamoeba histolytica*, *Trypanosoma cruzi*, and *Trypanosoma brucei* [56].

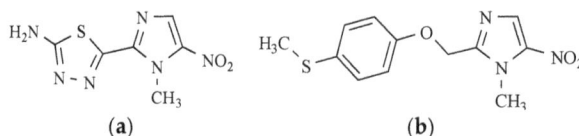

(a)   (b)

Figure 17. 5-Nitroimidazoles as antiprotozoal drugs: (a) Megazol; and (b) Fexinidazole.

The biologically relevant active metabolites in vivo are the sulfoxide and sulfone of the compound that is mentioned above. In another study, fexinidazole was established as a promising candidate for the acute and chronic stages of the African human trypanosomiasis. In 2009, this substance became the first new trypanosomatid illness clinical candidate for three decades. Currently, it is undergoing Phase III clinical trials [57].

Now, the drugs of choice for the treatment of infections that are caused by *Trichomonas vaginalis* are analogues of 5-nitroimidazole. The most essential connections from this group include metronidazole, ornidazole, tinidazole, nimorazole and azanidazole (see: Table 3). These drugs act against *Entamoeba histolytica*, *Lamblia intestinalis* and the majority of absolute anaerobic bacteria, as mentioned before. Nitroimidazoles easily penetrate the single-celled organisms of protozoans. The action of these drugs is associated with a reduction in the nitro group and the formation of cytotoxic agents for protozoa. The products of this reduction are formed within cells involving ferredoxin, which is the electron transport protein and only occurring in organisms with anaerobic metabolism or those deficient in oxygen. The source of electrons that are needed for the reduction may also be endogenous substances, such as reduced nicotinamide adenine dinucleotide phosphate (NADPH). The reduced form of the drug acts on microbial DNA by breaking the chain and then causes a protozoan cell damage.

Metronidazole and other derivatives of the 5-nitroimidazole administered orally are readily absorbed from the gastrointestinal tract. Moreover, they can be used vaginally and percutane ointment, thus also reaching high levels in the blood. In addition to treating infections that are caused by these protozoa, metronidazole is also used in the control *Giardia lamblia*, *Gardnerella vaginalis*, *Blastocystis hominis* [2]. 5-Nitroimidazole derivatives include secnidazole (see: Table 3), which has potent activity as a protozoonicidal. It is used in intestinal and hepatic amebiasis and trichomoniasis. It was also found that a combination of the nitroimidazole derivatives, i.e., metronidazole, tinidazole, or secnidazole with amphotericin B has high activity against *Candida albicans*.

Derivatives of the 5-nitroimidazole are widely used in veterinary medicine because they are useful agents for the treatment of protozoa invasion and infections that are caused by anaerobic bacteria. However, due to their genotoxic and carcinogenic potential, their use in food-producing animals or products that are intended for human consumption is prohibited in many countries. Nitroimidazoles, which in the past were registered in the European Union (EU) as veterinary drugs or food additives include metronidazole, dimetridazole, ronidazole, and ipronidazole. They were used because of their effectiveness in treating histomoniasis found in the poultry, which is caused by the flagellate *Histomonas meleagridis* [58].

9.2. 5-Nitrofuran Derivatives

This group includes nifurtimox (see: Table 2), which is used in the treatment of American trypanosomiasis, a disease occurring mostly in the rural areas of the South America carried by bugs [30,59] and nifursol, which acts against histomoniasis (Figure 18).

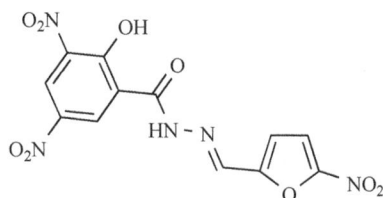

Figure 18. Nifursol as anti-trypanosomiasis drug.

Nifurtimox was used in the treatment of acute Chagas disease when it was identified by Bayer in in vitro screens against *Trypanosoma cruzi*. For many years, nifurtimox was considered to be the front-line therapy for this indication. Nifurtimox is also effective against *Trypanosoma brucei gambiense* infection.

9.3. 2-Nitroimidazole Derivatives

The current drug of choice for acute-stage Chagas disease is benznidazole, which is a derivative of 2-nitroimidazole (Figure 19). Benznidazole has been used in the treatment of Chagas disease for about 40 years. Unfortunately, a range of serious side effects is associated with its use, including dermatological reactions, agranulocytosis, and polyneuropathy [56].

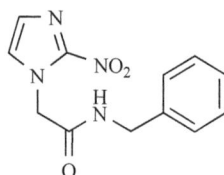

Figure 19. Benznidazole.

9.4. 5-Nitrothiazole Derivatives

Aminitrozole, nithiazide, nitazoxanide, tenonitrozole, and tizoxanide are drugs from the 5-nitrothiazole group, which act as antifungals and antiprotozoals, especially in the treatment of trichomoniasis (Table 5).

Table 5. Antiprotozoal 5-nitrothiazole derivatives.

Main Structure Caption	Derivative	R
	Aminitrazole	-CH$_3$
	Nithiazide	-NH-CH$_2$-CH$_3$
	Tenonitrozole	
	Tizoxanide	
	Nitazoxanide	

Formulations containing nitazoxanide are indicated in the treatment of diarrhea that is caused by *Cryptosporidium parvum* or *Giardia lamblia*. Nitazoxanide is an anti-infective prodrug, which very quickly converts to an active metabolite tizoxanide. The parent nitazoxanide is not detected in plasma. Tizoxanide is active against anaerobic bacteria, protozoan parasites, and viruses [60].

9.5. Others Antiprotozoal Drugs

Etofamide and clefamide are other antiprotozoal drugs that are effective in combating intestinal amebiasis. These are compounds that are derived from dichloroacetamide containing a nitrophenoxyphenyl substituent as a side moiety (Figure 20).

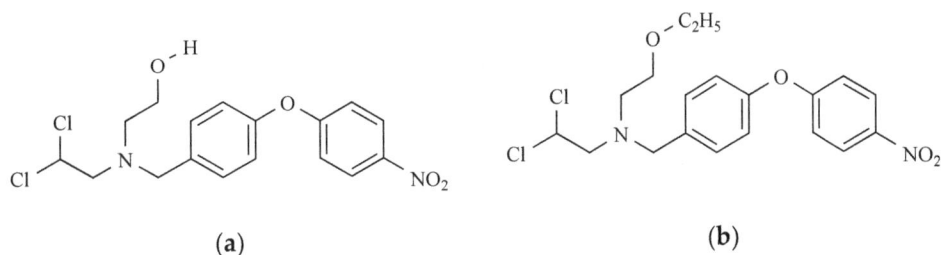

Figure 20. Nitrophenyl derivatives as antiprotozoal drugs: (a) Clefamide; and (b) Etofamide.

10. Radiosensitizers

Knowledge of oxygen's effect led to the development of compounds that mimic its radiosensitizing property. The radiosensitizing capabilities of the hypoxic cell sensitizers have been found to connect with electron affinity [61]. 2-Nitroimidazoles play a great role as bioreductive markers for tumour hypoxia and as radiosensitizers [35]. It is known that 2-nitroimidazoles (e.g., misonidazole, etanidazole) are more active than 5-nitroimidazoles (e.g., metronidazole, nimorazole) as hypoxic cell radiosensitizers. The differences in their activity in vitro correlate most closely with alterations in redox properties, especially in their electron-affinity [62].

The mechanism of action of this class of sensitizers is based on the "oxygen fixation" hypothesis [63]. They fix radiation damage by preventing the chemical restitutions of free radicals. Misonidazole has been observed to deplete -SH groups in cells, and to inhibit both glycolysis and the repair of potentially lethal radiation-induced cellular damage [64]. Clinical trials with misonidazole have shown undesirable effects, such as peripheral neuropathy, convulsions, and encephalopathy, and therefore its use is severely limited [65].

Etanidazole has been analyzed with perspective results in early phase II and III clinical trials. It appears to be less toxic to CNS tissue than misonidazole and crosses the blood-brain barrier in limited quantities. A phase III study of this agent showed increased survival in the two-year local control in N0 and N1 disease with 55% in the etanidazole arm and 37% in the radiation-alone arm [66].

Nimorazole is a member of the same structural class as metronidazole. However, it is less toxic, thus allowing for higher doses to be administered. A phase III study of nimorazole versus a placebo in subjects with squamous cell carcinoma of the supraglottic larynx and pharynx demonstrated a statistically significant difference regarding improvements in loco-regional control at five-year post-treatment [67]. In phase II, a study of nimorazole was conducted in patients with stage 3 or 4 squamous cell carcinoma of the head and neck who received continuous hyperfractionated accelerated radiation therapy (CHART). It was found that local control rates were higher than in other studies using CHART, suggesting the positive effect of nimorazole.

11. Drugs with Others Effects

Medications that do not belong to any of the above-described families and contain the nitro group are also present on the pharmaceuticals market. One such medicine is dantrolene, whose structure includes the hydantoin system, furan, and p-nitrophenol rings (Figure 21).

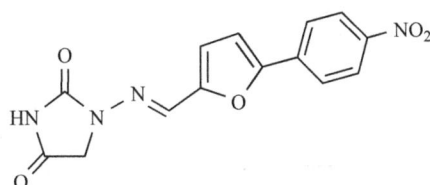

Figure 21. Dantrolene.

This is a drug acting as a striated muscle relaxant and that distorts the contraction of the muscle cell by inhibiting the intracellular movements of calcium ions [68] (Scheme 5). Dantrolene is used to treat post-stroke spasticity, resulting in the brain, spinal cord injury, cerebral palsy, multiple sclerosis running with paresis, and anesthesia for the prevention and treatment of malignant hyperthermia [69,70].

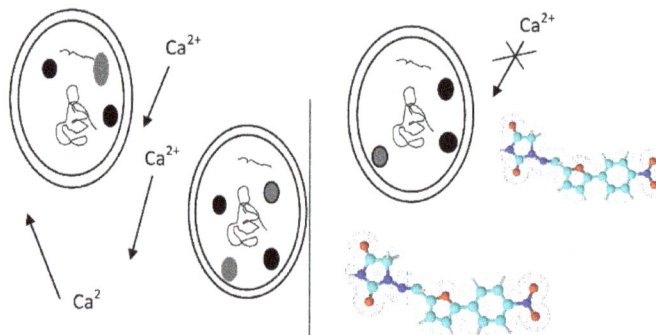

Scheme 5. The mechanism of action of dantrolene.

Next, nimesulide is a non-steroidal anti-inflammatory drug, analgesic, and antipyretic, belonging to the sulfonanilide group containing a diphenyl ether skeleton substituted with methanesulphonamide and nitro groups (Figure 22).

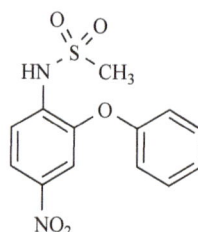

Figure 22. Nimesulide.

It inhibits the formation of free radical peroxide and it also blocks the activity of specific cyclooxygenase, thereby reducing prostaglandin synthesis (Scheme 6). The indication for nimesulide use is pain that is associated with bone diseases and joint pain, neuralgic, postoperative pain, and trauma [71,72]. Unfortunately, nimesulide had to be withdrawn in many countries due to the serious risk of fatal hepatic disorders.

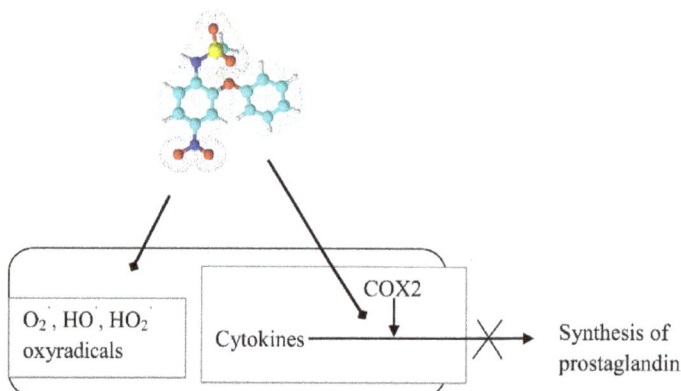

Scheme 6. Sites of action of nimesulide in cellular inflammation.

Nitromersol is a bicyclic compound that is used as an antiseptic and disinfectant for surgical and dental use (Figure 23). However, the presence of mercury in its structure has led to its limited use.

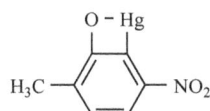

Figure 23. Nitromersol.

Moreover, two more compounds with the nitro group also exhibit pharmacological activity. For the treatment of alcoholism, nitrefazole, which is a nitrophenyl derivative of 4-nitroimidazole, is used, while nizofenone, which has nootropic activity, is a derivative of nitrobenzophenone comprising a substituted imidazole ring (Figure 24).

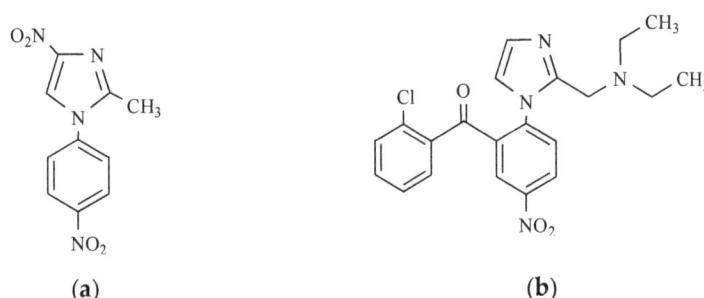

(a) (b)

Figure 24. The 4-nitroimidazole derivatives as nootropic: (a) Nitrefazole; and (b) Nizofenone.

Among the group of the nuclear receptors family (REV-ERB) activity modulators, a nitro compound called SR9009 can be found (Figure 25).

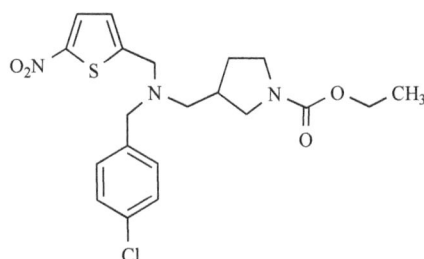

Figure 25. The structure of SR9009.

It alters the expression of genes that are involved in lipid and glucose metabolism, and therefore, it plays an essential role in maintaining the energy homeostasis [73,74]. Additionally, this substance increases basal oxygen consumption, decreases lipogenesis, cholesterol and bile acid synthesis in the liver, increases mitochondrial content, glucose and fatty acid oxidation in the skeletal muscle, and decreases lipid storage in the white adipose tissue. These observations make SR9009 a promising drug for the treatment of several metabolic disorders [73,74].

12. Drugs of the Future

Among exciting nitro compounds, a group of nitro-fatty acids (NO_2-FAs) can be found. They are formed in human plasma, cell membranes, and tissue by redox reactions of unsaturated fatty acids with secondary products of NO oxidation, e.g., NO_2, NO_2^-, NO_3^- [75]. This process occurs under physiological conditions—during digestion, where nitration is favored by the low pH of gastric juice in the stomach, and metabolism catalyzed by peroxidases, globins, and nitric oxide autooxidation [76].

However, the correct mechanism in vivo remains unknown [77]. Nitro-fatty acids are transported back into blood circulation in the form of conjugates that are synthesized by covalent adduction with glutathione (GSH) (Michael reaction) [78]. These reactions between proteins and NO_2-FAs are significant in the context of cell signaling, as this reaction is reversible. Protein adduction by NO_2-FAs is detected clinically, thus representing a metabolic and redox-sensitive mechanism for regulating protein distribution and function [79]. Other mechanisms are associated with hepatic β-oxidation and double-bond saturation (Scheme 7) [80].

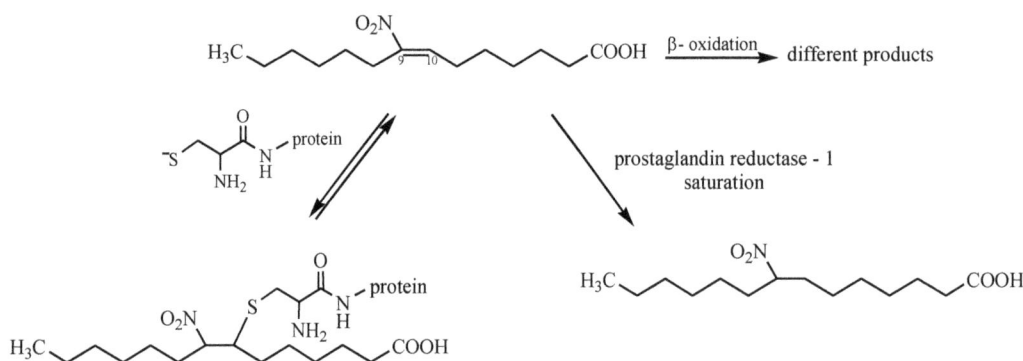

Scheme 7. Mechanism of action of nitro-fatty acids.

Furthermore, nitro-fatty acids can release nitric oxide [81]. They can be used as the source of NO in the organism. These compounds have full potential in medicine. They exert a long-term cardioprotective effect in experimental models of metabolic and cardiovascular diseases. They reduce lipid accumulation and promote plaque stability in atherosclerosis. As is shown in the literature [82], acute administration of NO_2-FAs is effective to minimize vascular inflammation in vivo. They act as disruptors of the TLR4 signaling complex in lipid rafts, leading to the resolution of pro-inflammatory activation. Moreover, nitro-fatty acids reduce blood pressure in an angiotensin II infusion model of hypertension. They interfere with angiotensin II signaling, thus causing limited calcium mobilization in vascular smooth muscle cells. This is the main cause of blood pressure reduction [83]. Considerable therapeutic potential is observed for the use of NO_2-FAs in renal inflammation and kidney diseases. Preliminary studies revealed that treatment with nitro-fatty acids significantly reduces creatinine levels, urinary lipid peroxidation products, and renal inflammation [84]. Nowadays, the active NO_2-FAs compound, named CXA-10 (10-nitro-oleic acid), undergo phase II clinical trials [84].

13. Conclusions

A great deal of research and medical use has revealed the huge potential of nitro compounds to treat different diseases and has eroded the long-held prejudice against them. In many cases, these drugs are essential in combating some types of ailments. There is still a need to search for novel, safe, and effective connections with potential medicinal properties resulting from the presence of the molecule with the nitro group in their structure. This task can be performed by the synthesis of new hybrid combinations of drugs containing the nitro group with fragments of macromolecular structures. During the drug design process, it should be remembered that the inclusion of the nitro group in a molecule alters the physicochemical and electronic properties, and is connected with increased mutagenicity and carcinogenicity [85]. Such hybrids appear in the initial phase of the trial. Treatment should take into account the risk that is associated with toxicity, acquired drug resistance, or cost of production. Currently, it seems that the most promising nitro-compounds with biological activity are nitro-fatty acids. Identification of their metabolism can lead to the discovery of new nitrated unsaturated acids, which are as yet unknown. Work on nitro-fatty acids significantly expanded the knowledge of biological redox processes, which can prove fruitful in the future.

Author Contributions: D.O. and J.Ż. wrote the paper. L.Z. contributed valuable discussion and revision of the manuscript.

References

1. Williams, M. *The Merck Index: An Encyclopedia of Chemicals, Drugs, and Biologicals*, 15th ed.; Royal Society of Chemisry: Cambridge, UK, 2013.

2. Brayfield, A. *Martindale: The Complete Drug Reference*, 39th ed.; Pharmaceutical Press: London, UK, 2017.

3. PDR Staff. *2017 Physicians' Desk Reference*, 71st ed.; PDR Network: Montvale, NJ, USA, 2016.

4. Klabunde, R.E. Cardiovascular Physiology Concepts. Available online: www.cvpharmacology.com (accessed on 23 June 2017).

5. Isaeva, E.V. Effect of nifedipine in high concentrations on inhibitory synaptic transmission. *Neurophys* **1999**, *31*, 63–65. [CrossRef]

6. Metra, M.; Nodari, S.; Nordio, G.; Bonandi, L.; Raddino, R.; Feroldi, P.; Dei Cas, L.; Visioli, O. A randomized double-blind crossover study of nicardipine and nifedipine in patients with angina pectoris and concomitant essential hypertension. *Cardiovasc. Drug Ther.* **1988**, *1*, 513–521. [CrossRef]

7. Van Geijn, H.P.; Lenglet, J.E.; Bolte, A.C. Nifedipine trials: effectiveness and safety aspects. *BJOG Int. J. Obstet. Gynaecol.* **2005**, *112*, 79–83. [CrossRef] [PubMed]

8. Van Schie, R.M.F.; Wessels, J.A.M.; le Cessie, S.; de Boer, A.; Schalekamp, T.; van der Meer, F.J.M.; Verhoef, T.I. Loading and maintenance dose algorithms for phenprocoumon and acenocoumarol using patient characteristics and pharmacogenetic data. *Eur. Heart J.* **2011**, *32*, 1909–1917. [CrossRef] [PubMed]

9. Trailokya, A.; Hiremath, J.S.; Sawhney, J.P.S.; Mishra, Y.K.; Kanhere, V.; Srinivasa, R.; Tiwaskar, M. Acenocoumarol: A review of anticoagulant efficacy and safety. *JAPI* **2016**, *64*, 88–93. [PubMed]

10. Mets, M.A.J.; Volkerts, E.R.; Olivier, B.; Verster, J.C. Effect of hypnotic drugs on body balance and standing steadiness. *Sleep Med. Rev.* **2010**, *14*, 259–267. [CrossRef] [PubMed]

11. Maltby, J.R.; Hamilton, R.C.; Phillips, R. Comparison of flunitrazepam and thiopentone for induction of general anaesthesia. *Can. Anesth. J. Soc.* **1980**, *27*, 331–337. [CrossRef]

12. Jenner, P.; Pratt, J.A.; Marsden, C.D. Mechanism of action of clonazepam in myoclonus in relation to effects on GABA and 5-HT. *Adv. Neurol.* **1986**, *43*, 629–643. [PubMed]

13. Buscemi, N.; Vandermeer, B.; Friesen, C.; Bialy, L.; Tubman, M.; Ospina, M.; Klassen, T.P.; Witmans, M. The efficacy and safety of drug treatments for chronic insomnia in adults: A meta-analysis of RCTs. *J. Gen. Int. Med.* **2007**, *22*, 1335–1350. [CrossRef] [PubMed]

14. Gordin, A.; Kaakkola, S.; Teräväinen, H. Clinical advantages of COMT inhibition with entacapone—A review. *J. Neural Trans.* **2004**, *111*, 1343–1363. [CrossRef] [PubMed]

15. Truong, D.D. Tolcapone: Review of its pharmacology and use as adjunctive therapy in patients with Parkinson's disease. *Clin. Interv. Aging* **2009**, *4*, 109–113. [CrossRef] [PubMed]

16. Leegwater-Kim, J.; Waters, C. Role of tolcapone in the treatment of Parkinson's disease. *Expert Rev. Neurother.* **2007**, *7*, 1649–1657. [CrossRef] [PubMed]

17. Futagami, S.; Shimpuku, M.; Kawagoe, T.; Kusunoki, M.; Ueki, N.; Miyake, K.; Iwakiri, K.; Sakamoto, C. Nizatidine administration improves clinical symptoms and gastric emptying of the patients with functional dyspepsia accompanying with impaired gastric emptying. *Gastroenterology* **2011**, *140*, S230. [CrossRef]

18. Law, R.; Maltepe, C.; Bozzo, P.; Einarson, A. Treatment of the heartbum and acid reflux associated with nausea and vomiting during pregnancy. *Can. Fam. Phys.* **2010**, *56*, 143–144.

19. Koskenpato, J.; Punkkinen, J.N.; Kairemo, K.; Färkkilä, M. Nizatidine and gastric emptying in functional dyspepsia. *Dig. Dis. Sci.* **2008**, *53*, 352–357. [CrossRef] [PubMed]

20. Noguchi, K.; Uemura, H.; Harada, M.; Miura, T.; Moriyama, M.; Fukuoka, H.; Kitami, K.; Hosaka, M. Inhibition of PSA flare in prostate cancer patients by administration of flutamide for 2 weeks before initiation of treatment of slow-releasing LH-RH agonist. *Int. J. Clin. Oncol.* **2001**, *6*, 29–33. [CrossRef] [PubMed]

21. Sufrin, G.; Coffey, D.S. Flutamide. Mechanism of action of a new nonsteroidal antiandrogen. *Investig. Urol.* **1976**, *13*, 429–434.

22. Ask, K.; Décologne, N.; Ginies, C.; La, M.; Boucher, J.L.; Holmec, J.A.; Pelczar, H.; Camus, P. Metabolism of nilutamide in rat lung. *Biochem. Pharmacol.* **2006**, *71*, 377–385. [CrossRef] [PubMed]

23. La Mantia, L.; Mascoli, N.; Milanese, C. Azathioprine. Safety profile in multiple sclerosis patients. *Neurol. Sci.* **2007**, *28*, 299–303. [CrossRef] [PubMed]

24. Patel, A.A.; Swerlick, R.A.; McCall, C.O. Azathioprine in dermatology: the past, the present, and the future. *J. Am. Acad. Dermatol.* **2006**, *55*, 369–389. [CrossRef] [PubMed]

25. Fontana, G.; Bombardelli, E.; Manzotti, C.; Battaglia, A.; Samori, C. Camptothecin derivatives with antitumor activity. EP Patent 2010/38 EP 2044078 B1, 22 September 2010.

26. Clark, J.W. Rubitecan. *Exp. Opin. Investig. Drugs* **2006**, *15*, 71–79. [CrossRef] [PubMed]

27. Bains, A.; Buna, D.; Hoag, N.A. A retrospective review assessing the efficacy and safety of nitrofurantoin in renal impairment. *Can. Pharm. J.* **2009**, *142*, 248–252. [CrossRef]

28. Cunha, B.A.; Schoch, P.E.; Hage, J.R. Nitrofurantoin: preferred empiric therapy for community-acquired lower urinary tract infections. *Mayo Clin. Proc.* **2011**, *86*, 1243–1244. [CrossRef] [PubMed]

29. El-Zaher, A.A.; Mahrouse, M.A. A validated spectrofluoremetric method for the determination of nifuroxazide through coumarin formation using experimental design. *Chem. Cent. J.* **2013**, *7*, 90. [CrossRef] [PubMed]

30. O'Neil, M.J.; Smith, A.; Heckelman, P.E. *Merck Index: An Encyclopedia of Chemicals, Drugs, and Biologicals*, 13th ed.; Merck: Whitehouse Station, NJ, USA, 2001.

31. Gagliardi, S.; Consonni, S.; Ronzoni, A.; Bulgheroni, A.; Ceriani, D. Nifuratel Sulfoxide for Use in the Treatment of Bacterial Infections. EP Patent EP 2797914 B1, 16 September 2015.

32. Yan, X.D.; Zhang, L.J.; Wang, J.P. Residue depletion of nitrovin in chicken after oral administration. *J. Agric. Food Chem.* **2011**, *59*, 3414–3419. [CrossRef] [PubMed]

33. Bot, C.; Hall, B.S.; Alvarez, G.; Di Maio, R.; González, M.; Cerecetto, H.; Wilkinson, S.R. Evaluating nitrofurans as trypanocidal agents. *Antimicrob. Agents Chemother.* **2013**, *57*, 1638–1647. [CrossRef] [PubMed]

34. Mukherjee, T.; Boshoff, H. Nitroimidazoles for the treatment of TB: Past, present, and future. *Future Med. Chem.* **2011**, *3*, 1427–1454. [CrossRef] [PubMed]

35. Mital, A. Synthetic nitroimidazoles: Biological activities and mutagenicity relationships. *Sci. Pharm.* **2009**, *77*, 497–520. [CrossRef]

36. Schwebke, J.R.; Desmond, R.A. Tinidazole vs metronidazole for the treatment of bacterial vaginosis. *Am. J. Obstet. Gynecol.* **2011**, *204*, 211.e1–211.e6. [CrossRef] [PubMed]

37. Ratnaparkhi, M.P.; Dhiwar, S.B.; Gurav, R.R.; Bhore, S.S. Formulation and In-Vitro Characterization of Nimorazole Mouth Dissolving Tablets. *Res. J. Pharm. Biol. Chem. Sci.* **2012**, *3*, 303–308.

38. Patel, P.; Patel, K.; Bhatt, K.; Patel, S. New improved RP-HPLC method for determination of norfloxacin and ornidazole in their combined dosage form. *Int. J. Res. Pharm. Biomed. Sci.* **2011**, *2*, 710–713.

39. Ashtekar, D.R.; Costa-Pereira, R.; Nagarajan, K.; Vishvanathan, N.; Bhatt, A.D.; Rittel, W. In vitro and in vivo activities of the nitroimidazole CGI 17341 against Mycobacterium tuberculosis. *Antimicrob. Agents Chemother.* **1993**, *37*, 183–186. [CrossRef] [PubMed]

40. Barry, C.E., 3rd; Boshoff, H.I.M.; Dowd, C.S. Prospects for clinical introduction of nitroimidazole antibiotics for the treatment of tuberculosis. *Curr. Pharm. Des.* **2004**, *10*, 3239–3269. [CrossRef] [PubMed]

41. Matsumoto, M.; Hashizume, H.; Tomishige, T.; Kawasaki, M.; Tsubouchi, H.; Sasaki, H.; Shimokawa, Y.; Komatsu, M. OPC 67683. A nitro-dihydro-imidazooxazole derivative with promising action against tuberculosis in vitro and in mice. *PLoS Med.* **2006**, *3*, e466. [CrossRef] [PubMed]

42. Sotgiu, G.; Pontali, E.; Centis, R.; D'Ambrosio, L.; Migliori, G.B. Delamanid (OPC 67683) for treatment of multi-drug resistant tuberculosis. *Expert Rev. Anti-Infect. Ther.* **2015**, *13*, 305–315. [CrossRef] [PubMed]

43. Wyllie, S.; Roberts, A.J.; Norval, S.; Patterson, S.; Foth, B.J.; Berriman, M.; Read, K.D.; Fairlamb, A.H. Activation of bicyclic nitro-drugs by a novel nitroreductase (NTR2) in leishmania. *PLOS Pathog.* **2016**, *12*, e1005971. [CrossRef] [PubMed]

44. Diacon, A.H.; Dawson, R.; Hanckom, M.; Narunsky, K.; Venter, A.; Hittel, N.; Geiter, L.J.; Wells, C.D.; Paccaly, A.J.; Donald, P.R. Early bactericidal activity of delamanid (OPC-67683) in smear-positive pulmonary tuberculosis patients. *Int. J. Tuberc. Lung Dis.* **2011**, *15*, 949–954. [CrossRef] [PubMed]

45. Stover, C.K.; Warrener, P.; Van Devanter, D.R.; Sherman, D.R.; Arain, T.M.; Langhorne, M.H.; Anderson, S.W.; Towell, J.A.; Yuan, Y.; McMurray, D.N.; et al. A small molecule nitroimidazopyran drug candidate for the treatment of tuberculosis. *Nature* **2000**, *405*, 962–966. [CrossRef] [PubMed]

46. Singh, R.; Manjunatha, U.; Boshoff, H.I.M.; Ha, Y.H.; Niyomrattanakit, P.; Ledwidge, R.; Dowd, C.S.; Lee, I.Y.; Kim, P.; Zhang, L.; et al. PA-824 kills nonreplicating Mycobacterium tuberculosis by intracellular NO release. *Science* **2008**, *322*, 1392–1395. [CrossRef] [PubMed]

47. Kim, P.; Zhang, L.; Manjunatha, U.H.; Singh, R.; Patel, S.; Jiricek, J.; Keller, T.H.; Boshoff, H.I.M.; Barry, C.E., 3rd; Dowd, C.S. Structure-activity relationships of antitubercular nitroimidazoles. I. Structural features associated with aerobic and anaerobic activities of 4- and 5-nitroimidazoles. *J. Med. Chem.* **2009**, *52*, 1317–1328. [CrossRef] [PubMed]

48. Kim, P.; Kang, S.; Boshoff, H.I.M.; Jiricek, J.; Collins, M.; Singh, R.; Manjunatha, U.H.; Niyomrattanakit, P.; Zhang, L.; Goodwin, M.; et al. Structure-activity relationships of antitubercular nitroimidazoles. 2. Determinants of aerobic activity and quantitative structure-activity relationships. *J. Med. Chem.* **2009**, *52*, 1329–1344. [CrossRef] [PubMed]

49. Naber, K.G.; Niggemann, H.; Stein, G.; Stein, G. Review of the literature and individual patients' data meta-analysis on efficacy and tolerance of nitroxoline in the treatment of uncomplicated urinary tract infections. *BMC Infect. Dis.* **2014**, *14*, 628–644. [CrossRef] [PubMed]

50. Zhang, Q.; Wang, S.; Yang, D.; Pan, K.; Li, L.; Yuan, S. Preclinical pharmacodynamic evaluation of antibiotic nitroxoline for anticancer drug repurposing. *Oncol. Lett.* **2016**, *11*, 3265–3272. [CrossRef] [PubMed]

51. Mitrović, A.; Sosič, I.; Kos, Š.; Tratar, U.L.; Breznik, B.; Kranjc, S.; Mirković, B.; Gobec, S.; Lah, T.; Serša, G.; et al. Addition of 2-(ethylamino)acetonitrile group to nitroxoline results in significantly improved anti-tumor activity in vitro and in vivo. *Oncotarget* **2017**, *8*, 59136–59147. [CrossRef] [PubMed]

52. Kostopoulou, N.; Kourelis, T.G.; Mamos, P.; Magoulas, G.E.; Kalpaxis, D.L. Insights into the chloramphenicol inhibition effect on peptidyl transferase activity, using two new analogs of the drug. *Open Enzyme Inhib. J.* **2011**, *4*, 1–10. [CrossRef]

53. Liaqat, J.; Sumbal, F.; Sabri, A.N. Tetracycline and chloramphenicol efficiency against selected biofilm forming bacteria. *Curr. Microbiol.* **2009**, *59*, 212–220. [CrossRef] [PubMed]

54. Bustos, J.A.; Rodriguez, S.; Jimenez, J.A.; Moyano, L.M.; Castillo, Y.; Ayvar, V.; Allan, J.C.; Craig, P.S.; Gonzales, A.E.; Gilman, R.H.; et al. Detection of Taenia solium taeniasis coproantigen is an early indicator of treatment failure for taeniasis. *Clin. Vaccine Immunol.* **2012**, *19*, 570–573. [CrossRef] [PubMed]

55. Salvana, E.M.T.; King, C.H. Schistosomiasis in travelers and immigrants. *Curr. Inf. Dis. Rep.* **2008**, *10*, 42–49. [CrossRef]

56. Patterson, S.; Wyllie, S. Nitro drugs for the treatment of trypanosomatid diseases: Past, present and future prospects. *Trends Parasitol.* **2014**, *30*, 289–298. [CrossRef] [PubMed]

57. Wyllie, S.; Foth, B.J.; Kelner, A.; Sokolova, A.Y.; Berriman, M.; Fairlamb, A.H. Nitroheterocyclic drug resistance mechanisms in Trypanosoma brucei. *J. Antimicrob. Chemother.* **2016**, *71*, 625–634. [CrossRef] [PubMed]

58. Mitrowska, K. Przyczyny i skutki zakazu stosowania 5-nitroimidazoli u zwierząt, których tkanki lub produkty przeznaczone są do spożycia przez ludzi. *Med. Weter.* **2015**, *71*, 736–742.

59. Franco, J.R.; Simarro, P.P.; Diarra, A.; Ruiz-Postigo, J.A.; Samo, M.; Jannin, J.G. Monitoring the use of nifurtimox-eflornithine combination therapy (NECT) in the treatment of second stage gambiense human African trypanosomiasis. *Res. Rep. Trop. Med.* **2012**, *3*, 93–101. [CrossRef]

60. Mullokandov, E.; Ahn, J.; Szalkiewicz, A.; Babayeva, M. Protein binding drug-drug interaction between warfarin and tizoxanide in human plasma. *Austin J. Pharmacol. Ther.* **2014**, *2*, 1038.

61. Raviraj, J.; Bokkasam, V.K.; Kumar, V.S.; Reddy, U.S.; Suman, V. Radiosensitizers, radioprotectors, and radiation mitigators. *Indian J. Dent. Res.* **2014**, *25*, 83–90. [CrossRef] [PubMed]

62. Asquith, J.C.; Foster, J.L.; Willson, R.L.; Ings, R.; McFadzean, J.A. Metronidazole ("Flagyl"), a radiosensitizer of hypoxic cells. *Br. J. Radiol.* **1974**, *47*, 474–481. [CrossRef] [PubMed]

63. Chapman, J.D.; Greenstock, C.L.; Reuvers, A.P.; McDonald, E.; Dunlop, I. Radiation chemical studies with nitrojurazone as related to its mechanism of radiosensitization. *Radiat. Res.* **1973**, *53*, 190–203. [CrossRef] [PubMed]

64. Guichard, M.; Malaise, E.P. Radiosensitizing effects of misonidazole and SR 2508 on a human melanoma transplanted in nude mice: influence on repair of potentially lethal damage. *Int. J. Radiat. Oncol. Biol. Phys.* **1982**, *8*, 465–468. [CrossRef]

65. Dische, S.; Saunders, M.I.; Lee, M.E.; Adams, G.E.; Flockhart, I.R. Clinical testing of the radiosensitizer Ro 07–0582: experience with multiple doses. *Br. J. Cancer* **1977**, *35*, 567–579. [CrossRef] [PubMed]

66. Lee, D.J.; Cosmatos, D.; Marcial, V.A.; Fu, K.K.; Rotman, M.; Cooper, J.S.; Ortiz, H.G.; Beitler, J.J.; Abrams, R.A.; Curran, W.J. Results of an RTOG phase III trial (RTOG 85–27) comparing radiotherapy plus etanidazole with radiotherapy alone for locally advanced head and neck carcinomas. *Int. J. Radiat. Oncol. Biol. Phys.* **1995**, *32*, 567–576. [CrossRef]

67. Overgaard, J.; Hansen, H.S.; Overgaard, M.; Bastholt, L.; Berthelsen, A. A randomized double-blind phase III study of nimorazole as a hypoxic radiosensitizer of primary radiotherapy in supraglottic larynx and pharynx carcinoma. Results of the Danish Head and Neck cancer Study (DAHANCA) Protocol 5–85. *Radiother. Oncol.* **1998**, *46*, 135–146. [CrossRef]

68. Kendall, G.C.; Mokhonova, E.I.; Moran, M.; Sejbuk, N.E.; Wang, D.W.; Silva, O.; Wang, R.T.; Martinez, L.; Lu, Q.L.; Damoiseaux, R.; et al. Dantrolene enhances antisense-mediated exon skipping in human and mouse models of Duchenne muscular dystrophy. *Sci. Transl. Med.* **2012**, *4*, 164ra160. [CrossRef] [PubMed]

69. Muehlschlegel, S.; Rordorf, G.; Bodock, M.; Sims, J.R. Dantrolene mediates vasorelaxation in cerebrial vasoconstriction: a case series. *Neurocrit. Care* **2009**, *10*, 116–121. [CrossRef] [PubMed]

70. Oo, Y.W.; Gomez-Hurtado, N.; Walweel, K.; van Helden, D.F.; Imtiaz, M.S.; Knollmann, B.C.; Laver, D.R. Essential role of calmodulin in RyR inhibition by dantrolene. *Mol. Pharmacol.* **2015**, *88*, 57–63. [CrossRef] [PubMed]

71. Rainsford, K.D. Nimesulide—A multifactorial approach to inflammation and pain. *Curr. Med. Res. Opin.* **2006**, *22*, 1161–1170. [CrossRef] [PubMed]

72. Al-Abd, A.M.; Al-Abbasi, F.A.; Nofal, S.M.; Khalifa, A.E.; Williams, R.O.; El-Eraky, W.I.; Nagy, A.A.; Abdel-Nain, A.B. Nimesulide improves the symptomatic and disease modifying effects of leflunomide in collagen induced arthritis. *PLoS ONE* **2014**, *9*, e111843. [CrossRef] [PubMed]

73. Banerjee, R.R.; Rangwala, S.M.; Shapiro, J.S.; Rich, A.S.; Rhoades, B.; Qi, Y.; Wang, J.; Rajala, M.W.; Pocai, A.; Scherer, P.E.; et al. Regulation of fasted blood glucose by resistin. *Science* **2004**, *303*, 1195–1198. [CrossRef] [PubMed]

74. Berg, A.H.; Combs, T.P.; Scherer, P.E. ACRP30/adiponectin: An adipokine regulating glucose and lipid metabolism. *Trends Endocrinol. Metab.* **2002**, *13*, 84–89. [CrossRef]

75. Villacorta, L.; Gao, Z.; Schopfer, F.J.; Freeman, B.A.; Chen, Y.E. Nitro-fatty acids in cardiovascular regulation and diseases: Characteristics and molecular mechanisms. *Front. Biosci.* **2016**, *21*, 873–889. [CrossRef]

76. Pereira, C.; Ferreira, N.R.; Rocha, B.S.; Barbosa, R.M.; Laranjinha, J. The redox interplay between nitrite and nitric oxide: From the gut to the brain. *Redox Biol.* **2013**, *1*, 276–284. [CrossRef] [PubMed]

77. Rubbo, H. Nitro-fatty acids: novel anti-inflammatory lipid mediators. *Braz. J. Med. Biol. Res.* **2013**, *46*, 728–734. [CrossRef] [PubMed]

78. Alvarez, B.; Turell, L.; Vitturi, D.A.; Coitino, E.L.; Lebrato, L.; Moller, M.N.; Sagasti, C.; Salvatore, S.R.; Woodcock, S.R.; Schopfer, F.J. Thiol addition to conjugated nitrolinoleic acid. *FASEB J.* **2017**, *31* (Supl. 1), 605.1.

79. Freeman, B.A.; Baker, P.R.S.; Schopfer, F.J.; Woodcock, S.R.; Napolitano, A.; d'Ischia, M. Nitro-fatty acid formation and signaling. *J. Biol. Chem.* **2008**, *283*, 15515–15519. [CrossRef] [PubMed]

80. Rudolph, V.; Schopfer, F.J.; Khoo, N.K.H.; Rudolph, T.K.; Cole, M.P.; Woodcock, S.R.; Bonacci, G.; Groeger, A.L.; Golin-Bisello, F.; Chen, C.S.; et al. Nitro-fatty acid metabolome: saturation, desaturation, β-oxidation, and protein adduction. *J. Biol. Chem.* **2009**, *284*, 1461–1473. [CrossRef] [PubMed]

81. Mata-Perez, C.; Sanchez-Calvo, B.; Begara-Moralez, J.C.; Padilla, M.N.; Valderrama, R.; Corpas, F.J.; Barroso, J.B. Nitric oxide release from nitro-fatty acids in Arabidopsis roots. *Plant Signal Behav.* **2016**, *11*, e1154255. [CrossRef] [PubMed]

82. Villacorta, L.; Chang, L.; Salvatore, S.R.; Ichikawa, T.; Zhang, J.; Petrovic-Djergovic, D.; Jia, L.; Carlsen, H.; Schopfer, F.J.; Freeman, B.A.; et al. Electrophilic nitro-fatty acids inhibit vascular inflammation by disrupting LPS-dependent TLR4 signaling in lipid rafts. *Cardiovasc. Res.* **2013**, *98*, 116–124. [CrossRef] [PubMed]

83. Wynne, B.M.; Chiao, C.W.; Webb, R.C. Vascular smooth muscle cell signaling mechanisms for contraction to angiotensin II and endothelin-1. *J. Am. Soc. Hypertens.* **2009**, *3*, 84–95. [CrossRef] [PubMed]

84. Wang, W.; Li, C.; Yang, T. Protection of nitro-fatty acids against kidney diseases. *Am. J. Physiol. Renal. Physiol.* **2016**, *310*, F697–F704. [CrossRef] [PubMed]

85. Chung, M.C.; Bosquesi, P.L.; dos Santos, J.L. A prodrug approach to improve the physico-chemical properties and decrease the genotoxicity of nitro compounds. *Curr. Pharm. Des.* **2011**, *17*, 3515–3526. [CrossRef] [PubMed]

6

Application of Nanoparticle Technology to Reduce the Anti-Microbial Resistance through β-Lactam Antibiotic-Polymer Inclusion Nano-Complex

Constain H. Salamanca [1,]* ⓘ, **Cristhian J. Yarce** [1], **Yony Roman** [1], **Andrés F. Davalos** [1] **and Gustavo R. Rivera** [2]

[1] Facultad de Ciencias Naturales, Universidad Icesi, Calle 18 No. 122-135, Cali 760031, Colombia; cjyarce@icesi.edu.co (C.J.Y.); yonyroa@yahoo.com (Y.R.); afdavalos@icesi.edu.co (A.F.D.).
[2] SIT Biotech GmbH, BMZ 2 Otto-Hahn-Str. 15, 44227 Dortmund, Germany; gunam04@gmail.com
* Correspondence: chsalamanca@icesi.edu.co

Abstract: Biocompatible polymeric materials with potential to form functional structures in association with different therapeutic molecules have a high potential for biological, medical and pharmaceutical applications. Therefore, the capability of the inclusion of nano-Complex formed between the sodium salt of poly(maleic acid-*alt*-octadecene) and a β-lactam drug (ampicillin trihydrate) to avoid the chemical and enzymatic degradation and enhance the biological activity were evaluated. PAM-18Na was produced and characterized, as reported previously. The formation of polymeric hydrophobic aggregates in aqueous solution was determined, using pyrene as a fluorescent probe. Furthermore, the formation of polymer-drug nano-complexes was characterized by Differential Scanning Calorimetry-DSC, viscometric, ultrafiltration/centrifugation assays, zeta potential and size measurements were determined by dynamic light scattering-DLS. The PAM-18Na capacity to avoid the chemical degradation was studied through stress stability tests. The enzymatic degradation was evaluated from a pure β-lactamase, while the biological degradation was determined by different β-lactamase producing *Staphylococcus aureus* strains. When ampicillin was associated with PAM-18Na, the half-life time in acidic conditions increased, whereas both the enzymatic degradation and the minimum inhibitory concentration decreased to a 90 and 75%, respectively. These results suggest a promissory capability of this polymer to protect the β-lactam drugs against chemical, enzymatic and biological degradation.

Keywords: polymer-drug association; inclusion nano-complex; an amphiphilic polymer; polysoaps; antibiotic resistance; ampicillin trihydrate

1. Introduction

Nowadays, bacterial antibiotic resistance stands as a significant public health problem in our society and, the considerable challenge of finding new antibiotic molecules or improving the activity of the existing ones demands a joint effort of multiple disciplines [1–3]. Antibiotic resistance results naturally from the inherent ability of bacteria to multiply rapidly and mutate as an adaptation strategy. However, patient misuse, the doctors' mis-prescription and their overuse in the food industry have exacerbated the problem of antibiotic resistance [2]. This issue is becoming even more significant due to the recent decrease in research efforts to produce new antibiotics [4]. Pharmaceutical companies, government agencies and academia are not investing enough resources to face the emerging strains of multidrug-resistant "superbugs". Many bacteria show resistance to antibiotics but *Staphylococcus aureus* stands as one of the most relevant due to the high morbidity and mortality due to its bacteremia [5,6]. The high prevalence of *S. aureus* in nosocomial infections and its high rate of penicillin resistance makes this pathogen the primary cause of resistant bacteria-related diseases, worldwide. The mechanisms of bacterial resistance are multiple and can be conjugate but the most common one involves the production of β-lactamases. These are a series of enzymes, which can hydrolyze the β-lactam ring present in the penicillin-like antibiotics [7].

Several alternatives have been developed to treat infections with antibiotics resistant to *S. aureus*. Initially, the first line of defense was the use of β-lactamase resistant molecules like methicillin and oxacillin. However, only two years after their introduction a *S. aureus* strain resistant to methicillin (MRSA) emerged [8–10]. Today, MRSA strains are endemic in hospitals worldwide. MRSA infections are commonly treated with non-β-lactam antibiotics like clindamycin but there are resistant strains as well. These strategies involve the use of new molecules that merely test the refined ability of the microbes to evolve and adapt. The continuous emergence of resistant strains highlights the need for the development of new strategies to treat bacterial infections. Recent plans that seek to improve the effectiveness of conventional antibiotics against resistant bacteria include their use along with inhibitors of β-lactamases [11,12] and, to a lesser extent, the control of β-lactamase expression [13,14]. However, there is few available information on the use of polymeric materials to avoid antibiotic biological degradation [15–17]. In aqueous solution, some amphiphilic polymers like polysoaps, hydrophobically modified polymers and block polymers may form hydrophobic pseudo-phases capable of solubilizing organic molecules [18–24].

The sodium salt of poly(maleic acid-*alt*-octadecene), named here as PAM-18Na, can form different hydrophobic "pseudo-phases" in a concentration-dependent way. At very low concentrations, PAM-18Na forms unimolecular aggregates, i.e. each polymer chain collapses forming a compact coil. Whereas, in more concentrated solutions, PAM-18Na forms multimolecular aggregates. This polymer has also been able to solubilize different organic molecules such as alkyl-phenols [25] and *N*-alkyl-nitroimidazoles [22]. Based on these observations we hypothesized that PAM-18Na polymer could be useful to protect β-lactam antibiotics from the action of β-lactamases and thus improves their effect on antibiotic-resistant bacteria. In this work, we evaluated the ability of the PAM-18Na polymer to prevent the chemical and enzymatic degradation of ampicillin trihydrate when subjected to severe acid conditions and purified β-lactamase obtained from *P. fluorescens*, respectively. Likewise, we compared the effect of the PAM-18Na polymer on the antibiotic activity of AT over several *S. aureus* strains. Our results suggest a promissory capability the polymer PAM-18Na to protect the β-lactam drugs against chemical and biological degradation through the formation of a polymer-drug inclusion nano-complex in aqueous media.

2. Materials and Methods

2.1. Materials

Poly(maleic anhydride-*alt*-octadecene) denominated like PAM-18 with average Mw 30,000–50,000 and Lucifer yellow were obtained from Sigma-Aldrich®, ampicillin trihydrate—here referred to as AT—was from Fersinsa Gb® (Coahuila, Mexico), recombinant β-lactamase from *Pseudomonas fluorescens* was obtained from Sigma® (Saint Louis, MO, USA). It was received lyophilized and suspended according to manufacturer indications. Ultrapure water was obtained with an Elix Essential Millipore® (Darmstadt, Germany) purification system. All other reagents were from Merck® (Kenilworth, NJ, USA). *Bacterial strains: S. aureus* strains ATCC 25923, ATCC 29213 y ATCC 43300 were purchased from Microbiologics Inc.© (St Cloud, MN, USA) and were reconstituted according to the instructions.

2.2. Obtention and FTIR Characterization of PAM-18Na Polymer

PAM-18Na was obtained as previously described [22]. Briefly, 100 g of PAM-18 was hydrolyzed in 2 L of ultrapure water mixed with NaOH in a 1:1 molar ratio (according to PAM-18 copolymer unit), where the polymeric material obtained was named PAM-18Na. The modification was carried out at room temperature for 24 h under moderate agitation (200 rpm). Subsequently, the polymer solution was dialyzed using cellulose membrane (12 kD cut off size) and pre-concentrated through a stirred ultrafiltration cell (Amicon® cells 8400, Merk-Millipore, Billerica, MA, USA) with a 12-kDa cut-off polyethersulfone (PES) membrane. Subsequently, the polymer solution was lyophilized (model FDU 1110, Eyela, Tokyo Rikakikai, Tokyo, Japan) until obtaining solid materials with a yield greater than 90%, which was sieved with 75 μm mesh (number 200).

2.3. Preparation of Inclusion Nano-Complexes in Aqueous Media

The inclusion nano-complexes between TA and the PAM-18Na polymer were formed in situ. For this, a defined amount of PAM-18Na polymer was added in ultra-pure water until reaching a homogeneous dispersion with desired concentration. Then, the β-lactam drug was added "little by little" to the polymeric dispersion, using moderate magnetic stirring (200 rpm) at room temperature until obtaining a translucent dispersion.

2.4. Steady-State Fluorescence Assay

The presence of polymeric hydrophobic aggregates in aqueous media formed by the PAM-18Na was evidenced through by the steady-state fluorescence study using a microplate reader (Synergy h1 hybrid multi-mode) and pyrene as a fluorescent probe. A stock solution of pyrene (2.66×10^{-5} M) was prepared to which micro-volumes of PAM-18Na polymeric solution (1 mg/mL) were added until a pyrene concentration of 1.33×10^{-6} M was obtained. The excitation wavelength was set at 337 nm and the intensities of the third (I_3) and first (I_1) peaks of the pyrene emission spectrum, (at 382 nm and 373 nm, respectively) were measured.

2.5. Characterization of Drug-Polymer Inclusion Complex

2.5.1. Thermal Characterization of the Polymer-Drug Blend

PAM-18Na polymer, AT and polymer-drug solid mixture in different proportions was studied on a DSC Q2000 (TA Instruments) calibrated with indium $T_m = 155.78$ °C, $\Delta H_m = 28.71$ J/g. The DSC analysis was performed using three cycles of heating and cooling from -90 °C (183.15 ° K) to 200 °C (523.15 ° K) with a heating rate of 20 °C/min.

2.5.2. Association Efficiency

Independent solutions of AT and PAM-18Na polymer were prepared using several phosphate buffer solutions, having pH values of 4.0, 7.0 and 10.0. Each solution was fixed to an ionic strength of 10 mM. For AT, the solution concentration was 40 μg/mL, while the PAM-18Na amount was set to form a 1:1 polymer-drug molar ratio according to PAM-18Na co-monomeric unit. Equal volumes of both solutions were mixed by ultrasonic stirring for 1 h. Then, each solution was settled inside an ultrafiltration tube (VWR, Modified PES 10 kDa, 500 μL) and centrifuged at 9000 G (10.000 rpm) for 7 min. From the filtrate obtained (lower fraction in the ultrafiltration tube), to quantify the amount of AT. The absorbance was measured in a microplate reader (Synergy h1 hybrid multi-mode) at a wavelength of 256 nm and the amount of AT was determined by interpolation from the calibration curve built at concentrations of 2, 5, 10, 20 y 40 μg/mL. The amount of AT encapsulated or contained in the PAM-18Na polymeric hydrophobic aggregates was calculated using the following expression:

$$AE = \left[\frac{(Q_t - Q_s)}{Q_t} \right] \times 100\% \tag{1}$$

where AE corresponds to the association efficiency, Q_t is the initial total amount of added AT and Q_s is the filtrated amount after centrifugation.

2.5.3. Zeta Potential and Size Measurements

Each of the zeta measures was performed in triplicate using a Zetasizer Nano ZSP (Malvern Instrument, Malvern, UK) at 25 °C. The first part of the study was focused on characterizing PAM-18Na polymer in aqueous media regarding the pH of the media. In this case, 40 μg/mL polymer solutions were prepared, where the pH was adjusted with concentrated solutions of NaOH and HCl and slightly shaken for 48 h. The second study was focused on the characterization of the drug-polymer interactions between PAM18-Na and ampicillin trihydrate in aqueous media. In this case, each solution was prepared using several phosphate buffer solutions, with different pH values of 4.0, 7.0 and 10.0 and was fixed to the ionic strength of 10 mM. Each measurement was performed with freshly prepared samples. To the aim of evaluating the impact of AT loading into the hydrophobic polymeric aggregates formed by PAM-18Na, different amounts of AT were added until achieving a final concentration of 0.23 μg/mL, corresponding to 1:1 polymer-drug molar ratio according to the PAM-18Na co-monomeric unit. Each of these studies was carried out by auto-titration with independent cells, where measurements of size were carried out using a quartz flow cell (ZEN0023), while the zeta potential was carried out with a disposable folded capillary cell (DTS1070).

2.5.4. Viscometric Measurements

The characterization of the polymer-drug interactions was also studied by viscosimetry. A viscometer (microVisc TC, RheoSense, San Francisco, CA, USA) coupled to a low viscosity chip (16HA05100243) was used. Each measurement was performed using a 1:1 polymer-drug molar ratio according to a co-monomeric unit of PAM-18Na at 25 °C and at different pH values (1, 4, 7 and 10), with freshly prepared samples and in triplicate as described above.

2.6. Degradation Assays

2.6.1. Chemical Degradation Assay

Due to the remarkable degradability of the beta-lactam ring in AT respect to temperature and media pH [26], a stability test to stress conditions, in the presence and absence of the PAM-18Na polymer was performed to evaluate the potential of this polymer as protector of the β-lactam drugs. For this, different initial concentrations of AT (1, 3 and 5 mg/mL) in a strong acidic media (pH 1.2) were prepared and stirred for 6 h at 40 °C. Consecutively, each sample was taken every 10 min and analyzed by UHPLC with a photo-diode-array detector (Lachrom ultra Hitachi, VWR, Tokio, Japon). This assay was performed by in triplicate.

2.6.2. Enzymatic Degradation Assay

The β-Lactamase activity was monitored by measuring the hydrolysis of the β–lactam ring of ampicillin at 204 nm, as reported previously [27,28]. The assays were carried out by mixing 125 μL of a β-Lactamase solution (38 μg/mL) with a solution containing 800 μL of AT (81.25 μM) and 1325 μL of phosphate buffer 50 mM (pH 7.0) in a quartz cell. The reactions were carried out at 25 °C for 20 min, measuring the absorbance every 2 min using a UV spectrophotometry (Shimadzu UV model 1800) coupled to a temperature control system). Initial rates (v_0) were calculated using the linear portion of the absorbance vs. time plot for each enzymatic reaction. The β-Lactamase activity units (U) were defined as the amount of enzyme that hydrolyzes 1.0 nmol of AT per minute at 25 °C and pH 7.0. The AT concentration in the enzymatic assay was calculated using a standard curve made by measuring the absorbance at 204 nm of standard solutions ranging from 8.13 to 81.25 μM. The β-Lactamase activity in the presence of the PAM-18Na polymer was calculated as described above but using a solution prepared by mixing ampicillin and the polymer in a 1:1 molar ratio in phosphate buffer 50 mM (pH 7.0).

2.6.3. Biological Degradation Assays

Ampicillin Susceptibility

AT susceptibility for each of the *S. aureus* strains used in this study (*S. aureus* ATCC 25923, *S. aureus* ATCC 29213 and *S. aureus* ATCC 43300) was measured following the guidelines of the Clinical and Laboratory Standards Institute (CLSI) [29]. In brief, a culture was grown in a petri dish using Mueller-Hinton (Scharlab®, Barcelona, Spain) agar and the diameter of the inhibition halo around an ampicillin Sensi-Disc (BD) was measured. For each bacterial strain, the average of four replicates was used in the analysis.

β-Lactamase Production

The β-Lactamase production, in each of the four *S. aureus* strains, was assayed by the chromogenic cephalosporin nitrocefin [30,31]. For each strain, three colonies were inoculated on top of a Nitrocefin disc (Abtek Biologicals, Liverpool, UK) and a color change was monitored as an indicator of β-Lactamase enzymatic activity according to manufacturer instructions.

Minimum Inhibitory Concentration (MIC)

Ampicillin trihydrate MIC was determined by the broth microdilution method according to the CLSI guidelines [32]. In each case, the MIC was determined for AT, PAM-18Na polymer and the mix of PAM-18Na and AT, in a 1:1 ratio (based on the copolymer unit), as previously described. The concentrations evaluated were 0.0625, 0.125, 0.25, 0.35, 0.5, 2, 8, 32, 128, 192, 256 µg/mL, respectively. The assays were performed in 96 round bottom well plates (BD) using 500 µL of the appropriate *S. aureus* strain grown in Mueller-Hinton broth (Scharlau®) at a turbidity of 0.1 absorbance units. Twenty-four replicates were performed for each concentration and visually inspected for the presence of a bacterial cell pellet.

2.7. Data Analysis

Data analysis for MIC was carried out using the Microsoft® Excel and Statgraphics Centurion XV (Version 15.2.06 software). The effect of ampicillin, PAM-18Na polymer and polymer-drug mix, on culture growth, was determined with a 95% confidence interval.

3. Results and Discussion

3.1. Obtention and FTIR Characterization of PAM-18Na Polymer

Formation of PAM-18Na polymer was evidenced by a physical change. The solution passes from a heterogeneous mixture to an utterly homogenous solution with a yellowish color, due to the opening of the maleic group in PAM-18 which produces carboxylic acid and carboxylate groups in the polymer backbone. This structural modification was inferred by comparing the FTIR spectra of both PAM-18 and PAM-18Na polymers according to previous reports (Supplementary Materials). The results showed the typical symmetric and asymmetric stretching values characteristic of the hydro-carbonated alkyl chain at 2920 and 2848 cm^{-1}. Upon the reaction, two new signals of the maleic anhydride carbonyl groups at 1773 and 1704 cm^{-1} to 1706 and 1556 cm^{-1} supports the formation of the carboxylic acid and carboxylate species. Likewise, the typical broad signal of the hydroxyl group of carboxylic acid at 3110 cm^{-1} is observed, corroborating that PAM-18Na polymer presents both the carboxylic acid and carboxylate form.

3.2. Steady-State Fluorescence Assay

The I_3/I_1 pyrene ratio of emission spectra is strongly dependent on the medium polarity and it has been used to establish an empirical polarity scale that is widely used in the study of microheterogeneous systems [33]. The I_3/I_1 pyrene ratio in aqueous solutions of PAM-18Na at different pH is shown in

Figure 1. For the sake of comparison, the spectra were normalized using the intensity of the peak located at 373 nm. The results show that PAM-18Na might create aggregates in aqueous media with a similar polarity like that described by pyrene in butanol (~0.95). However, this effect is trivial to those previously found in a similar polymer [34]. On the other hand, the I_3/I_1 ratio does not show a considerable change concerning the media pH, suggesting that the hydrophobicity of polymeric aggregates tends to remain constant independently of the pH. Hence is possible to solubilize or contain small organic molecules.

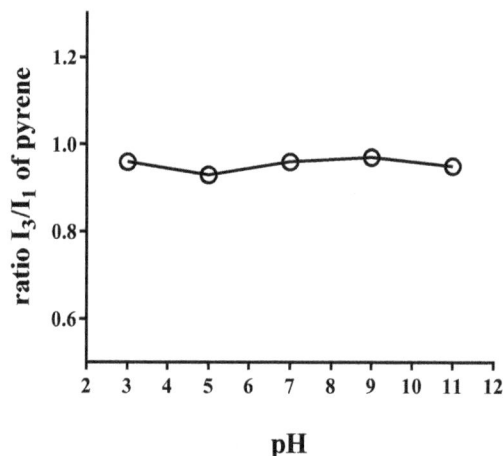

Figure 1. I_3/I_1 pyrene ratio of emission spectra in aqueous solutions of PAM-18Na at different pH and solvent with different polarity degree.

3.3. Characterization of the Drug-Polymer Inclusion Complex

3.3.1. Thermal Characterization of the Polymer-Drug Blend

The analysis of thermal characterization for ampicillin trihydrate in different proportions of PAM-18Na polymer is shown in Figure 2.

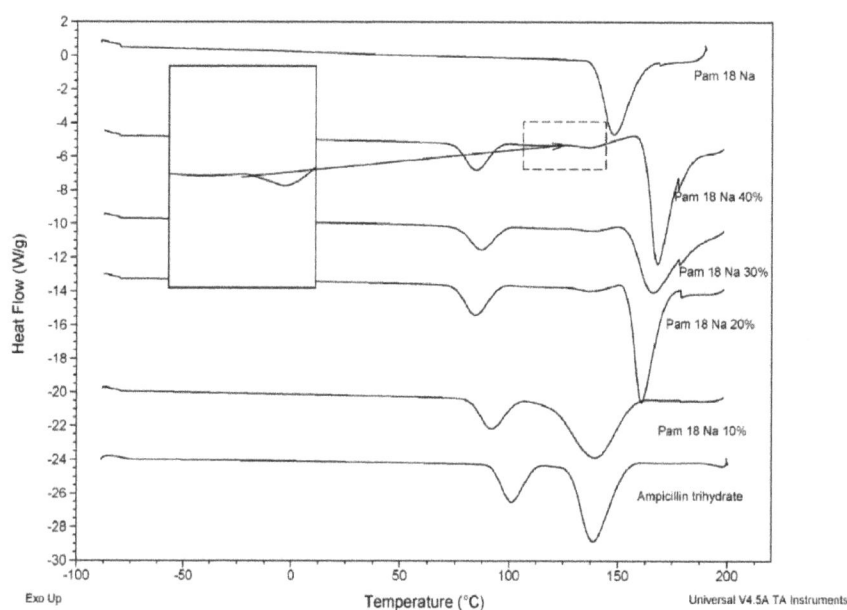

Figure 2. DSC Thermograms of ampicillin trihydrate and PAM-18Na polymer in solid blends at different proportions.

From the DCS thermograms, it is possible to observe two phenomena: (i) a decrease in the thermal transition temperature of the PAM-18Na polymer around 175 °C and a higher thermal transition temperature of AT around 137.5 °C, which becomes stronger with the increase of the polymer amount; (ii) The appearance of a new thermal signal that increases its intensity and energy with the rise in the polymer amount. These results suggest an intense interaction between the PAM-18Na polymer and AT.

3.3.2. Encapsulation Efficiency

The results of ampicillin trihydrate associated or contained into the PAM-18Na polymeric hydrophobic aggregates are shown in Figure 3, where the results shown a dependence of the AT association efficiency regarding media pH, being higher at pH 7.0 than pH 4.0 and 12.0, respectively. The above mentioned is a fascinating result because the PAM-18Na polymer has shown the capacity to form hydrophobic aggregates or "hydrophobic domains" independent of pH. Therefore, a high association degree should be expected, as has been observed in similar studies [21,22]. On the other hand, these differences can be explained according to (i) the amphoteric nature of ampicillin and (ii) the type of polymer-drug complex formed at each pH. In the first case, the ability of AT to transfer from aqueous phase to the polymeric hydrophobic pseudo-phase will depend on its ionization degree, where at pH close to 7.0, the AT tends a neutral form, favoring its incorporation into the PAM-18Na polymeric pseudo-phase. Based on the measured value of ~0.95 in the I_3/I_1 pyrene ratio of, the polarity of the pseudo-phases presents a favorable environment to incorporate organic molecules like ampicillin. Therefore, our results also suggest that hydrophobic domains are formed by the PAM-18Na might associate or contain a significant amount of AT.

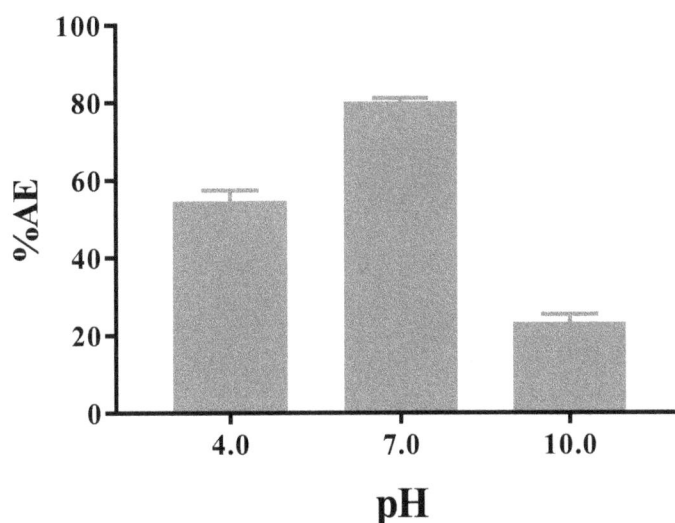

Figure 3. Association efficiency of ampicillin trihydrate by the PAM-18Na polymer in aqueous media to different pH values at 25 °C.

Also, it was possible to appreciate a very interesting situation related to the organoleptic characteristics of AT, which has a typical strong smell. This effect was a considerable loss of such characteristic odor in the presence of polymer PAM-18Na, disappeared almost entirely at pH: 7.4. This result suggests indirectly, the formation of a complex between the PAM-18Na polymer and the drug. Regarding the type of polymer-drug complex formed at each pH, it is necessary to consider the effects of size, zeta potential and viscosity of the PAM-18Na system with and without drug at different pH, which is explained as follows. Finally, we must comment that the evaluations at pH values of 1.2 and 12 were not possible because the integrity of the ultrafiltration membrane was affected by those pH values.

3.3.3. Zeta Potential and Size Measurements

It is imperative to highlight that it is common to assume that all association processes between organic substrates and polymers, such as PAM18Na, occur through solubilization within the polymer hydrophobic domain formed in aqueous media. However, there is another possibility of an association—such as the adsorption on the polymer-solvent interface—as we have already demonstrated for ampicillin with a cationic polymer, such as Eudragit E, where the drug-polymer association is mainly given on this interface [35]. The first study was focused on evaluating the effect of pH on the size and zeta potential of PAM-18Na polymer in solution with the aim of elucidating the association mechanism. These results are shown in Figure 4. In the case of size measurements, a bimodal size distribution was observed, in the range of pH between 3 and ~11. Here, the first population was around 20 nm (Figure 4A), while the second population was approximately 200 nm (Figure 4B). When there was pH below ~3, an increase of both size populations was observed, the first one went from ~20 nm to ~600 nm and the second from ~200 to ~6000 nm. Also, the signal intensity of size and polydispersity (Figure 4C,D) in both populations were strongly affected by extreme acidic conditions. In the case of the first population, an increase in signal intensity from ~60% to almost ~95% occurs; here the particles ranging from ~20 nm to ~200 nm possibly corresponds to individual polymer coiled chains that begin to several polymer chains. This result is consistent with the fluorescence studies, using the pyrene probe, where a hydrophobic environment at such pH was observed. In the case second population, a decrease in the signal intensity of size from ~40% to almost ~5% occurs, suggesting the formation of a heterogeneous system like "coarse colloid," with particles ranging from ~200 nm to ~6000 nm. According to the zeta potential measurements (Figure 4E), the expected behavior was observed because PAM18Na is a polyanion the charges of which can be neutralized due to high proton concentration, as reflected in the values of zeta potential.

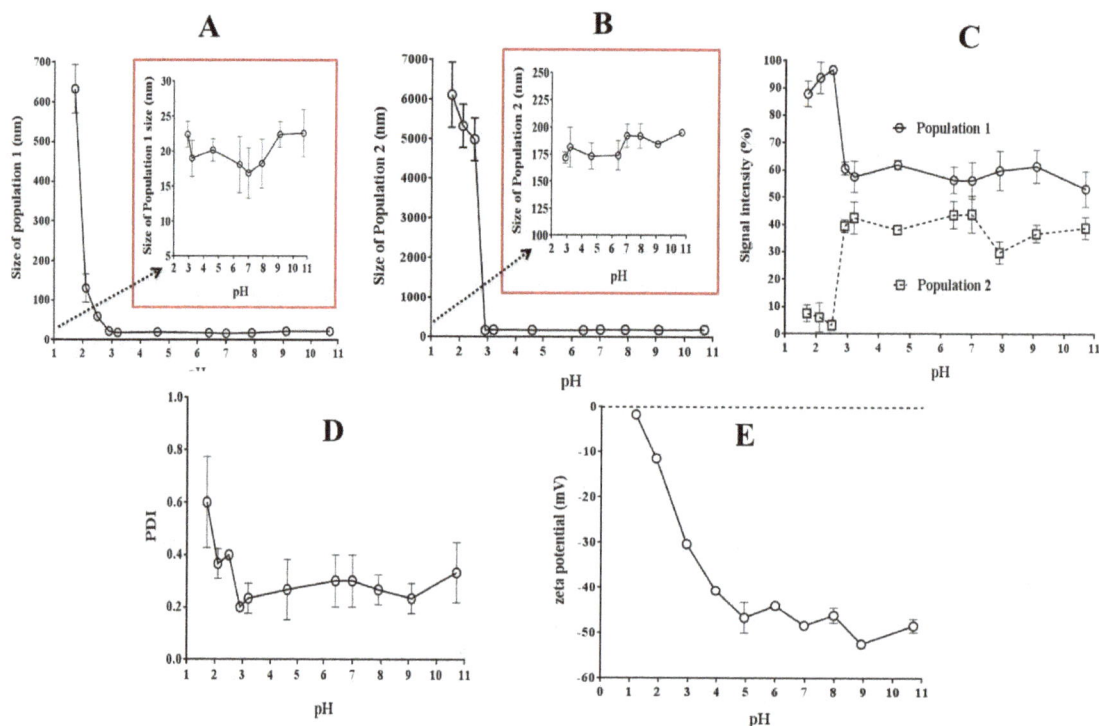

Figure 4. Size, signal intensity, polydispersity (PDI) and zeta potential of PAM-18Na in aqueous media regarding media pH at 25 °C.

On the other hand, the second study was a focus on the characterization of the drug-polymer complex between PAM18-Na and AT in aqueous media at 25 °C and different pH values. The results are shown in Figure 5. The results showed that addition of stoichiometric amounts of AT to the PAM-18Na does not affect either the size or the zeta potential in solution. In fact, for the second population, there is a slight change from ~250nm to ~320 nm. Since no relevant differences on the surface properties of the nanoparticles were observed, it is possible to indicate that the association mechanisms between PAM-18Na and AT were driven by the incorporation of the drug within the hydrophobic core of the nano-aggregate formed by the polymer. This result is a similar phenomenon as solubilization in an inclusion nano-complex.

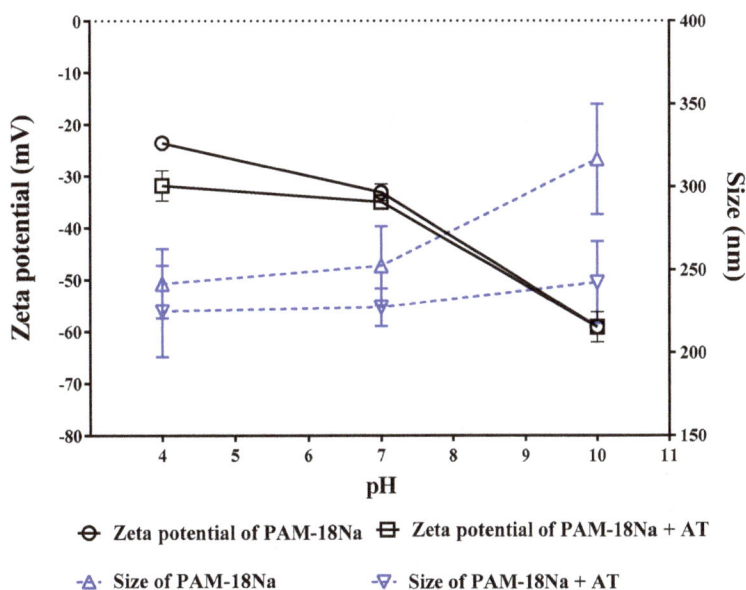

Figure 5. Influence of pH on size and zeta potential values of PAM-18Na in aqueous media in absence and presence of 1:1 molar ratio of Ampicillin Trihydrate at 25 °C.

3.3.4. Viscometric Measurements

The viscometric study of PAM-18Na polymeric solutions in the absence and presence of ampicillin trihydrate at different pH values are shown in Figure 6. In the case of PAM-18Na polymer alone in aqueous media with pH values from 1 to 4, the viscosities varied between 1.31 and 1.41 Cp, whereas at pH values from 4 to 7, viscosity decreased to 0.95 at which point it remained constant. Under acidic conditions, PAM-18Na is practically neutral (zeta potential ~0) forming a heterogeneous system like a coarse colloid, where aggregation is highly favored thermodynamically and thus affecting the fluidity of the dispersion media. Otherwise, at pH values from 4 to 7, the PAM-18Na polymer begins to change from a coarse colloid to a nano-dispersion and at pH above 7, the system turns into the polymer solution, where the aqueous media might flow more smoothly. In the case of the polymer-drug mixture at pH values from 1 to 4, the viscosity is lower than that shown by the PAM-18Na polymer alone. This effect could be due to the AT entails a more structured organization in the system avoiding aggregation among particles in the coarse colloid. In the case of pH values above 7, the system becomes a polymeric solution, where AT might be solubilized into the hydrophobic or adsorbed to the polymer/solvent interface, acting as a cross-linker forming a gel and then increasing the viscosity. These results are consistent with the slight increase in size observed in the second population of particles.

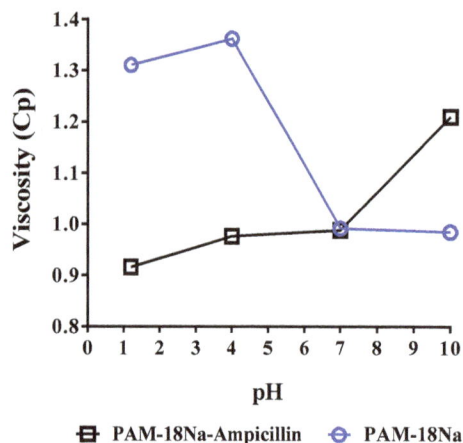

Figure 6. Viscometric Profile of PAM-18 aqueous at different pH in the absence and presence of Ampicillin trihydrate in 1:1 molar ratio at 25 °C.

3.4. Degradation Assays

3.4.1. Chemical Stability

The chemical degradation profile of AT in presence and absence of PAM-18Na polymer, using several initial concentrations of ampicillin to stress conditions are shown in Figure 7. The kinetic analysis of the degradation profiles was analyzed by using an integral method, where each model was fixed to a second-order equation.

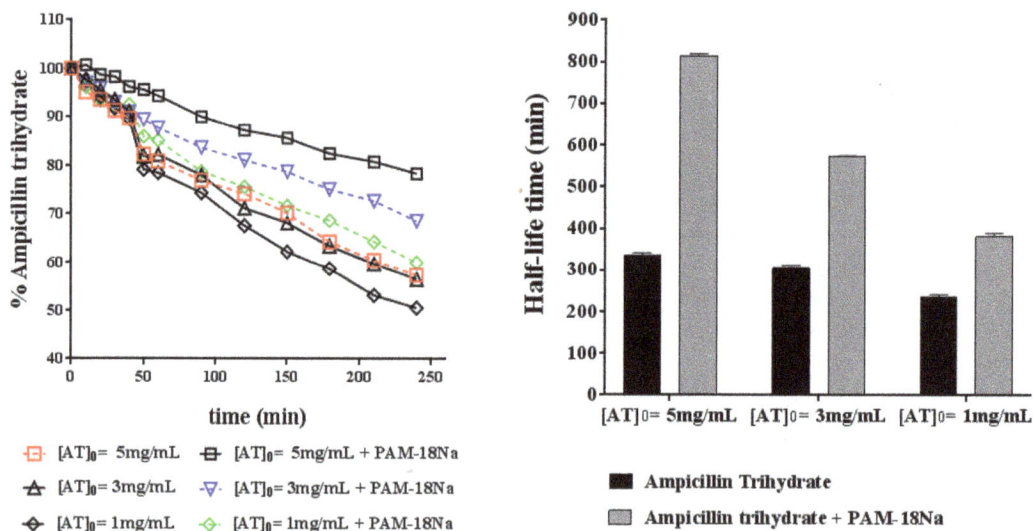

Figure 7. (**Left**) degradation profile of ampicillin trihydrate (AT) at different concentrations under acidic conditions, pH: 1.2 at 40 °C. (**Right**) calculated half-life of AT under same conditions.

The results show that the half-life increases in the presence of PAM-18Na polymer. It is also noted that, as the initial amount of the drug increased, the average half-life time increased, which is a very interesting, because it has been reported that this drug accelerates the hydrolytic degradation concerning its concentration [26]. Therefore, these results suggest that degradation of this drug that is highly susceptible to the acid hydrolysis is avoided by its incorporation into PAM-18Na polymeric nano-aggregates.

3.4.2. β-Lactamase Activity Assay

Based on the previous results suggesting the formation of an inclusion nano-complex between PAM-18Na polymer and AT, the capability of this polymer to protect the antibiotic against the enzymatic activity of a β-Lactamase was tested. The ability of the class C β-Lactamase (obtained from *P. fluorescens*) to hydrolyze ampicillin has been well established [28]. In our study, the β-Lactamase from *P. fluorescens* showed an enzymatic activity of 0.207 ± 0.039 U/mL over the substrate (ampicillin trihydrate). Remarkably, the enzymatic activity significantly decreased to 0.029 ± 0.001 U/mL when the AT was incorporated into the polymer PAM-18Na. This result represents an 86% decrease in the capacity of the β-Lactamase to hydrolyze AT once is encapsulated in PAM-18Na (Figure 8).

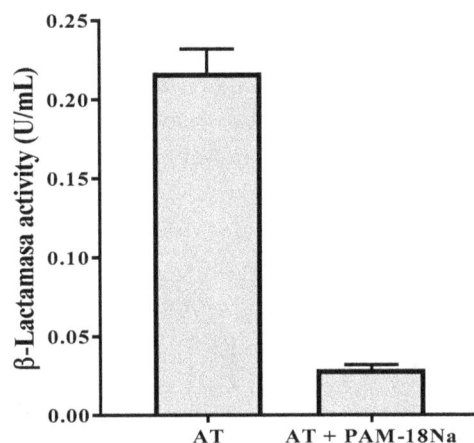

Figure 8. Effect of the polymer PAM-18Na on the activity of the *P. fluorescens* β-lactamase.

3.4.3. Antimicrobial Activity Assays

Strains Characterization

The *S. aureus* strains used in this study were classified as ampicillin resistant or susceptible according to the parameters reported in the M100 guide from the CLSI [36]. According to this guide, a strain is classified as resistant when the diameter of the halo around a 10-µg ampicillin Sensi-Disc is ≤ 28 mm, or sensitive when this width is ≥ 29 mm. Based on the results reported in Table 1, *S. aureus* strain ATCC 25923 is susceptible to ampicillin. Whereas, *S. aureus* strains ATCC 29213 and ATCC 43300 are resistant to the antibiotic.

Table 1. Ampicillin disk diffusion tests for various *S. aureus* strains.

Strain	Average Diameter (mm)	Standard Deviation
S. aureus ATCC 25923 (sensitive)	33.99	0.52
S. aureus ATCC 29213 (resistant)	20.15	0.93
S. aureus ATCC 43300 (resistant)	12.19	0.51

We evaluated the effect of the polymer PAM-18Na on the ampicillin MIC for the three *S. aureus* strains described here. In the case of the sensitive strain, the presence of the polymer did not affect the ampicillin MIC. On the other hand, when PAM-18Na was used in a 1:1 ratio with ampicillin the MIC decreased to 75% for both resistant strains (Figure 9). In all cases, PAM-18Na by itself showed no antibiotic effect up to the maximum concentration evaluated (256 µg/mL).

The ampicillin resistance in the strains evaluated arises mainly from β-Lactamase secretion. Thus, the improvement in antibiotic activity observed for the combination of PAM-18Na and ampicillin can be explained by the capacity of the polymer to interact with the antibiotic and protect it from enzymatic cleavage. Complementary, the ATCC 43300 strain showed a higher ampicillin-PAM-18Na tolerance than that of ATCC 29213. This observation might be a consequence of the second resistance mechanism present in the former strain, which involves penicillin-binding protein modification. In the resistant strains tested the β-Lactamase is secreted by the media. Therefore, PAM-18Na protection is most likely taking place outside the microorganism. Future studies are undertaken to a better understanding of the way the polymer delivers its cargo to complete the picture of pharmacological activity for the PAM-18Na-ampicillin association.

Altogether, the results presented here support the association of the polymer PAM-18Na and ampicillin in solution. Also, they suggest that this polymer can be useful to improve the antibiotic activity of traditional drugs against their resistant bacteria. Similar results, with chemically related polymers, have been reported previously. For example, β–lactam antibiotics in association with polyacrylate nanoparticles [37,38] or vehiculated in liposomes [39,40] showed increased effectiveness against methicillin-resistant *S. aureus* strains. Likewise, ampicillin associated with amphiphilic polymers, made by maleic acid and 2-vinylpyrrolidone, showed a marked increment of the antimicrobial activity of ampicillin on clinical isolates of resistant *S. aureus* [16]. Overall, these results highlight the ability of amphiphilic polymers, like PAM-18Na, to increase the antibiotic effect of ampicillin on resistant bacterial strains.

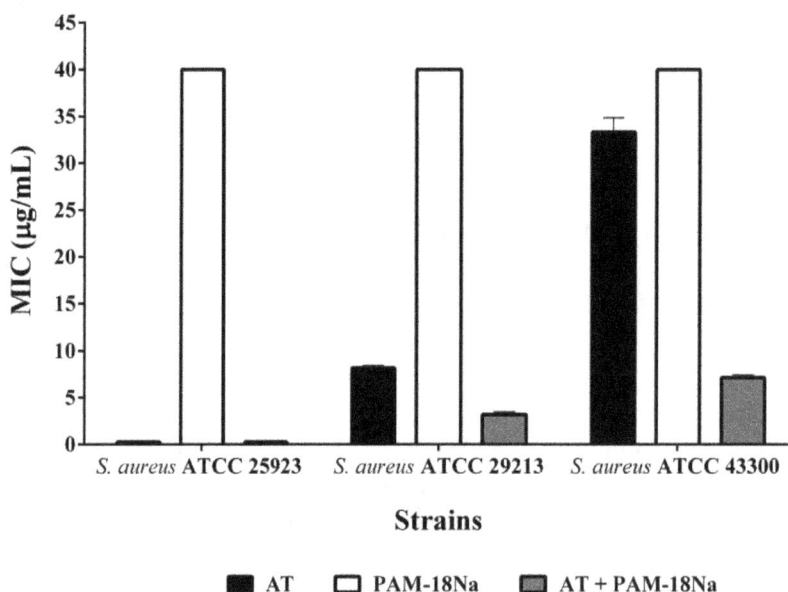

Figure 9. Minimum Inhibitory Concentration (MIC) of ampicillin trihydrate (AT) in the absence and presence of the PAM-18Na polymer in different *S. aureus* Strains.

On the other hand, the high MIC values for PAM-18Na polymer alone, indicate that it has no antimicrobial properties and possibly is a biocompatible material since its chemical characteristics are very similar to others [41,42]. However, this is an effect that will need to be assessed given its potential. Finally, due to the current problem of antimicrobial resistance to antibiotic drugs, the polymer PAM-18Na might be an exciting alternative to improve this effect. Also, it might be a very interesting alternative for those antibiotic β-lactams that are becoming obsolete, where their activity can be enhanced with the development of "smart pharmaceutical formulations."

4. Conclusions

Here we demonstrated the formation of hydrophobic nano-aggregates in aqueous media by PAM-18Na, which could generate nanoparticles as polymeric intra-aggregates that efficiently incorporated ampicillin trihydrate, leading to the loss of organoleptic characteristics, as well as the avoidance of its degradation by: (i) extreme acidic conditions and (ii) several enzyme beta-lactamases. Furthermore, the complex formed has a size of around 200 nm and a slightly negative neutral surface charge. Finally, our results suggest that the polymer PAM-18Na can be a useful alternative to increase the effectiveness of conventional antibiotics against resistant bacterial strains.

Acknowledgments: The authors wish to thank ICESI University for the internal grant 041312, and Tecnoquimicas S.A. for providing the ampicillin material.

Author Contributions: Constain H. Salamanca, Cristhian J. Yarce and Gustavo R. Rivera obtained the polymer and carried out all the physicochemical characterizations, while Yony Roman did the enzymatic assay and Andrés F. Davalos performed the entire microbiological test.

References

1. Fauci, A.; Marston, H. The Perpetual Challenge of Antimicrobial Resistance. *J. Am. Med. Assoc.* **2014**, *311*, 1853–1854. [CrossRef] [PubMed]

2. Alanis, A.J. Resistance to Antibiotics: Are We in the Post-Antibiotic Era? *Arch. Med. Res.* **2005**, *36*, 697–705. [CrossRef] [PubMed]

3. Demain, A.; Sanchez, S. Microbial drug discovery: 80 Years of progress. *J. Antibiot.* **2009**, *62*, 5–16. [CrossRef] [PubMed]

4. Katz, M.; Mueller, L.; Polyakov, M.; Weinstock, S. Where have all the antibiotic patents gone. *Nat. Biotechnol.* **2006**, *24*, 1529–1531. [CrossRef] [PubMed]

5. Naber, C.K. *Staphylococcus aureus* bacteremia: Epidemiology, pathophysiology, and management strategies. *Clin. Infect. Dis. Oxf. J.* **2009**, *48*, S231–S237. [CrossRef] [PubMed]

6. Valaperta, R.; Tejada, M.; Frigerio, M. *Staphylococcus aureus* nosocomial infections: The role of a rapid and low-cost characterization for the establishment of a surveillance system. *New Microbiol.* **2010**, *33*, 223–232. [PubMed]

7. Stratton, C.W. The clinical implications of ß-lactamases. *Antimicrob. Infect. Dis. Newsl.* **1996**, *15*, 67–72. [CrossRef]

8. Mediavilla, J.R.; Chen, L.; Mathema, B.; Kreiswirth, B.N. Global epidemiology of community-associated methicillin resistant *Staphylococcus aureus* (CA-MRSA). *Curr. Opin. Microbiol.* **2012**, *15*, 588–595. [CrossRef] [PubMed]

9. Enright, M.C.; Robinson, D.A.; Randle, G.; Feil, E.J.; Grundmann, H.; Spratt, B.G. The evolutionary history of methicillin-resistant *Staphylococcus aureus* (MRSA). *Proc. Natl. Acad. Sci. USA* **2002**, *99*, 7687–7692. [CrossRef] [PubMed]

10. Grema, H.A. Methicillin Resistant *Staphylococcus aureus* (MRSA): A Review. *Adv. Anim. Vet. Sci.* **2015**, *3*, 79–98. [CrossRef]

11. Papp-Wallace, K.M.; Bethel, C.R.; Gootz, T.D.; Shang, W.; Stroh, J.; Lau, W.; McLeod, D.; Price, L.; Marfat, A.; Distler, A.; et al. Inactivation of a class A and a class C β-lactamase by 6β-(hydroxymethyl)penicillanic acid sulfone. *Biochem. Pharmacol.* **2012**, *83*, 462–471. [CrossRef] [PubMed]

12. Fast, W.; Sutton, L.D. Metallo-β-lactamase: Inhibitors and reporter substrates. *Biochim. Biophys. Acta Proteins Proteom.* **2013**, *1834*, 1648–1659. [CrossRef] [PubMed]

13. Zeng, X.; Lin, J. Beta-lactamase induction and cell wall metabolism in Gram-negative bacteria. *Front. Microbiol.* **2013**, *4*, 128. [CrossRef] [PubMed]

14. Stubbs, K.; Balcewich, M.; Mark, B.; Vocadlo, D. Small molecule inhibitors of a glycoside hydrolase attenuate inducible AmpC-mediated beta-lactam resistance. *J. Biol. Chem.* **2007**, *282*, 21382–21391. [CrossRef] [PubMed]

15. Kalhapure, R.S.; Suleman, N.; Mocktar, C.; Seedat, N.; Govender, T. Nanoengineered drug delivery systems for enhancing antibiotic therapy. *J. Pharm. Sci.* **2015**, *104*, 872–905. [CrossRef] [PubMed]

16. Arenas, T.; Mora, C.; Salamanca, C.H.; Jaramillo, M.C. Actividad del (2E)-3-(2, 3-dimetoxifenil)-1-(4-metilfenil) prop-2-en-1-ona en presencia del poli(ácido maleico-co-2-vinil-pirrolidona) sobre un aislamiento clínico de *Staphylococcus aureus* productor de β-lactamasas. *Iatreia* **2012**, *25*, 12–19.

17. Xiong, M.H.; Bao, Y.; Yang, X.Z.; Zhu, Y.H.; Wang, J. Delivery of antibiotics with polymeric particles. *Adv. Drug Deliv. Rev.* **2014**, *78*, 63–76. [CrossRef] [PubMed]

18. Bezzaoucha, F.; Lochon, P.; Jonquières, A.; Fischer, A.; Brembilla, A.; Aïnad-Tabet, D. New amphiphilic polyacrylamides: Synthesis and characterisation of pseudo-micellar organisation in aqueous media. *Eur. Polym. J.* **2007**, *43*, 4440–4452. [CrossRef]

19. Salamanca, C.; Urbano, B.; Olea, A.F. Potential drug delivery system: Study of the association of a model nitroimidazole drug with aggregates of amphiphilic polymers on aqueous solution. *Braz. J. Pharm. Sci.* **2011**, *47*, 6. [CrossRef]

20. Wang, Y.; Grayson, S.M. Approaches for the preparation of non-linear amphiphilic polymers and their applications to drug delivery. *Adv. Drug Deliv. Rev.* **2012**, *64*, 852–865. [CrossRef] [PubMed]

21. Barraza, R.G.; Olea, A.F.; Valdebenito, C.E.; Dougnac, V.; Fuentes, I. Solubilization of p-nitrophenol in aggregates formed by hydrophobically modified polyelectrolytes. *J. Colloid Interface Sci.* **2004**, *275*, 434–438. [CrossRef] [PubMed]

22. Salamanca, C.; Barraza, R.G.; Acevedo, B.; Olea, A.F. Hydrophobically modified polyelectrolytes as potential drugs reservoirs of N-alkyl-nitroimidazoles. *J. Chil. Chem. Soc.* **2007**, *52*. [CrossRef]

23. Anton, P.; Laschewsky, A. Solubilization by polysoaps. *Colloid Polym. Sci.* **1994**, *272*, 1118–1128. [CrossRef]

24. Bayoudh, S.; Laschewsky, A.; Wischerhoff, E. Amphiphilic hyperbranched polyelectrolytes: A new type of polysoap. *Colloid Polym. Sci.* **1999**, *277*, 519–527. [CrossRef]

25. Olea, A.F.; Barraza, R.; Fuentes, I.; Acevedo, B. Solubilization of Phenols by Intramolecular Micelles Formed by Copolymers of Maleic Acid and Olefins. *Macromolecules* **2002**, *35*, 1049–1053. [CrossRef]

26. Mitchell, S.M.; Ullman, J.L.; Teel, A.L.; Watts, R.J. PH and temperature effects on the hydrolysis of three β-lactam antibiotics: Ampicillin, cefalotin and cefoxitin. *Sci. Total Environ.* **2014**, *466–467*, 547–555. [CrossRef] [PubMed]

27. Galleni, M.; Frere, J. A survey of the kinetic parameters of class C beta-lactamases. Penicillins. *Biochem. J.* **1988**, *255*, 119–122. [CrossRef] [PubMed]

28. Michaux, C.; Massant, J.; Kerff, F. Crystal structure of a cold-adapted class C β-lactamase. *FEBS J.* **2012**, *275*, 1687–1697. [CrossRef] [PubMed]

29. Clinical and Laboratory Standards Institute. *M02-A11. Performance Standards for Antimicrobial Disk Susceptibility Tests*; Clinical and Laboratory Standards Institute: Wayne, PA, USA, 2012.

30. Marshall, S.A.; Sutton, L.D.; Jones, R.N. Evaluation of S1 chromogenic cephalosporin??-lactamase disk assay tested against Gram-positive anaerobes, coagulase-negative staphylococci, *Prevotella* spp. and *Enterococcus* spp. *Diagn. Microbiol. Infect. Dis.* **1995**, *22*, 353–355. [CrossRef]

31. Yu, S.; Vosbeek, A.; Corbella, K.; Severson, J.; Schesser, J.; Sutton, L.D. A chromogenic cephalosporin for β-lactamase inhibitor screening assays. *Anal. Biochem.* **2012**, *428*, 96–98. [CrossRef] [PubMed]

32. Clinical and Laboratory Standards Institute. *M07-A9. Methods for Dilution Antimicrobial Susceptibility Tests for Bacteria That Grow Aerobically*; Clinical and Laboratory Standards Institute: Wayne, PA, USA, 2012; Volume 32.

33. Kalyanasundaram, K.; Thomas, J.K. Environmental effects on vibronic band intensities in pyrene monomer fluorescence and their application in studies of micellar systems. *J. Am. Chem. Soc.* **1977**, *99*, 2039–2044. [CrossRef]

34. W. Binana-Limbele, R.Z. Fluorescence probing of microdomains in aqueous solutions of polysoaps. 1. Use of pyrene to study the conformational state of polysoaps and their comicellization with cationic surfactants. *Macromolecules* **1987**, *20*, 1331–1335. [CrossRef]

35. Salamanca, C.H.; Castillo, D.F.; Villada, J.D.; Rivera, G.R. Physicochemical characterization of in situ drug-polymer nanocomplex formed between zwitterionic drug and ionomeric material in aqueous solution. *Mater. Sci. Eng. C* **2017**, *72*. [CrossRef] [PubMed]

36. Clinical and Laboratory Standards Institute. *CLSI Document M100-S24. Performance Standards for Antimicrobial Susceptibility Testing*; Clinical and Laboratory Standards Institute: Wayne, PA, USA, 2012.

37. Turos, E.; Reddy, G.; Greenhalgh, K. Penicillin-Bound Polyacrylate Nanoparticles: Restoring the Activity of β-Lactam Antibiotics Against MRSA. *Bioorg. Med. Chem. Lett.* **2007**, *17*, 3468–3472. [CrossRef] [PubMed]

38. Turos, E.; Shim, J.-Y.; Wang, Y.; Greenhalgh, K.; Reddy, G.S.K.; Dickey, S.; Lim, D.V. Antibiotic-conjugated

polyacrylate nanoparticles: New opportunities for development of anti-MRSA agents. *Bioorg. Med. Chem. Lett.* **2007**, *17*, 53–56. [CrossRef] [PubMed]

39. Colzi, I.; Troyan, A.N.; Perito, B.; Casalone, E.; Romoli, R.; Pieraccini, G.; Škalko-Basnet, N.; Adessi, A.; Rossi, F.; Gonnelli, C.; et al. Antibiotic delivery by liposomes from prokaryotic microorganisms: Similia cum similis works better. *Eur. J. Pharm. Biopharm.* **2015**, *94*, 411–418. [CrossRef] [PubMed]

40. Muppidi, K.; Pumerantz, A.; Wang, J.; Betageri, G. Development and stability studies of novel liposomal vancomycin formulations. *Arch. ISRN Pharm.* **2012**, *2012*, 636743. [CrossRef] [PubMed]

41. Salvage, J.P.; Rose, S.F.; Phillips, G.J.; Hanlon, G.W.; Lloyd, A.W.; Ma, I.Y.; Armes, S.P.; Billingham, N.C.; Lewis, A.L. Novel biocompatible phosphorylcholine-based self-assembled nanoparticles for drug delivery. *J. Control. Release* **2005**, *104*, 259–270. [CrossRef] [PubMed]

42. Ma, Y.; Tang, Y.; Billingham, N.C.; Armes, S.P. Synthesis of Biocompatible, Stimuli-Responsive, Physical Gels Based on ABA Triblock Copolymers. *Biomacromolecules* **2003**, *4*, 864–868. [CrossRef] [PubMed]

7

Role of Microbiota and Tryptophan Metabolites in the Remote Effect of Intestinal Inflammation on Brain and Depression

Barbora Waclawiková and Sahar El Aidy * ⓘ

Department of Molecular Immunology and Microbiology, Groningen Biomolecular Sciences and Biotechnology Institute (GBB), University of Groningen, Nijenborgh 7, 9747 AG Groningen, The Netherlands;
b.waclawikova@rug.nl
* Correspondence: sahar.elaidy@rug.nl

Abstract: The human gastrointestinal tract is inhabited by trillions of commensal bacteria collectively known as the gut microbiota. Our recognition of the significance of the complex interaction between the microbiota, and its host has grown dramatically over the past years. A balanced microbial community is a key regulator of the immune response, and metabolism of dietary components, which in turn, modulates several brain processes impacting mood and behavior. Consequently, it is likely that disruptions within the composition of the microbiota would remotely affect the mental state of the host. Here, we discuss how intestinal bacteria and their metabolites can orchestrate gut-associated neuroimmune mechanisms that influence mood and behavior leading to depression. In particular, we focus on microbiota-triggered gut inflammation and its implications in shifting the tryptophan metabolism towards kynurenine biosynthesis while disrupting the serotonergic signaling. We further investigate the gaps to be bridged in this exciting field of research in order to clarify our understanding of the multifaceted crosstalk in the microbiota–gut–brain interphase, bringing about novel, microbiota-targeted therapeutics for mental illnesses.

Keywords: microbiota; kynurenine pathway; serotonin; inflammation; gut motility

1. Introduction

The complex communities of the microbiota that inhabit the mammalian gut have a significant impact on the health of their host. These gut bacteria has coevolved with the human body to perform numerous beneficial functions ranging from being simple fermenters of food to having profound effects on the host immune development, metabolism and food preferences, brain development, stress responses, pain, and behavior [1–5]. Consequently, disruptions or alterations in this resilient relationship are a significant factor in many diseases such as inflammatory gastrointestinal diseases and neuropsychiatric disorders, including depression [1,6–8].

Depression is a severe neuropsychiatric disease with multiple comorbidities in play. According to the World Health Organization (WHO), this longstanding mental disorder affects more than 300 million people of all ages worldwide [9]. Moreover, it is the leading cause of disability in modern society, and approximately one million people suffering from depression commit suicide every year [9]. It is widely recognized now that depression is closely linked with inflammation, and disrupted serotonergic systems throughout the human body, including the gut [10–16]. In fact, in a state of inflammation, not only high levels of proinflammatory cytokines are produced but also altered levels of neurotransmitters, such as serotonin, a derivative of tryptophan metabolism, are detected in the gut [17–19]. The presence of vast majority of bodily serotonin and immune cells in the gut in close proximity to the trillion of the gut-associated microbes implies the gut microbiota is likely to be an orchestrator in this multifaceted crosstalk between inflammation, serotonin, and depression, as will be discussed in this review article.

2. Gastrointestinal Inflammation and Depression

In a state of intestinal inflammation, the immune system responds by producing various proinflammatory cytokines and metabolites, several of which are detected in the systemic blood circulation [20]. The fact that these molecules can cross the blood–brain barrier suggests that they can signal to the brain to ultimately result in serious changes in behavior [21]. Several routes, by which cytokines and metabolites present in the gut can influence the brain and behavior, have been described; (1) neural, (2) humoral, (3) cellular, and (4) carrier route [22] (Figure 1A). In the neural route, afferent nerves, such as the vagus nerve, are involved. Vagal nerves are activated by proinflammatory cytokines and other metabolites released by immune cells, neurons or intestinal bacteria during intestinal inflammation or infections [23] (Figure 1A$_a$). This cascade leads to activation of the hypothalamus–pituitary–adrenal axis, thus increased levels of cortisol (stress hormone) and decreased levels of brain-derived neurotrophic factor [21]. The humoral route involves signaling via the circumventricular organs (CVOs), which have been described as a way by which leukocytes can reach the central nervous system [24]. CVOs are areas in the brain that lack an intact blood–brain barrier, thus allow molecules with limited access to the brain to migrate [25] (Figure 1A$_b$). The carrier route includes cytokine transporters at the blood–brain barrier, where circulating cytokines can access the brain via the energy- and carrier-dependent active transport system or via no energy-dependent carrier-mediated facilitated diffusion system, commonly called saturable transport systems [26] (Figure 1A$_c$). Finally, the cellular route involves cytokine receptors, such as receptors for tumor necrosis factor α (TNF-α) and interleukin (IL)-1β, expressed on non-neuronal cells in the brain, such as microglia and astrocytes [27–29]. Binding of TNF-α and IL-1β to their receptors in the brain activates cerebral NF-κB signaling pathway and induces the production of secondary cytokines, which can promote a depressed mood [29,30] (Figure 1A$_d$). Indeed, proinflammatory cytokines, such as interferon-γ (IFN-γ), IL-2, TNF-α, and inflammatory markers such as C reactive protein (CRP), have been linked to higher risk of depression [31,32]. All together, these pathways show a number of sophisticated signaling mechanisms in the brain, which when stimulated by molecules produced during intestinal inflammation could lead to altered brain functionality, potentially leading to progression of depression.

2.1. A Gut Perspective on the Role of Tryptophan Metabolites in Depression

Tryptophan is an essential amino acid, derived from the diet [33]. Apart from its role in protein synthesis, tryptophan and its metabolites are associated with numerous physiological functions, such as immune homeostasis, but also with inflammatory response [34]. Once absorbed in the gut, tryptophan can cross the blood–brain barrier to participate in serotonin synthesis [35]. However, there are many other pathways through which tryptophan can be readily metabolized in the gut, thereby influencing its availability to pass the blood–brain barrier. Among these pathways are the kynurenine [36] and the serotonin synthesis pathways within the gut [37,38]. Kynurenine and serotonin are vital signaling molecules in immune response and gut–brain communication [34,39,40]. Most of the digested tryptophan (about 90%) is metabolized along the kynurenine biosynthesis pathways [41], while only approximately 3% is metabolized into serotonin throughout the body, and the rest is degraded by the gut microbiota to produce indole and its derivatives [42]. This implies a strong competition between serotonin and the first downstream metabolites from the kynurenine pathway, kynurenine, for the available tryptophan, as described below. In inflammatory conditions, more kynurenine is produced on the expenses of serotonin [43,44], which, if happens also in the brain, results in behavioral changes including persistent sadness, loss of interest, and decreased energy levels [45] (Figure 1A).

2.2. Gut Inflammation-Induced Kynurenine Biosynthesis; Possible Cause of Altered Kynurenine Pathway in the Brain during Depression?

Tryptophan forms kynurenine via the rate-limiting enzyme, indoleamine-2,3-dioxygenase (IDO) enzyme, found ubiquitously in all tissues, including the gut, and tryptophan-2,3-dioxygenase (TDO), which is localized in the liver [41]. The activity of TDO and IDO is uniquely induced by different stimuli; while TDO is induced by stress-elevated glucocorticoids, such as cortisol [46], IDO is induced during intestinal inflammation [47] by proinflammatory stimuli, with interferon γ (IFN-γ) being the most potent inducer [48]. Induction of IDO results in a shift in the tryptophan metabolism towards the production of kynurenine and its downstream metabolites; kynurenic acid, anthranilic acid, and quinolinic acid rather than serotonin synthesis [47,49] (Figure 1A,B). Moreover, activated IDO accelerates the degradation of serotonin into formyl-5-hydroxykynuramine [50,51]. Degradation of serotonin yields reactive oxygen species byproducts and subsequently inflammation [52]. This further intensifies serotonin deficiency, leading to the disruption in neurotransmission and consequently causes depression.

In contrast to kynurenic acid and quinolinic acid, kynurenine and anthranilic acid can cross the blood–brain barrier via the saturable transfer [53]. This suggests that inflammatory-induced altered levels of kynurenine in the gut may transfer to the blood circulation and ultimately to the brain, resulting in altered levels of kynurenine and its metabolites, kynurenic acid, and quinolinic acid (Figure 1A). In fact, during inflammation, the enzymes of the kynurenine pathway are activated leading to changed production of kynurenic and quinolinic acids. Depression is believed to arise from the excessive production of the neurotoxic quinolinic acid together with a reduction in kynurenic acid [54]. Reduced levels of kynurenic acid have been correlated with severe depressive and suicidal symptoms [55,56], and decreased blood levels of this molecule has been detected in the patients with major depressive disorder [57]. Quinolinic acid is a neurotoxic agent, and its production is significantly enhanced by proinflammatory cytokines through their stimulation of the rate limiting step enzyme in the quinolinic acid pathway, kynurenine-3-monooxygenase (KMO) enzyme [58,59]. For instance, levels of quinolinic acid in the cerebrospinal fluids of suicide attempters showed around 300% increase compared to healthy controls [60]. In the brain, quinolinic acid acts as an agonist of *N*-methyl-D-aspartate (NMDA) receptors, which play a key role in the regulation of synaptic function [61]. Activation of NMDA receptors upon binding to quinolinic acid has been described to be another mechanism involved in promotion of depression [49]. Specifically, when microglia are stimulated by proinflammatory cytokines, glutamate, another agonist of NMDA receptors, and the main excitatory neurotransmitter in the central nervous system, is released leading to additional activation of NMDA receptors [61]. Therefore, quinolinic acid alone or in combination with glutamate, can enhance NMDA receptor activation and subsequently lead to depression [49]. Intriguingly, a high proportion of the enteric neurons in the gut express the NMDA-type glutamate receptors [62,63]. In line with these observations, previous data have suggested that enhanced activation of NMDA receptors maybe involved in altered inflammation-linked motility and in inflammatory-induced nociception [64,65] as a remote consequence of intestinal inflammation on the brain [66] (Figure 1B). In contrast to quinolinic acid, kynurenic acid is an indigenous antagonist of the enteric NMDA receptors, thereby suppressing the hypermobility of the gut associated with the activated NMDA receptors and excitability of the enteric neurons during an intestinal inflammatory response. Collectively, the current data support an effect of intestinal inflammation on redirecting the tryptophan metabolic pathway towards kynurenine rather that serotonin biosynthesis. Kynurenine metabolites have a profound effect on the enteric nervous system and intestinal motility alteration. Whether altered gut motility can stimulate a state of depression and whether changes in intestinal kynurenine metabolism could be the source of altered levels of these metabolites in the brain, warrant more investigation.

2.3. Intestinal Inflammation and Disrupted Serotonin Signaling System: From Altered Gut Functionality to Development of Depression

Serotonin is a key-signaling regulator that modulates a wide range of effects on host physiology, including the control of gut motility, secretory reflexes, platelet aggregation, regulation of immune responses, and regulation of mood and behavior [67]. Once tryptophan is absorbed in the gut, it crosses the blood–brain barrier to be partially metabolized into serotonin in the raphe nuclei within the brain stem [34]. However, the majority (~95%) of serotonin in the body is synthesized, stored, and released in the gut, mainly from a subset of enteroendocrine cells called enterochromaffin cells in the intestinal mucosa [19]. The small amount of serotonin that is not in enterochromaffin cells is in the enteric nervous system, in particular, the myenteric plexus, which contains descending serotonergic interneurons [68] (Figure 1B).

Enterochromaffin cells, also known as epithelial sensory transducers, secrete serotonin in response to mucosal stimuli, such as microbiota metabolites as discussed below. Once synthesized, serotonin is secreted in the lamina propria, where it has access to the nerve fibers. This implies a large amount of serotonin is secreted in the extracellular space. Thus, to avoid receptors' desensitization by their contact with excessive amounts of serotonin, which is toxic [69], serotonin overflow must be efficiently controlled. One important player in serotonin uptake by gut epithelial cells, thus serotonergic termination, is the Na^+/Cl^- dependent, serotonin transporter (SERT). SERT, is a recently crystallized protein [70] comprised of 12 transmembrane domains, and is a member of a large superfamily of sodium/chloride dependent transporters, which also contain transporters for other neurotransmitters, such as dopamine and norepinephrine [71].

Secreted serotonin mediates its actions via several receptor subtypes [72], where it has been observed to affect epithelial cells' proliferation and secretion [73], but mainly acts as a regulator of the gut motility. Secretion of serotonin by enterochromaffin cells activates intrinsic primary afferent neurons (IPANs) in the submucosal plexus via its action on $5\text{-}HT_{1P}$ receptor. These cells initiate peristaltic and secretory reflexes, which influences gut motility (Figure 1C). Moreover, intestinal serotonin activates extrinsic sensory nerves via its action on $5\text{-}HT_3$, which are postsynaptic receptors found on the terminals of extrinsic sensory neurons terminal in the gut and transmit noxious signals to the brain [74] (Figure 1B). Though it does not initiate peristaltic movement, $5\text{-}HT_3$ conveys any kind of change in gut motility to the brain via its presence on myenteric IPANs and in the myenteric plexus, where they mediate fast excitatory neurotransmission [75]. Similarly, $5\text{-}HT_4$ receptors themselves do not initiate peristaltic reflexes, but because of their location at the terminals of submucosal IPANs, at synapses within the myenteric plexus, and at the neuromuscular junction, stimulation of $5\text{-}HT_4$ receptors is critical for these reflexes [76]. $5\text{-}HT_4$ receptors work through stimulating the production of the neurotransmitters acetylcholine and calcitonin gene-related peptide, which enhances the spread of stimuli around and through the gut wall, to ultimately enhance and maintain a normal gut motility [77,78].

The strong link between inflammation, and disruptions of serotonin metabolism has been well established. Immune cells including lymphocytes, mast cells, dendritic cells and monocytes have all been reported to express SERT, serotonin receptors and enzymes involved in the production and metabolism of serotonin [79,80] (Figure 1C). T lymphocytes express the main components of serotonin metabolism, i.e., tryptophan hydroxylase (TPH), the first rate limiting enzyme involved in serotonin production, SERT, monoamine oxidase (MAO) [80], which breaks down serotonin into its metabolite 5-HIAA, and 5-HT receptors [80]. While resting, naïve T cells express very little TPH1, the TPH isoform present in the intestinal enterochromaffin cells, where intestinal serotonin is synthesized, activated T cells show approximately 30-fold higher expression of TPH1, suggesting increased levels of serotonin in activated T cells [81], and 5-HT receptors, including $5\text{-}HT_{1B}$, $5\text{-}HT_{2A}$, and $5\text{-}HT_7$ receptors [81]. However, expression of SERT in T cells is still questionable; León-Ponte et al. shows that neither naïve nor activated T cells express high-affinity SERT [81], however another study claims that SERT is present in T cells membranes [82] (Figure 1C). Thus, these contradictory conclusions warrant further investigation. B lymphocytes are also known to express 5-HT receptors, including

5-HT$_{1A}$, 5-HT$_{2A}$, 5-HT$_{3A}$ and 5-HT$_7$ [80], and activated B cells exhibit a significant increase in SERT expression [83] (Figure 1C). Whether B cells express other components of serotonin machinery and thus influencing serotonin signaling, it is still unknown. Like T cells, monocytes, the immature leukocytes that eventually differentiate into macrophages or dendritic cells, express the complete set of components needed for serotonin production [80]. Dendritic cells, have also been found to mediate the release of proinflammatory cytokines, IL-1β and IL-8 via 5-HT$_3$, 5-HT$_4$, and 5-HT$_7$ receptor subtypes [84]. In fact, serotonin has been demonstrated as an important regulator of the immune system. For example, serotonin has been described to modulate proinflammatory cytokines production in human monocytes via stimulation of different 5-HT receptor subtypes, particularly 5-HT$_3$, 5-HT$_4$, and 5-HT$_7$ receptors [85] (Figure 1C). Interestingly, deletion of 5-HT$_4$ receptors in mice results in inflammatory response, slowed colonic motility, and behavioral abnormalities [86,87]. Similarly, reduced expression of SERT and subsequent altered serotonin levels, have been associated with different inflammatory and diarrheal disorders [15,16,88]. Targeted deletion of the SERT in mice led to increased colonic motility and increased water in stools [89] in a similar manner to that observed in inflammatory bowel disorders, where SERT expression is also reduced [18,90]. That the altered structure or expression of SERT leads to disrupted serotonin transmission [91], the current data point to a strong link between intestinal inflammation, disruption of serotonin signaling and the consequent alteration in gut motility, and development of depression. Whether the altered gut motility [14,16,88,89,92,93] is the driving factor in inducting depression in this cascade is unclear. One plausible mechanism is via the gut motility-mediated changes in the microbial population complexity, which might exert detrimental effects on enteric and central neurons leading to a state of depression.

3. Microbiota as an Orchestrator in the Crosstalk between Inflammation and Serotonin Imbalances

The presence of vast number of gut microbiota in close proximity to serotonin and immune cells in the gut, makes it plausible to consider these bacteria as a conductor in the orchestra of intestinal inflammation and serotonin, to remotely result in a state of altered mood and depression in the brain (Figure 1).

3.1. Gut Microbiota and Intestinal Immune (Hyper)-Stimulation

It is well-established that the gut microbiota plays a critical role in both innate and adaptive immunity, where it mediates the formation, maturation, and function of several immune cells [94]. Interactions between the gut bacteria and gut mucosa regulate the production of numerous proinflammatory cytokines [95–97]. Several species within the gut bacteria have been shown to be essential in the development and maturation of the immune response. For example, a monocolonization of germ-free mice with the ubiquitous gut bacterium, *Bacteroides fragilis*, shows immunomodulatory activities of this bacterium, including correction of T cell deficiencies and T$_H$1/T$_H$2 imbalances [98]. Segmented filamentous bacteria, the epithelial-associated bacteria, stimulate the maturation of proinflammatory IL-17A-producing T helper 17 (T$_H$17) cells in the mouse small intestine [99,100]. Though considered as commensals, these bacteria have pathogenic properties and are referred to as pathobionts due to their capacity to induce a profound inflammatory state if an imbalance within the microbial population (also known as dysbiosis) occurs [101]. Microbial dysbiosis has been strongly linked to inflammatory bowel disease, a comorbidity of anxiety and depression [102]. Increased relative abundance of *Escherichia coli* and *Enterococcus faecalis* have been described to induce intestinal inflammation and bacterial-antigen specific cytokine production (IFN-γ and IL-4) in a well-characterized murine colitis model *IL10$^{-/-}$* [103]. Several *Bacteroides* genera have been recognized to be important for induction of inflammatory bowel disease in *IL-10r2$^{-/-}$ × Tgfbr2$^{-/-}$* mouse colitis model [104]. *Klebsiella pneumoniae* and *Proteus mirabilis*, has been positively correlated with colitis in *Tbx21$^{-/-}$ × Rag2$^{-/-}$* mouse inflammatory bowel disease model [105]. A common resident of the human mouth and gut, *Fusobacterium nucleatum*, when isolated from the inflamed gut of Crohn's disease patients evoked significantly greater TNF-α gene expression [106]. Finally, in experimental autoimmune encephalomyelitis, a mouse model of multiple sclerosis, germ-free or antibiotic-treated mice exhibited reduced inflammation and disease scores compared to conventional mice, suggesting a role for gut microbes on peripheral immune response, leading to brain inflammation [107,108]. Overall, these data suggest gut microbiota as an important immunomodulatory player in the gut–inflammation–brain crosstalk (Figure 1D).

3.2. Gut Microbiota and Serotonin Production

Recently, it has been shown that gut microbiota plays an important role in the regulation of the host serotonin levels [109]. Particular microbial metabolites, namely short chain fatty acids, have been shown to promote serotonin production from enterochromaffin cells in the epithelia via induction of TPH1 gene expression [109,110] (Figure 1D), most likely, due to their acidic pH. The effect of gut microbiota on intestinal serotonin levels expands beyond the gut. Plasma serotonin levels were in germ-free mice compared to conventional mice [111]. On the other hand, levels of hippocampal serotonin were significantly increased in germ-free and colonized germ-free mice compared to conventional mice [112]. However, a causation of differences in serotonin levels in germ-free mice still needs to be explained. Yano et al., further showed that SERT expression is increased in germ-free mice, suggesting its regulation by gut microbiota [109]. Indeed, SERT genotype has been linked to altered gut microbiota composition in young rats [88], where SERT knock out rats showed imbalanced microbial community dominated by members of the gut microbiota previously reported to be associated with a state of intestinal inflammation, and brain disorders including multiple depressive disorders [106,113–118]. Of note, the observed microbial imbalance was magnified when young rats were exposed to another stimulus, maternal separation [88], implying that the absence or domination of certain bacterial members in the gut of early-life stressed individuals may represent risk factors for the development of depression during later life stages.

Gut produced serotonin has been the target of several antidepressants, such as fluoxetine, which block its transport into the plasma via targeting SERT, thus named selective serotonin reuptake inhibitors (SSRIs). Administration of these antidepressants has been also successfully used as a treatment for gastrointestinal diseases, such as motility disorder and gastrointestinal bleeding [92,119], confirming comorbidity of these disorders, but exert a puzzling effect on the intestinal bacterial composition. Fluoxetine has an antimicrobial activity against Gram-positive bacteria such as *Staphylococcus* and *Enterococcus* and some anaerobic bacteria such as *Clostridium difficile* and *Clostridium perfringens* [3,120–122]. Similarly, Gram-negative bacteria such as *Citrobacter* spp., *Pseudomonas aeruginosa*, *Klebsiella pneumoniae* and *Morganella morganii* have been proven to be susceptible to SSRIs [120,123]. Notably, most of these bacteria are key players in induction of inflammation in the gut [99,100,103–108]. This suggests that through their antimicrobial activity, antidepressants might restore a balanced composition of the gut microbiota, and immune response, hence re-establish homeostasis at the gut–brain interphase. Deciphering the actual contribution of the antimicrobial effects of antidepressants for treatment of depression as well as determining the long-term consequences of these effects to gut microbiota composition and their implications to clinical outcomes is crucial for the development of microbiota derived therapeutic alternatives [3,8,120,123].

Taken together, game-changing science is suggesting that depression is not only a result of a deficiency of serotonin and other neurotransmitters in the brain, but could rather start in the gut, via changing the microbiota composition through consumption of processed, nutrient poor diet, which in turn, leads to a state of inflammation, imbalanced levels of neurotransmitters, and eventually depression.

3.3. The Dual Effect of Gut Microbiota and Its Metabolites in Depression

Recently, changes in the composition of the gut microbiota have been associated with depressive-like behavior in humans and animal models [124,125]. Decreased levels of bacterial genera

Bifidobacterium and *Lactobacillus* and increased levels of Streptococcaceae, Clostridiales, Eubacteriaceae and Ruminococcaceae, have been positively correlated with depressive symptoms [124,126]. Kelly et al. have shown that fecal microbiota transplantation from depressed patients to microbiota-depleted rats induced behavioral and physiological changes, leading to anxiety-like behaviors in the recipient animals, as well as alterations in tryptophan metabolism [125]. This suggests that changes in gut microbiota composition could play a causative role in the onset of depression.

Probiotic therapies have been applied in an attempt to correct for the possible absence of microbiota species capable of exhibiting suitable drivers of a "healthy" behavior. For example, the classical probiotics, Bifidobacteria and Lactobacilli, have been recently suggested as an alternative treatment for anxiety and depressive-like behaviors. Oral administration of a combination of *Lactobacillus helveticus* R0052 and *Bifidobacterium longum* R0175 (Probio'Stick®, Lallemand, Montreal, QC, Canada) for a period of one month, has been reported to improve depression, anxiety, and lower the level of the stress hormone cortisol in humans ($n = 26$) [127]. A three-week consumption of a probiotic-containing milk drink that contained *Lactobacillus casei* Shirota, showed improved mood in healthy volunteers ($n = 124$) [128]. Similarly, when healthy male and female participants ($n = 20$) were administered with, either a placebo product or a mixture of several probiotics strains of Bifidobacteria and Lactobacilli over a period of 4 weeks, they exhibited substantially reduced reactivity to sad mood compared to control group [129]. Another small ($n = 12$) placebo-controlled study involving functional magnetic imaging has also demonstrated that a one-month consumption of a fermented food containing *Bifidobacterium animalis* subsp. *lactis*, *Streptococcus thermophilus*, *Lactobacillus bulgaricus*, and *Lactococcus lactis* subsp. *lactis* can influence brain activity as compared to baseline [130]. More recently, *Lactobacillus reuteri* has been described to reduce despair like behavior in mice by inhibiting elevated levels of IDO and reducing peripheral levels of kynurenine [131]. Whether the observed antidepressant effect of probiotics is due to their modulation of an intestinal inflammatory state, restoration of tryptophan metabolism, or reduction in serotonin turnover is still unclear.

Important to consider is indeed the influence of altered IDO activity and kynurenine pathway metabolism induced by gut microbiota [132]. In the germ-free state, microbial colonization induced the expression of genes encoding IDO, suggesting that gut microbiota activates this enzyme [17,96,132]. Moreover, other bacteria that flourish in an inflammatory environment, in particular *Pseudomonas* genera, can catabolize tryptophan into kynurenine via tryptophan 2,3-dioxygenase, *kynA* and kynurenine formamidase, *kynB* [133] (Figure 1D). Whether intestinal proinflammatory cytokines or any other metabolites have similar effect on induction of *kynA* and *kynB* expression in this bacterium, and subsequent increased levels of downstream metabolites, is still unknown. Additionally, in *Pseudomonas aeruginosa*, kynurenine acts as the main precursor of the *Pseudomonas* quinolone signal, a quorum-sensing signal that regulates numerous virulence genes in these bacteria [133]. This suggests that shifting tryptophan metabolism towards kynurenine during inflammation might result in inducing virulence in *Pseudomonas*, which in turn, causes imbalance in the microbial population, and disruption in the kynurenine and serotonin signaling systems, eventually leading to a state of depression.

Besides the kynurenine and serotonin arms within tryptophan metabolism, indole represents another important product in this metabolic pathway. Indole and its derivatives are exclusively produced by gut bacterial metabolism of tryptophan, via the tryptophanase (*tnaA*) enzyme [111,134,135]. In their recent rodent study, Jaglin et al. suggested that human subjects, who carry microbiota type dominated by species capable of overproducing indole may be more prone to develop anxiety and mood disorders [136]. The authors mimicked this situation by injecting indole in the cecum of conventional rats. The treated rats showed a dramatic decrease of motor activity, and higher levels of the indole-derivatives oxindole and isatin were detected in the brain. When germ-free rats were colonized with the indole-producing bacterial species *E. coli* to mimic a state of a chronic and moderate overproduction of indole and compared their behavior with that observed in germ-free counterparts mono-colonized with a mutant strain $E.$ $coli^{-\Delta tnaA}$, which is unable to produce indole, only rats colonized with wild-type strain showed anxiety-like behavior suggesting that indole and its metabolites might play a role in developing depression [136]. This study implies a direct mechanism by which the gut microbiota can influence the brain, and result in a state of depression, in this case via the production of the neuro-suppressive indole-derivatives; oxindole and isatin, which are products of gut epithelial or hepatic xenobiotic metabolizing enzymes (Figure 1D). However, another plausible mechanism could be through activation of the vagal afferent fibers in the intestinal mucosa either directly by indole or indirectly via secondary signals whose production could be triggered by indole. Another indole derivative, indole pyruvic acid, was shown to normalize the level of corticosterone in rodent model of depression and this effect was suggested to be due to the production of kynurenic acid in the brain [137]. Altogether, further studies are warranted for a comprehensive understanding of the mechanisms governing the beneficial or detrimental effects of gut microbiota and its metabolites on mood and behavior.

4. Conclusions and Future Perspectives

Given the mounting evidence over the past five years that microbiota play a key role at the gut–brain interphase shows a need to reveal the mechanisms that underpin this interaction in order to close the gap between therapeutic strategies and fundamental science. That the metabolites of the gut microbiota is evident to have a substantial effect on the regulation of immune response, tryptophan metabolism, and serotonin production, a diet characterized by nutrient-poor, energy-dense processed foods can well explain the strong link between depression and this multifaceted crosstalk. Restoring the gut microbiota composition via nutritional interventions could be an indirect strategic tool to treat depression. The use of selective dietary microbial growth substrates could be as beneficial but may result in long-lasting changes of the microbiome compared to the application of probiotic therapies.

Achieving a better understanding of the role of the complex triggers of depression requires further development of analytical approaches, including, metabolomics, to allow unraveling the metabolic dialogue between the microbiota and gut–brain axis. Equally important is the development of reliable models to decipher the complex interactions between the gut microbiota and its products, disruptions in immune response and dietary metabolism, all of which ultimately affect brain functionality, mood and behavior. The use of reductionist animal models has been very helpful in identifying underlying mechanisms in the host–microbe cross talk. However, it is increasingly clear that animal models fall short in translation to humans. Data acquired from large longitudinal human cohorts followed over long period of time, is essential to understand the real-world complexity of these interactions. Currently, there is an exponential growth of large bio-banks holding vast amounts of information about the same individual [138–140]. If combined with the state-of-art technologies including bacterial culturomics and individualized organs-on-chips to further understand the underlying causalities and mechanisms, only then we can bridge the gap between basic science and clinical practice and make major advances in personalized medicine.

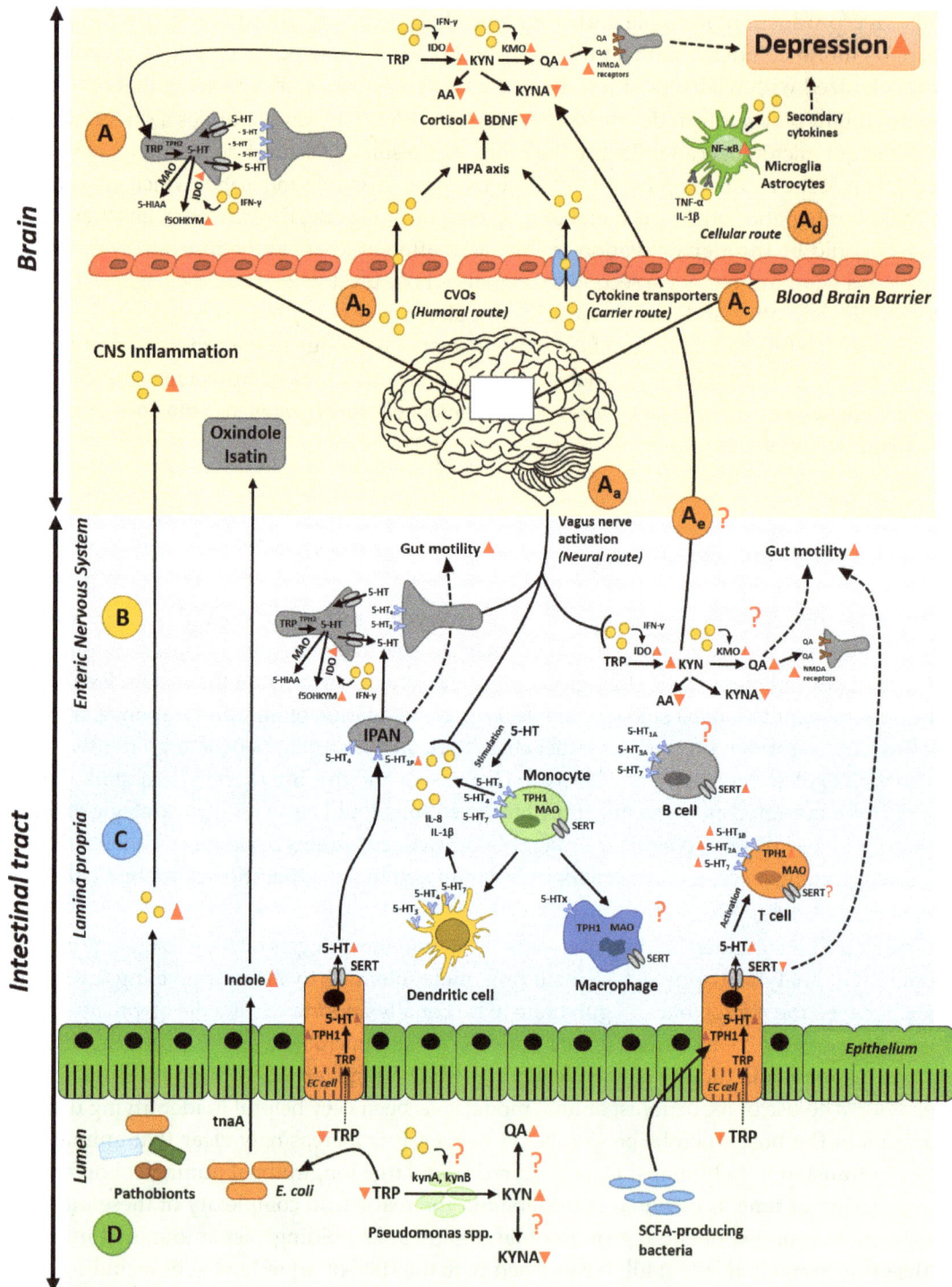

Figure 1. Gut microbiota remotely influences brain and depression. Potential routes by which the gut microbiota could govern the comorbidity of gut inflammation, disruption in tryptophan metabolism, and induction of depression. (**A**) Signaling mechanisms in the brain stimulated by inflammatory molecules in the gut; (**B**) molecular mechanisms by which the enteric nervous system affects gut motility and tryptophan metabolism during intestinal inflammation; (**C**) possible alterations of serotonin signaling in lamina propria resulting in gut hypermobility and inflammatory response; (**D**) influence of the gut microbiota and its secreted compounds on disruption on tryptophan metabolism and gut inflammation. Red triangles represent decreased/increased production or expression. Red question marks indicate missing links in this multi-faceted crosstalk. Dotted lines depict effects on gut motility. Abbreviations: 5-HIAA = 5-hydroxyindoleacetic acid; 5-HT = serotonin; 5-HT$_x$ = serotonin receptors;

AA = anthranilic acid; BDNF = brain-derived neurotrophic factor; CVOs = circumventricular organs; EC cell = enterochromaffin cell; HPA axis = hypothalamus-pituitary adrenal axis; IDO = indoleamine-2,3-dioxygenase; IFN-γ = interferon γ; IPAN = intrinsic primary afferent neuron; KMO = kynurenine-3-monooxygenase; KYN = kynurenine; KYNA = kynurenic acid; MAO = monoamine oxidase; NMDA receptors = N-methyl-D-aspartate receptors; QA = quinolinic acid; SCFAs = short-chain fatty acids; SERT = serotonin transporter; TNF-α = tumor necrosis factor α; TPH1 = tryptophan hydroxylase; TRP = tryptophan; f5OHKYM = formyl-5-hydroxykynuramine; kynA = tryptophan-2,3-dioxygenase from Pseudomonas spp.; kynB = kynurenine formamidase from Pseudomonas spp.; tnaA = tryptophanase.

Author Contributions: Conceptualization, B.W., S.E.A.; Writing-Original draft, B.W., S.E.A.; Writing-Review and Editing, B.W., S.E.A.; Funding Acquisition, S.E.A.

Funding: This research was funded by Rosalind Franklin Fellowships, co-funded by the European Union and University of Groningen.

References

1. El Aidy, S.; Stilling, R.; Dinan, T.G.; Cryan, J.F. Microbiome to Brain: Unravelling the Multidirectional Axes of Communication. In *Microbial Endocrinology: Interkingdom Signaling in Infectious Disease and Health. Advances in Experimental Medicine and Biology*; Springer: Cham, Switzerland, 2016; pp. 301–336. ISBN 978-3-319-20214-3.

2. Shepherd, E.S.; DeLoache, W.C.; Pruss, K.M.; Whitaker, W.R.; Sonnenburg, J.L. An Exclusive Metabolic Niche Enables Strain Engraftment in the Gut Microbiota. *Nature* **2018**, *557*, 434–438. [CrossRef] [PubMed]

3. Maier, L.; Pruteanu, M.; Kuhn, M.; Zeller, G.; Telzerow, A.; Anderson, E.E.; Brochado, A.R.; Fernandez, K.C.; Dose, H.; Mori, H.; et al. Extensive Impact of Non-Antibiotic Drugs on Human Gut Bacteria. *Nature* **2018**, *555*, 623–628. [CrossRef] [PubMed]

4. Dodd, D.; Spitzer, M.H.; Van Treuren, W.; Merrill, B.D.; Hryckowian, A.J.; Higginbottom, S.K.; Le, A.; Cowan, T.M.; Nolan, G.P.; Fischbach, M.A.; et al. A Gut Bacterial Pathway Metabolizes Aromatic Amino Acids into Nine Circulating Metabolites. *Nature* **2017**, *551*, 648–652. [CrossRef] [PubMed]

5. Blander, J.M.; Longman, R.S.; Iliev, I.D.; Sonnenberg, G.F.; Artis, D. Regulation of Inflammation by Microbiota Interactions with the Host. *Nat. Immunol.* **2017**, *18*, 851–860. [CrossRef] [PubMed]

6. Berk, M.; Williams, L.J.; Jacka, F.N.; O'Neil, A.; Pasco, J.A.; Moylan, S.; Allen, N.B.; Stuart, A.L.; Hayley, A.C.; Byrne, M.L.; et al. So Depression Is an Inflammatory Disease, but Where Does the Inflammation Come From? *BMC Med.* **2013**, *11*, 200. [CrossRef] [PubMed]

7. Kiecolt-Glaser, J.K.; Derry, H.M.; Fagundes, C.P. Inflammation: Depression Fans the Flames and Feasts on the Heat. *Am. J. Psychiatry* **2015**, *172*, 1075–1091. [CrossRef] [PubMed]

8. Koopman, M.; El Aidy, S. Depressed Gut? The Microbiota-Diet-Inflammation Trialogue in Depression. *Curr. Opin. Psychiatry* **2017**, *30*, 369–377. [CrossRef] [PubMed]

9. World Health Organization. Depression. Available online: http://www.who.int/en/news-room/fact-sheets/detail/depression (accessed on 20 June 2018).

10. Raison, C.L.; Borisov, A.S.; Majer, M.; Drake, D.F.; Pagnoni, G.; Woolwine, B.J.; Vogt, G.J.; Massung, B.; Miller, A.H. Activation of Central Nervous System Inflammatory Pathways by Interferon-Alpha: Relationship to Monoamines and Depression. *Biol. Psychiatry* **2009**, *65*, 296–303. [CrossRef] [PubMed]

11. Thomas, J.; Khanam, R.; Vohora, D. Augmentation of Effect of Venlafaxine by Folic Acid in Behavioral Paradigms of Depression in Mice: Evidence of Serotonergic and pro-Inflammatory Cytokine Pathways. *Pharmacol. Rep.* **2016**, *68*, 396–403. [CrossRef] [PubMed]

12. Lebeña, A.; Vegas, O.; Gómez-Lázaro, E.; Arregi, A.; Garmendia, L.; Beitia, G.; Azpiroz, A. Melanoma Tumors Alter Proinflammatory Cytokine Production and Monoamine Brain Function, and Induce Depressive-like Behavior in Male Mice. *Behav. Brain Res.* **2014**, *272*, 83–92. [CrossRef] [PubMed]

13. Wang, J.; Jia, Y.; Li, G.; Wang, B.; Zhou, T.; Zhu, L.; Chen, T.; Chen, Y. The Dopamine Receptor D3 Regulates Lipopolysaccharide-Induced Depressive-Like Behavior in Mice. *Int. J. Neuropsychopharmacol.* **2018**, *21*, 448–460. [CrossRef] [PubMed]

14. Coates, M.D.; Johnson, A.C.; Greenwood-van Meerveld, B.; Mawe, G.M. Effects of Serotonin Transporter Inhibition on Gastrointestinal Motility and Colonic Sensitivity in the Mouse. *Neurogastroenterol. Motil.* **2006**, *18*, 464–471. [CrossRef] [PubMed]

15. Coates, M.D.; Mahoney, C.R.; Linden, D.R.; Sampson, J.E.; Chen, J.; Blaszyk, H.; Crowell, M.D.; Sharkey, K.A.; Gershon, M.D.; Mawe, G.M. Molecular Defects in Mucosal Serotonin Content and Decreased Serotonin Reuptake Transporter in Ulcerative Colitis and Irritable Bowel Syndrome. *Gastroenterology* **2004**, *126*, 1657–1664. [CrossRef] [PubMed]

16. Kidd, M.; Gustafsson, B.I.; Drozdov, I.; Modlin, I.M. IL1β- and LPS-Induced Serotonin Secretion Is Increased in EC Cells Derived from Crohn's Disease. *Neurogastroenterol. Motil.* **2009**, *21*, 439–450. [CrossRef] [PubMed]

17. El Aidy, S.; Dinan, T.G.; Cryan, J.F. Immune Modulation of the Brain-Gut-Microbe Axis. *Front. Microbiol.* **2014**, *5*, 146. [CrossRef] [PubMed]

18. Linden, D.R.; Chen, J.-X.; Gershon, M.D.; Sharkey, K.A.; Mawe, G.M. Serotonin Availability Is Increased in Mucosa of Guinea Pigs with TNBS-Induced Colitis. *Am. J. Physiol. Liver Physiol.* **2003**, *285*, G207–G216. [CrossRef] [PubMed]

19. Mawe, G.M.; Hoffman, J.M. Serotonin Signalling in the Gut—functions, Dysfunctions and Therapeutic Targets. *Nat. Rev. Gastroenterol. Hepatol.* **2013**, *10*, 473–486. [CrossRef] [PubMed]

20. Dantzer, R. Cytokine, Sickness Behavior, and Depression. *Immunol. Allergy Clin. N. Am.* **2009**, *29*, 247–264. [CrossRef] [PubMed]

21. Van Heesch, F. *Inflammation-Induced Depression. Studying the Role of Proinflammatory Cytokines in Anhedonia*; Utrecht University: Utrecht, The Netherlands, 2014.

22. Capuron, L.; Miller, A.H. Immune System to Brain Signaling: Neuropsychopharmacological Implications. *Pharmacol. Ther.* **2011**, *130*, 226–238. [CrossRef] [PubMed]

23. D'Mello, C.; Swain, M.G. Immune-to-Brain Communication Pathways in Inflammation-Associated Sickness and Depression. In *Inflammation-Associated Depression: Evidence, Mechanisms and Implications. Current Topics in Behavioral Neurosciences*; Springer: Cham, Switzerland, 2016; pp. 73–94.

24. Ransohoff, R.M.; Kivisäkk, P.; Kidd, G. Three or More Routes for Leukocyte Migration into the Central Nervous System. *Nat. Rev. Immunol.* **2003**, *3*, 569–581. [CrossRef] [PubMed]

25. Dantzer, R.; O'Connor, J.C.; Freund, G.G.; Johnson, R.W.; Kelley, K.W. From Inflammation to Sickness and Depression: When the Immune System Subjugates the Brain. *Nat. Rev. Neurosci.* **2008**, *9*, 46–56. [CrossRef] [PubMed]

26. Banks, W.A. The Blood–brain Barrier as a Regulatory Interface in the Gut–brain Axes. *Physiol. Behav.* **2006**, *89*, 472–476. [CrossRef] [PubMed]

27. Jensen, C.J.; Massie, A.; De Keyser, J. Immune Players in the CNS: The Astrocyte. *J. Neuroimmune Pharmacol.* **2013**, *8*, 824–839. [CrossRef] [PubMed]

28. Yang, I.; Han, S.J.; Kaur, G.; Crane, C.; Parsa, A.T. The Role of Microglia in Central Nervous System Immunity and Glioma Immunology. *J. Clin. Neurosci.* **2010**, *17*, 6–10. [CrossRef] [PubMed]

29. Nadeau, S.; Rivest, S. Effects of Circulating Tumor Necrosis Factor on the Neuronal Activity and Expression of the Genes Encoding the Tumor Necrosis Factor Receptors (P55 and P75) in the Rat Brain: A View from the Blood–brain Barrier. *Neuroscience* **1999**, *93*, 1449–1464. [CrossRef]

30. Rivest, S.; Lacroix, S.; Vallières, L.; Nadeau, S.; Zhang, J.; Laflamme, N. How the Blood Talks to the Brain Parenchyma and the Paraventricular Nucleus of the Hypothalamus during Systemic Inflammatory and Infectious Stimuli. *Proc. Soc. Exp. Biol. Med.* **2000**, *223*, 22–38. [CrossRef] [PubMed]

31. Capuron, L.; Gumnick, J.F.; Musselman, D.L.; Lawson, D.H.; Reemsnyder, A.; Nemeroff, C.B.; Miller, A.H. Neurobehavioral Effects of Interferon-α in Cancer Patients Phenomenology and Paroxetine Responsiveness of Symptom Dimensions. *Neuropsychopharmacology* **2002**, *26*, 643–652. [CrossRef]

32. Howren, M.B.; Lamkin, D.M.; Suls, J. Associations of Depression with C-Reactive Protein, IL-1, and IL-6: A Meta-Analysis. *Psychosom. Med.* **2009**, *71*, 171–186. [CrossRef] [PubMed]

33.　Kałużna-Czaplińska, J.; Gątarek, P.; Chirumbolo, S.; Chartrand, M.S.; Bjørklund, G. How Important Is Tryptophan in Human Health? *Crit. Rev. Food Sci. Nutr.* **2017**, 1–17. [CrossRef] [PubMed]

34.　Le Floc'h, N.; Otten, W.; Merlot, E. Tryptophan Metabolism, from Nutrition to Potential Therapeutic Applications. *Amino Acids* **2011**, *41*, 1195–1205. [CrossRef] [PubMed]

35.　Ruddick, J.P.; Evans, A.K.; Nutt, D.J.; Lightman, S.L.; Rook, G.A.W.; Lowry, C.A. Tryptophan Metabolism in the Central Nervous System: Medical Implications. *Expert Rev. Mol. Med.* **2006**, *8*, 1–27. [CrossRef] [PubMed]

36.　Kennedy, P.J.; Cryan, J.F.; Dinan, T.G.; Clarke, G. Kynurenine Pathway Metabolism and the Microbiota-Gut-Brain Axis. *Neuropharmacology* **2017**, *112*, 399–412. [CrossRef] [PubMed]

37.　Spiller, R. Serotonin and GI Clinical Disorders. *Neuropharmacology* **2008**, *55*, 1072–1080. [CrossRef] [PubMed]

38.　Gershon, M.D. 5-Hydroxytryptamine (Serotonin) in the Gastrointestinal Tract. *Curr. Opin. Endocrinol. Diabetes Obes.* **2013**, *20*, 14–21. [CrossRef] [PubMed]

39.　Nguyen, N.T.; Nakahama, T.; Le, D.H.; Van Son, L.; Chu, H.H.; Kishimoto, T. Aryl Hydrocarbon Receptor and Kynurenine: Recent Advances in Autoimmune Disease Research. *Front. Immunol.* **2014**, *5*, 551. [CrossRef] [PubMed]

40.　O'Mahony, S.M.; Clarke, G.; Borre, Y.E.; Dinan, T.G.; Cryan, J.F. Serotonin, Tryptophan Metabolism and the Brain-Gut-Microbiome Axis. *Behav. Brain Res.* **2015**, *277*, 32–48. [CrossRef] [PubMed]

41.　Badawy, A.A.-B. Tryptophan Availability for Kynurenine Pathway Metabolism across the Life Span: Control Mechanisms and Focus on Aging, Exercise, Diet and Nutritional Supplements. *Neuropharmacology* **2017**, *112*, 248–263. [CrossRef] [PubMed]

42.　Richard, D.M.; Dawes, M.A.; Mathias, C.W.; Acheson, A.; Hill-Kapturczak, N.; Dougherty, D.M. L-Tryptophan: Basic Metabolic Functions, Behavioral Research and Therapeutic Indications. *Int. J. Tryptophan Res.* **2009**, *2*, 45–60. [CrossRef] [PubMed]

43.　Keszthelyi, D.; Troost, F.J.; Jonkers, D.M.; van Donkelaar, E.L.; Dekker, J.; Buurman, W.A.; Masclee, A.A. Does Acute Tryptophan Depletion Affect Peripheral Serotonin Metabolism in the Intestine? *Am. J. Clin. Nutr.* **2012**, *95*, 603–608. [CrossRef] [PubMed]

44.　Gál, E.M.; Sherman, A.D. L-Kynurenine: Its Synthesis and Possible Regulatory Function in Brain. *Neurochem. Res.* **1980**, *5*, 223–239. [CrossRef] [PubMed]

45.　Catena-Dell'Osso, M.; Rotella, F.; Dell'Osso, A.; Fagiolini, A.; Marazziti, D. Inflammation, Serotonin and Major Depression. *Curr. Drug Targets* **2013**, *14*, 571–577. [CrossRef] [PubMed]

46.　Salter, M.; Pogson, C.I. The Role of Tryptophan 2,3-Dioxygenase in the Hormonal Control of Tryptophan Metabolism in Isolated Rat Liver Cells. Effects of Glucocorticoids and Experimental Diabetes. *Biochem. J.* **1985**, *229*, 499–504. [CrossRef] [PubMed]

47.　Yeung, A.W.S.; Terentis, A.C.; King, N.J.C.; Thomas, S.R. Role of Indoleamine 2,3-Dioxygenase in Health and Disease. *Clin. Sci.* **2015**, *129*, 601–672. [CrossRef] [PubMed]

48.　Jurgens, B.; Hainz, U.; Fuchs, D.; Felzmann, T.; Heitger, A. Interferon-γ-Triggered Indoleamine 2,3-Dioxygenase Competence in Human Monocyte-Derived Dendritic Cells Induces Regulatory Activity in Allogeneic T Cells. *Blood* **2009**, *114*, 3235–3243. [CrossRef] [PubMed]

49.　Dantzer, R. Role of the Kynurenine Metabolism Pathway in Inflammation-Induced Depression: Preclinical Approaches. In *Inflammation-Associated Depression: Evidence, Mechanisms and Implications. Current Topics in Behavioral Neurosciences*; Springer: Cham, Switzerland, 2016; pp. 117–138. ISBN 978-3-319-51152-8.

50.　Pertz, H.; Back, W. Synthesis and Resolution of Chiral Ring-Opened Serotonin Analogs of the 5-Hydroxykynuramine Type. *Pharm. Acta Helv.* **1988**, *63*, 128–131. [PubMed]

51.　Jeon, S.W.; Kim, Y.-K. Inflammation-Induced Depression: Its Pathophysiology and Therapeutic Implications. *J. Neuroimmunol.* **2017**, *313*, 92–98. [CrossRef] [PubMed]

52.　Keszthelyi, D.; Troost, F.J.; Masclee, A.A.M. Understanding the Role of Tryptophan and Serotonin Metabolism in Gastrointestinal Function. *Neurogastroenterol. Motil.* **2009**, *21*, 1239–1249. [CrossRef] [PubMed]

53.　Fukui, S.; Schwarcz, R.; Rapoport, S.I.; Takada, Y.; Smith, Q.R. Blood-Brain Barrier Transport of Kynurenines: Implications for Brain Synthesis and Metabolism. *J. Neurochem.* **1991**, *56*, 2007–2017. [CrossRef] [PubMed]

54.　Savitz, J.; Drevets, W.C.; Wurfel, B.E.; Ford, B.N.; Bellgowan, P.S.F.; Victor, T.A.; Bodurka, J.; Teague, T.K.;

Dantzer, R. Reduction of Kynurenic Acid to Quinolinic Acid Ratio in Both the Depressed and Remitted Phases of Major Depressive Disorder. *Brain Behav. Immun.* **2015**, *46*, 55–59. [CrossRef] [PubMed]

55. Bay-Richter, C.; Linderholm, K.R.; Lim, C.K.; Samuelsson, M.; Träskman-Bendz, L.; Guillemin, G.J.; Erhardt, S.; Brundin, L. A Role for Inflammatory Metabolites as Modulators of the Glutamate N-Methyl-D-Aspartate Receptor in Depression and Suicidality. *Brain Behav. Immun.* **2015**, *43*, 110–117. [CrossRef] [PubMed]

56. Bryleva, E.Y.; Brundin, L. Kynurenine Pathway Metabolites and Suicidality. *Neuropharmacology* **2017**, *112*, 324–330. [CrossRef] [PubMed]

57. Wurfel, B.E.; Drevets, W.C.; Bliss, S.A.; McMillin, J.R.; Suzuki, H.; Ford, B.N.; Morris, H.M.; Teague, T.K.; Dantzer, R.; Savitz, J.B. Serum Kynurenic Acid Is Reduced in Affective Psychosis. *Transl. Psychiatry* **2017**, *7*, e1115. [CrossRef] [PubMed]

58. Connor, T.J.; Starr, N.; O'Sullivan, J.B.; Harkin, A. Induction of Indolamine 2,3-Dioxygenase and Kynurenine 3-Monooxygenase in Rat Brain Following a Systemic Inflammatory Challenge: A Role for IFN-γ? *Neurosci. Lett.* **2008**, *441*, 29–34. [CrossRef] [PubMed]

59. Molteni, R.; Macchi, F.; Zecchillo, C.; Dell'Agli, M.; Colombo, E.; Calabrese, F.; Guidotti, G.; Racagni, G.; Riva, M.A. Modulation of the Inflammatory Response in Rats Chronically Treated with the Antidepressant Agomelatine. *Eur. Neuropsychopharmacol.* **2013**, *23*, 1645–1655. [CrossRef] [PubMed]

60. Erhardt, S.; Lim, C.K.; Linderholm, K.R.; Janelidze, S.; Lindqvist, D.; Samuelsson, M.; Lundberg, K.; Postolache, T.T.; Träskman-Bendz, L.; Guillemin, G.J.; et al. Connecting Inflammation with Glutamate Agonism in Suicidality. *Neuropsychopharmacology* **2013**, *38*, 743–752. [CrossRef] [PubMed]

61. Husi, H. NMDA Receptors, Neural Pathways, and Protein Interaction Databases. *Int. Rev. Neurobiol.* **2004**, *61*, 49–77. [CrossRef] [PubMed]

62. Giaroni, C.; Zanetti, E.; Chiaravalli, A.M.; Albarello, L.; Dominioni, L.; Capella, C.; Lecchini, S.; Frigo, G. Evidence for a Glutamatergic Modulation of the Cholinergic Function in the Human Enteric Nervous System via NMDA Receptors. *Eur. J. Pharmacol.* **2003**, *476*, 63–69. [CrossRef]

63. Kirchgessner, A. Glutamate in the Enteric Nervous System. *Curr. Opin. Pharmacol.* **2001**, *1*, 591–596. [CrossRef]

64. Zhou, Q.; Nicholas Verne, G. NMDA Receptors and Colitis: Basic Science and Clinical Implications. *Rev. Analg.* **2008**, *10*, 33–43. [CrossRef] [PubMed]

65. Varga, G.; Érces, D.; Fazekas, B.; Fülöp, M.; Kovács, T.; Kaszaki, J.; Fülöp, F.; Vécsei, L.; Boros, M. N-Methyl-D-Aspartate Receptor Antagonism Decreases Motility and Inflammatory Activation in the Early Phase of Acute Experimental Colitis in the Rat. *Neurogastroenterol. Motil.* **2010**, *22*, 217–e68. [CrossRef] [PubMed]

66. Coutinho, S.V.; Meller, S.T.; Gebhart, G.F. Intracolonic Zymosan Produces Visceral Hyperalgesia in the Rat That Is Mediated by Spinal NMDA and Non-NMDA Receptors. *Brain Res.* **1996**, *736*, 7–15. [CrossRef]

67. Berger, M.; Gray, J.A.; Roth, B.L. The Expanded Biology of Serotonin. *Annu. Rev. Med.* **2009**, *60*, 355–366. [CrossRef] [PubMed]

68. Wade, P.R.; Tamir, H.; Kirchgessner, A.L.; Gershon, M.D. Analysis of the Role of 5-HT in the Enteric Nervous System Using Anti-Idiotopic Antibodies to 5-HT Receptors. *Am. J. Physiol. Liver Physiol.* **1994**, *266*, G403–G416. [CrossRef] [PubMed]

69. Gershon, M.D.; Ross, L.L. Studies on the Relationship of 5-Hydroxytryptamine and the Enterochromaffin Cell to Anaphylactic Shock in Mice. *J. Exp. Med.* **1962**, *115*, 367–382. [CrossRef] [PubMed]

70. Coleman, J.A.; Green, E.M.; Gouaux, E. X-Ray Structures and Mechanism of the Human Serotonin Transporter. *Nature* **2016**, *532*, 334–339. [CrossRef] [PubMed]

71. Murphy, D.L.; Lerner, A.; Rudnick, G.; Lesch, K.-P. Serotonin Transporter: Gene, Genetic Disorders, and Pharmacogenetics. *Mol. Interv.* **2004**, *4*, 109–123. [CrossRef] [PubMed]

72. Hannon, J.; Hoyer, D. Molecular Biology of 5-HT Receptors. *Behav. Brain Res.* **2008**, *195*, 198–213. [CrossRef] [PubMed]

73. Tutton, P.J. The Influence of Serotonin on Crypt Cell Proliferation in the Jejunum of Rat. *Virchows Arch. B Cell Pathol.* **1974**, *16*, 79–87. [CrossRef] [PubMed]

74. Gershon, M.D. Nerves, Reflexes, and the Enteric Nervous System. *J. Clin. Gastroenterol.* **2005**, *39*, S184–S193. [CrossRef] [PubMed]

75. Mazzia, C.; Hicks, G.; Clerc, N. Neuronal Location of 5-Hydroxytryptamine$_3$ Receptor-like Immunoreactivity in the Rat Colon. *Neuroscience* **2003**, *116*, 1033–1041. [CrossRef]

76. Grider, J.R. Desensitization of the Peristaltic Reflex Induced by Mucosal Stimulation with the Selective 5-HT$_4$ Agonist Tegaserod. *Am. J. Physiol. Liver Physiol.* **2006**, *290*, G319–G327. [CrossRef] [PubMed]

77. Pan, H.; Galligan, J.J. 5-HT$_{1A}$ and 5-HT$_4$ Receptors Mediate Inhibition and Facilitation of Fast Synaptic Transmission in Enteric Neurons. *Am. J. Physiol.* **1994**, *266*, G230-8. [CrossRef] [PubMed]

78. Galligan, J.J.; Pan, H.; Messori, E. Signalling Mechanism Coupled to 5-Hydroxytryptamine$_4$ Receptor-Mediated Facilitation of Fast Synaptic Transmission in the Guinea-Pig Ileum Myenteric Plexus. *Neurogastroenterol. Motil.* **2003**, *15*, 523–529. [CrossRef] [PubMed]

79. Baganz, N.L.; Blakely, R.D. A Dialogue between the Immune System and Brain, Spoken in the Language of Serotonin. *ACS Chem. Neurosci.* **2013**, *4*, 48–63. [CrossRef] [PubMed]

80. Herr, N.; Bode, C.; Duerschmied, D. The Effects of Serotonin in Immune Cells. *Front. Cardiovasc. Med.* **2017**, *4*, 48. [CrossRef] [PubMed]

81. Leon-Ponte, M.; Ahern, G.P.; O'Connell, P.J. Serotonin Provides an Accessory Signal to Enhance T-Cell Activation by Signaling through the 5-HT$_7$ Receptor. *Blood* **2007**, *109*, 3139–3146. [CrossRef] [PubMed]

82. Medina-Martel, M.; Urbina, M.; Fazzino, F.; Lima, L. Serotonin Transporter in Lymphocytes of Rats Exposed to Physical Restraint Stress. *Neuroimmunomodulation* **2013**, *20*, 361–367. [CrossRef] [PubMed]

83. Meredith, E.J.; Holder, M.J.; Chamba, A.; Challa, A.; Drake-Lee, A.; Bunce, C.M.; Drayson, M.T.; Pilkington, G.; Blakely, R.D.; Dyer, M.J.S.; et al. The Serotonin Transporter (SLC6A4) Is Present in B-Cell Clones of Diverse Malignant Origin: Probing a Potential Anti-Tumor Target for Psychotropics. *FASEB J.* **2005**, *19*, 1187–1189. [CrossRef] [PubMed]

84. Idzko, M.; Panther, E.; Stratz, C.; Muller, T.; Bayer, H.; Zissel, G.; Durk, T.; Sorichter, S.; Di Virgilio, F.; Geissler, M.; et al. The Serotoninergic Receptors of Human Dendritic Cells: Identification and Coupling to Cytokine Release. *J. Immunol.* **2004**, *172*, 6011–6019. [CrossRef] [PubMed]

85. Dürk, T.; Panther, E.; Müller, T.; Sorichter, S.; Ferrari, D.; Pizzirani, C.; Di Virgilio, F.; Myrtek, D.; Norgauer, J.; Idzko, M. 5-Hydroxytryptamine Modulates Cytokine and Chemokine Production in LPS-Primed Human Monocytes via Stimulation of Different 5-HTR Subtypes. *Int. Immunol.* **2005**, *17*, 599–606. [CrossRef] [PubMed]

86. Fiorica-Howells, E.; Liu, M.-T.; Ponimaskin, E.G.; Li, Z.-S.; Compan, V.; Hen, R.; Gingrich, J.A.; Gershon, M.D. Distribution of 5-HT$_4$ Receptors in Wild-Type Mice and Analysis of Intestinal Motility in 5-HT$_4$ Knockout Mice. *Gastroenterology* **2003**, *124*, A342. [CrossRef]

87. Compan, V. Attenuated Response to Stress and Novelty and Hypersensitivity to Seizures in 5-HT$_4$ Receptor Knock-Out Mice. *J. Neurosci.* **2004**, *24*, 412–419. [CrossRef] [PubMed]

88. El Aidy, S.; Ramsteijn, A.S.; Dini-Andreote, F.; van Eijk, R.; Houwing, D.J.; Salles, J.F.; Olivier, J.D.A. Serotonin Transporter Genotype Modulates the Gut Microbiota Composition in Young Rats, an Effect Augmented by Early Life Stress. *Front. Cell. Neurosci.* **2017**, *11*, 222. [CrossRef] [PubMed]

89. Chen, J.J.; Li, Z.; Pan, H.; Murphy, D.L.; Tamir, H.; Koepsell, H.; Gershon, M.D. Maintenance of Serotonin in the Intestinal Mucosa and Ganglia of Mice That Lack the High-Affinity Serotonin Transporter: Abnormal Intestinal Motility and the Expression of Cation Transporters. *J. Neurosci.* **2001**, *21*, 6348–6361. [CrossRef] [PubMed]

90. Gershon, M.D.; Tack, J. The Serotonin Signaling System: From Basic Understanding To Drug Development for Functional GI Disorders. *Gastroenterology* **2007**, *132*, 397–414. [CrossRef] [PubMed]

91. Canli, T.; Lesch, K.-P. Long Story Short: The Serotonin Transporter in Emotion Regulation and Social Cognition. *Nat. Neurosci.* **2007**, *10*, 1103–1109. [CrossRef] [PubMed]

92. Scheerens, C.; Tack, J.; Rommel, N. Buspirone, a New Drug for the Management of Patients with Ineffective Esophageal Motility? *United Eur. Gastroenterol. J.* **2015**, *3*, 261–265. [CrossRef] [PubMed]

93. Di Sabatino, A.; Giuffrida, P.; Vanoli, A.; Luinetti, O.; Manca, R.; Biancheri, P.; Bergamaschi, G.; Alvisi, C.;

Pasini, A.; Salvatore, C.; et al. Increase in Neuroendocrine Cells in the Duodenal Mucosa of Patients with Refractory Celiac Disease. *Am. J. Gastroenterol.* **2014**, *109*, 258–269. [CrossRef] [PubMed]

94. Bruce-Keller, A.J.; Salbaum, J.M.; Berthoud, H.-R. Harnessing Gut Microbes for Mental Health: Getting From Here to There. *Biol. Psychiatry* **2018**, *83*, 214–223. [CrossRef] [PubMed]

95. Round, J.L.; O'Connell, R.M.; Mazmanian, S.K. Coordination of Tolerogenic Immune Responses by the Commensal Microbiota. *J. Autoimmun.* **2010**, *34*. [CrossRef] [PubMed]

96. El Aidy, S.; van Baarlen, P.; Derrien, M.; Lindenbergh-Kortleve, D.J.; Hooiveld, G.; Levenez, F.; Doré, J.; Dekker, J.; Samsom, J.N.; Nieuwenhuis, E.E.S.; et al. Temporal and Spatial Interplay of Microbiota and Intestinal Mucosa Drive Establishment of Immune Homeostasis in Conventionalized Mice. *Mucosal Immunol.* **2012**, *5*, 567–579. [CrossRef] [PubMed]

97. El Aidy, S.; Derrien, M.; Aardema, R.; Hooiveld, G.; Richards, S.E.; Dane, A.; Dekker, J.; Vreeken, R.; Levenez, F.; Doré, J.; et al. Transient Inflammatory-like State and Microbial Dysbiosis Are Pivotal in Establishment of Mucosal Homeostasis during Colonisation of Germ-Free Mice. *Benef. Microbes* **2014**, *5*, 67–77. [CrossRef] [PubMed]

98. Mazmanian, S.K.; Liu, C.H.; Tzianabos, A.O.; Kasper, D.L. An Immunomodulatory Molecule of Symbiotic Bacteria Directs Maturation of the Host Immune System. *Cell* **2005**, *122*, 107–118. [CrossRef] [PubMed]

99. Gaboriau-Routhiau, V.; Rakotobe, S.; Lécuyer, E.; Mulder, I.; Lan, A.; Bridonneau, C.; Rochet, V.; Pisi, A.; De Paepe, M.; Brandi, G.; et al. The Key Role of Segmented Filamentous Bacteria in the Coordinated Maturation of Gut Helper T Cell Responses. *Immunity* **2009**, *31*, 677–689. [CrossRef] [PubMed]

100. Ivanov, I.I.; Atarashi, K.; Manel, N.; Brodie, E.L.; Shima, T.; Karaoz, U.; Wei, D.; Goldfarb, K.C.; Santee, C.A.; Lynch, S.V.; et al. Induction of Intestinal Th17 Cells by Segmented Filamentous Bacteria. *Cell* **2009**, *139*, 485–498. [CrossRef] [PubMed]

101. Chow, J.; Mazmanian, S.K. A Pathobiont of the Microbiota Balances Host Colonization and Intestinal Inflammation. *Cell Host Microbe* **2010**, *7*, 265–276. [CrossRef] [PubMed]

102. Emge, J.R.; Huynh, K.; Miller, E.N.; Kaur, M.; Reardon, C.; Barrett, K.E.; Gareau, M.G. Modulation of the Microbiota-Gut-Brain Axis by Probiotics in a Murine Model of Inflammatory Bowel Disease. *Am. J. Physiol. Liver Physiol.* **2016**, *310*, G989–G998. [CrossRef] [PubMed]

103. Kim, S.C.; Tonkonogy, S.L.; Albright, C.A.; Tsang, J.; Balish, E.J.; Braun, J.; Huycke, M.M.; Sartor, R.B. Variable Phenotypes of Enterocolitis in Interleukin 10-Deficient Mice Monoassociated with Two Different Commensal Bacteria. *Gastroenterology* **2005**, *128*, 891–906. [CrossRef] [PubMed]

104. Bloom, S.M.; Bijanki, V.N.; Nava, G.M.; Sun, L.; Malvin, N.P.; Donermeyer, D.L.; Dunne, W.M.; Allen, P.M.; Stappenbeck, T.S. Commensal Bacteroides Species Induce Colitis in Host-Genotype-Specific Fashion in a Mouse Model of Inflammatory Bowel Disease. *Cell Host Microbe* **2011**, *9*, 390–403. [CrossRef] [PubMed]

105. Garrett, W.S.; Gallini, C.A.; Yatsunenko, T.; Michaud, M.; DuBois, A.; Delaney, M.L.; Punit, S.; Karlsson, M.; Bry, L.; Glickman, J.N.; et al. Enterobacteriaceae Act in Concert with the Gut Microbiota to Induce Spontaneous and Maternally Transmitted Colitis. *Cell Host Microbe* **2010**, *8*, 292–300. [CrossRef] [PubMed]

106. Dharmani, P.; Strauss, J.; Ambrose, C.; Allen-Vercoe, E.; Chadee, K. *Fusobacterium Nucleatum* Infection of Colonic Cells Stimulates MUC2 Mucin and Tumor Necrosis Factor Alpha. *Infect. Immun.* **2011**, *79*, 2597–2607. [CrossRef] [PubMed]

107. Lee, Y.K.; Menezes, J.S.; Umesaki, Y.; Mazmanian, S.K. Proinflammatory T-Cell Responses to Gut Microbiota Promote Experimental Autoimmune Encephalomyelitis. *Proc. Natl. Acad. Sci. USA* **2011**, *108*, 4615–4622. [CrossRef] [PubMed]

108. Ochoa-Reparaz, J.; Mielcarz, D.W.; Ditrio, L.E.; Burroughs, A.R.; Foureau, D.M.; Haque-Begum, S.; Kasper, L.H. Role of Gut Commensal Microflora in the Development of Experimental Autoimmune Encephalomyelitis. *J. Immunol.* **2009**, *183*, 6041–6050. [CrossRef] [PubMed]

109. Yano, J.M.; Yu, K.; Donaldson, G.P.; Shastri, G.G.; Ann, P.; Ma, L.; Nagler, C.R.; Ismagilov, R.F.; Mazmanian, S.K.; Hsiao, E.Y. Indigenous Bacteria from the Gut Microbiota Regulate Host Serotonin Biosynthesis. *Cell* **2015**, *161*, 264–276. [CrossRef] [PubMed]

110. Reigstad, C.S.; Salmonson, C.E.; Rainey, J.F.; Szurszewski, J.H.; Linden, D.R.; Sonnenburg, J.L.; Farrugia, G.;

Kashyap, P.C. Gut Microbes Promote Colonic Serotonin Production through an Effect of Short-Chain Fatty Acids on Enterochromaffin Cells. *FASEB J.* **2015**, *29*, 1395–1403. [CrossRef] [PubMed]

111. Wikoff, W.R.; Anfora, A.T.; Liu, J.; Schultz, P.G.; Lesley, S.A.; Peters, E.C.; Siuzdak, G. Metabolomics Analysis Reveals Large Effects of Gut Microflora on Mammalian Blood Metabolites. *Proc. Natl. Acad. Sci. USA* **2009**, *106*, 3698–3703. [CrossRef] [PubMed]

112. Clarke, G.; Grenham, S.; Scully, P.; Fitzgerald, P.; Moloney, R.D.; Shanahan, F.; Dinan, T.G.; Cryan, J.F. The Microbiome-Gut-Brain Axis during Early Life Regulates the Hippocampal Serotonergic System in a Sex-Dependent Manner. *Mol. Psychiatry* **2013**, *18*, 666–673. [CrossRef] [PubMed]

113. Rooks, M.G.; Veiga, P.; Wardwell-Scott, L.H.; Tickle, T.; Segata, N.; Michaud, M.; Gallini, C.A.; Beal, C.; van Hylckama-Vlieg, J.E.; Ballal, S.A.; et al. Gut Microbiome Composition and Function in Experimental Colitis during Active Disease and Treatment-Induced Remission. *ISME J.* **2014**, *8*, 1403–1417. [CrossRef] [PubMed]

114. Robertson, B.R. *Mucispirillum Schaedleri* Gen. Nov., Sp. Nov., a Spiral-Shaped Bacterium Colonizing the Mucus Layer of the Gastrointestinal Tract of Laboratory Rodents. *Int. J. Syst. Evol. Microbiol.* **2005**, *55*, 1199–1204. [CrossRef] [PubMed]

115. Berry, D.; Schwab, C.; Milinovich, G.; Reichert, J.; Ben Mahfoudh, K.; Decker, T.; Engel, M.; Hai, B.; Hainzl, E.; Heider, S.; et al. Phylotype-Level 16S RRNA Analysis Reveals New Bacterial Indicators of Health State in Acute Murine Colitis. *ISME J.* **2012**, *6*, 2091–2106. [CrossRef] [PubMed]

116. Carbonero, F.; Benefiel, A.C.; Gaskins, H.R. Contributions of the Microbial Hydrogen Economy to Colonic Homeostasis. *Nat. Rev. Gastroenterol. Hepatol.* **2012**, *9*, 504–518. [CrossRef] [PubMed]

117. Kostic, A.D.; Chun, E.; Robertson, L.; Glickman, J.N.; Gallini, C.A.; Michaud, M.; Clancy, T.E.; Chung, D.C.; Lochhead, P.; Hold, G.L.; et al. *Fusobacterium Nucleatum* Potentiates Intestinal Tumorigenesis and Modulates the Tumor-Immune Microenvironment. *Cell Host Microbe* **2013**, *14*, 207–215. [CrossRef] [PubMed]

118. Strauss, J.; Kaplan, G.G.; Beck, P.L.; Rioux, K.; Panaccione, R.; DeVinney, R.; Lynch, T.; Allen-Vercoe, E. Invasive Potential of Gut Mucosa-Derived *Fusobacterium Nucleatum* Positively Correlates with IBD Status of the Host. *Inflamm. Bowel Dis.* **2011**, *17*, 1971–1978. [CrossRef] [PubMed]

119. Wang, Y.-P.; Chen, Y.-T.; Tsai, C.-F.; Li, S.-Y.; Luo, J.-C.; Wang, S.-J.; Tang, C.-H.; Liu, C.-J.; Lin, H.-C.; Lee, F.-Y.; et al. Short-Term Use of Serotonin Reuptake Inhibitors and Risk of Upper Gastrointestinal Bleeding. *Am. J. Psychiatry* **2014**, *171*, 54–61. [CrossRef] [PubMed]

120. Macedo, D.; Filho, A.J.M.C.; Soares de Sousa, C.N.; Quevedo, J.; Barichello, T.; Júnior, H.V.N.; Freitas de Lucena, D. Antidepressants, Antimicrobials or Both? Gut Microbiota Dysbiosis in Depression and Possible Implications of the Antimicrobial Effects of Antidepressant Drugs for Antidepressant Effectiveness. *J. Affect. Disord.* **2017**, *208*, 22–32. [CrossRef] [PubMed]

121. Coban, A.Y.; Tanriverdi Cayci, Y.; Keleş Uludağ, S.; Durupinar, B. Investigation of Antibacterial Activity of Sertralin. *Mikrobiyol. Bul.* **2009**, *43*, 651–656. [PubMed]

122. Munoz-Bellido, J.; Munoz-Criado, S.; Garcìa-Rodrìguez, J. Antimicrobial Activity of Psychotropic Drugs: Selective Serotonin Reuptake Inhibitors. *Int. J. Antimicrob. Agents* **2000**, *14*, 177–180. [CrossRef]

123. Kruszewska, H.; Zaręba, T.; Tyski, S. Examination of Antimicrobial Activity of Selected Non-Antibiotic Medicinal Preparations. *Acta Pol. Pharm. Drug Res.* **2012**, *69*, 1368–1371.

124. Cenit, M.C.; Sanz, Y.; Codoñer-Franch, P. Influence of Gut Microbiota on Neuropsychiatric Disorders. *World J. Gastroenterol.* **2017**, *23*, 5486–5498. [CrossRef] [PubMed]

125. Kelly, J.R.; Borre, Y.; O'Brien, C.; Patterson, E.; El Aidy, S.; Deane, J.; Kennedy, P.J.; Beers, S.; Scott, K.; Moloney, G.; et al. Transferring the Blues: Depression-Associated Gut Microbiota Induces Neurobehavioural Changes in the Rat. *J. Psychiatr. Res.* **2016**, *82*, 109–118. [CrossRef] [PubMed]

126. Aizawa, E.; Tsuji, H.; Asahara, T.; Takahashi, T.; Teraishi, T.; Yoshida, S.; Ota, M.; Koga, N.; Hattori, K.; Kunugi, H. Possible Association of *Bifidobacterium* and *Lactobacillus* in the Gut Microbiota of Patients with Major Depressive Disorder. *J. Affect. Disord.* **2016**, *202*, 254–257. [CrossRef] [PubMed]

127. Messaoudi, M.; Lalonde, R.; Violle, N.; Javelot, H.; Desor, D.; Nejdi, A.; Bisson, J.-F.; Rougeot, C.; Pichelin, M.; Cazaubiel, M.; et al. Assessment of Psychotropic-like Properties of a Probiotic Formulation

(*Lactobacillus Helveticus* R0052 and *Bifidobacterium Longum* R0175) in Rats and Human Subjects. *Br. J. Nutr.* **2011**, *105*, 755–764. [CrossRef] [PubMed]

128. Benton, D.; Williams, C.; Brown, A. Impact of Consuming a Milk Drink Containing a Probiotic on Mood and Cognition. *Eur. J. Clin. Nutr.* **2007**, *61*, 355–361. [CrossRef] [PubMed]

129. Steenbergen, L.; Sellaro, R.; van Hemert, S.; Bosch, J.A.; Colzato, L.S. A Randomized Controlled Trial to Test the Effect of Multispecies Probiotics on Cognitive Reactivity to Sad Mood. *Brain Behav. Immun.* **2015**, *48*, 258–264. [CrossRef] [PubMed]

130. Tillisch, K.; Labus, J.; Kilpatrick, L.; Jiang, Z.; Stains, J.; Ebrat, B.; Guyonnet, D.; Legrain-Raspaud, S.; Trotin, B.; Naliboff, B.; et al. Consumption of Fermented Milk Product With Probiotic Modulates Brain Activity. *Gastroenterology* **2013**, *144*, 1394–1401.e4. [CrossRef] [PubMed]

131. Marin, I.A.; Goertz, J.E.; Ren, T.; Rich, S.S.; Onengut-Gumuscu, S.; Farber, E.; Wu, M.; Overall, C.C.; Kipnis, J.; Gaultier, A. Microbiota Alteration Is Associated with the Development of Stress-Induced Despair Behavior. *Sci. Rep.* **2017**, *7*, 43859. [CrossRef] [PubMed]

132. Gao, J.; Xu, K.; Liu, H.; Liu, G.; Bai, M.; Peng, C.; Li, T.; Yin, Y. Impact of the Gut Microbiota on Intestinal Immunity Mediated by Tryptophan Metabolism. *Front. Cell. Infect. Microbiol.* **2018**, *8*, 13. [CrossRef] [PubMed]

133. Genestet, C.; Le Gouellec, A.; Chaker, H.; Polack, B.; Guery, B.; Toussaint, B.; Stasia, M.J. Scavenging of Reactive Oxygen Species by Tryptophan Metabolites Helps Pseudomonas Aeruginosa Escape Neutrophil Killing. *Free Radic. Biol. Med.* **2014**, *73*, 400–410. [CrossRef] [PubMed]

134. Zheng, X.; Xie, G.; Zhao, A.; Zhao, L.; Yao, C.; Chiu, N.H.L.; Zhou, Z.; Bao, Y.; Jia, W.; Nicholson, J.K.; et al. The Footprints of Gut Microbial–Mammalian Co-Metabolism. *J. Proteome Res.* **2011**, *10*, 5512–5522. [CrossRef] [PubMed]

135. El Aidy, S.; Merrifield, C.A.; Derrien, M.; van Baarlen, P.; Hooiveld, G.; Levenez, F.; Doré, J.; Dekker, J.; Holmes, E.; Claus, S.P.; et al. The Gut Microbiota Elicits a Profound Metabolic Reorientation in the Mouse Jejunal Mucosa during Conventionalisation. *Gut* **2013**, *62*, 1306–1314. [CrossRef] [PubMed]

136. Jaglin, M.; Rhimi, M.; Philippe, C.; Pons, N.; Bruneau, A.; Goustard, B.; Daugé, V.; Maguin, E.; Naudon, L.; Rabot, S. Indole, a Signaling Molecule Produced by the Gut Microbiota, Negatively Impacts Emotional Behaviors in Rats. *Front. Neurosci.* **2018**, *12*, 216. [CrossRef] [PubMed]

137. Biagini, G.; Pich, E.M.; Carani, C.; Marrama, P.; Gustafsson, J.-Å.; Fuxe, K.; Agnati, L.F. Indole-Pyruvic Acid, a Tryptophan Ketoanalogue, Antagonizes the Endocrine but Not the Behavioral Effects of Repeated Stress in a Model of Depression. *Biol. Psychiatry* **1993**, *33*, 712–719. [CrossRef]

138. Tigchelaar, E.F.; Zhernakova, A.; Dekens, J.A.M.; Hermes, G.; Baranska, A.; Mujagic, Z.; Swertz, M.A.; Muñoz, A.M.; Deelen, P.; Cénit, M.C.; et al. Cohort Profile: LifeLines DEEP, a Prospective, General Population Cohort Study in the Northern Netherlands: Study Design and Baseline Characteristics. *BMJ Open* **2015**, *5*, e006772. [CrossRef] [PubMed]

139. Sudlow, C.; Gallacher, J.; Allen, N.; Beral, V.; Burton, P.; Danesh, J.; Downey, P.; Elliott, P.; Green, J.; Landray, M.; et al. UK Biobank: An Open Access Resource for Identifying the Causes of a Wide Range of Complex Diseases of Middle and Old Age. *PLoS Med.* **2015**, *12*, e1001779. [CrossRef] [PubMed]

140. Falony, G.; Joossens, M.; Vieira-Silva, S.; Wang, J.; Darzi, Y.; Faust, K.; Kurilshikov, A.; Bonder, M.J.; Valles-Colomer, M.; Vandeputte, D.; et al. Population-Level Analysis of Gut Microbiome Variation. *Science* **2016**, *352*, 560–564. [CrossRef] [PubMed]

8

Side Effects and Interactions of the Xanthine Oxidase Inhibitor Febuxostat

Andreas Jordan and Ursula Gresser *

Internal Medicine, Medical Faculty, Ludwig Maximilians University of Munich, 80539 Munich, Germany;
jordan.andreas@gmx.de
* Correspondence: ursulagresser@email.de

Abstract: The paper addresses the safety of febuxostat and summarizes reports on side effects and interactions of febuxostat published by the cut-off date (last day of literature search) of 20 March 2018. Publications on side effects and the interactions of febuxostat were considered. Information concerning the occurrence of side effects and interactions in association with the treatment with febuxostat was collected and summarized in the review. The incidence of severe side effects was much less frequent than mild side effects (1.2–3.8% to 20.1–38.7%). The rate and range of febuxostat side effects are low at doses of up to 120 mg and only increase with a daily dose of over 120 mg. The publications reveal no age-dependent increase in side effects for febuxostat. In patients with impaired renal function, no increase in adverse events is described with a dose of up to 120 mg of febuxostat per day. Patients with impaired liver function had no elevated risk for severe side effects. A known allopurinol intolerance increases the risk of skin reactions during treatment with febuxostat by a factor of 3.6. No correlation between treatment with febuxostat and agranulocytosis has been confirmed. Possible interactions with very few medications (principally azathioprine) are known for febuxostat. Febuxostat is well tolerated and a modern and safe alternative to allopurinol therapy.

Keywords: febuxostat; side effects; interactions

1. Introduction

Allopurinol (market launch in Germany 1964, [1]) and febuxostat (market launch in Germany 2010, [2]) are two inhibitors of the xanthine oxidase. Febuxostat is, other than allopurinol, a non-purine xanthine oxidase inhibitor (see Figure 1) [3].

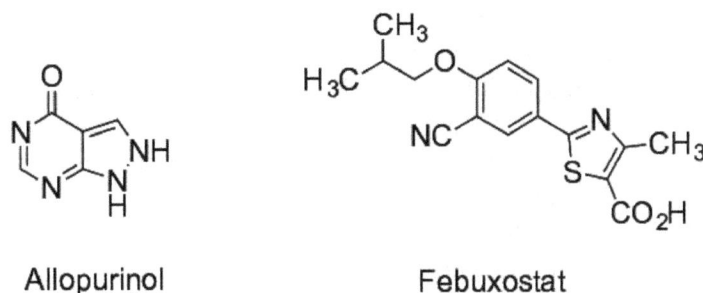

Figure 1. Chemical structures of allopurinol and febuxostat [3].

Spiekermann showed, that the xanthine oxidase is also located in the vessel wall [4]. There is evidence for a connection between the activity of xanthine oxidase and vasodilation as well as endothelial function [5]. The free oxygen radicals formed during xanthine oxidase play an important pathophysiological role in this context [6]. It was demonstrated that—in contrast to allopurinol—febuxostat has a positive impact on stress parameters and vascular elasticity [7].

The present review addresses the following questions:

1.   What is known from scientific publications with regard to side effects and interactions during treatment with the xanthine oxidase inhibitor febuxostat?
2.   Febuxostat's safety profile in comparison and contrast to allopurinol.

2. Results

2.1. Findings in Original Works and Secondary Analyses

Tables A1 and A2 present the original works and secondary analyses with the respective events that occurred.

The results of the evaluation of the stated publications are summarized below by content. The administered daily febuxostat dose in the reviewed papers was between 10 mg and 240 mg.

In the original papers and secondary analyses, at least one side effect (without severe side effects) occurred in 20.1% and 39.7% of the patients and at least one severe side effect in 1.2% and 3.8%, respectively. The five most frequently reported side effects were musculoskeletal symptoms (7.7% of the patients who received febuxostat); upper respiratory tract symptoms (5.4%); changes in liver function values (4.7%); diarrhea (3.6%); headache (2.8%). Of the patients in the original papers and secondary analyses, 2.9% and 1.0%, respectively, dropped out of the study prematurely due to side effects. The most frequent side effect reported in the original papers that resulted in a patient dropping out of the study prematurely was an increase in liver values (20.9%) [8–12]. Other reasons were diarrhea (12.0%), rash (1.7%), as well as cardiac symptoms (1.7%). The latter were three patients with unspecified cardiovascular symptoms [9], one patient with precordial pain [13], one patient with palpitations and chest pain [14], as well as one patient with acute heart failure [15]. In the CARES-study from White et al., the incidence of major cardiovascular events was similar in both groups [16]. "Sudden cardiac death was [. . .] occuring in [. . .] 2.7% [of the patients] in the febuxostat group and [. . .] 1.8% [of the patients] in the allopurinol group" [16]. The risk of cardiovascular death was higher under febuxostat therapy compared to allopurinol in patients with gout [16]. The overall mortality in both groups was similar [16].

2.1.1. Duration of therapy and dosage

An increase in the occurrence of events with the increasing duration of the therapy was shown for severe side effects (see Figure 2). The share of patients affected increased from 0.6% (up to one week) to 3.5% (more than one year). The share of patients with at least one side effect (without severe side effects) was in a range between 4.7% (duration of therapy over one week to one month) and 53.3% (duration of therapy over six months to one year) during the therapy periods considered. The share of these patients in the periods considered were the lowest for a duration of therapy over one week to one month (4.7%) and over one year (26.9%). The share of patients who dropped out of the study prematurely due to side effects increased from 0.9% (duration of therapy up to 1 week) to 6.4% (duration of therapy of more than one year).

As the dose increased, the share of patients with at least one side effect (without severe side effects) was 72% at a daily dose of febuxostat of more than 120 mg (see Figure 3). At lower doses, this share was a maximum of 41.8%. In the dose group of 81 to 120 mg/day compared with the dose group of 51 to 80 mg/day, an increase in the share of patients with at least one severe side effect due to febuxostat from 2.6% to 4.8% was observed. The share of patients who dropped out of the study prematurely increased to a maximum of 9% in the highest dose group (121 and more mg/day).

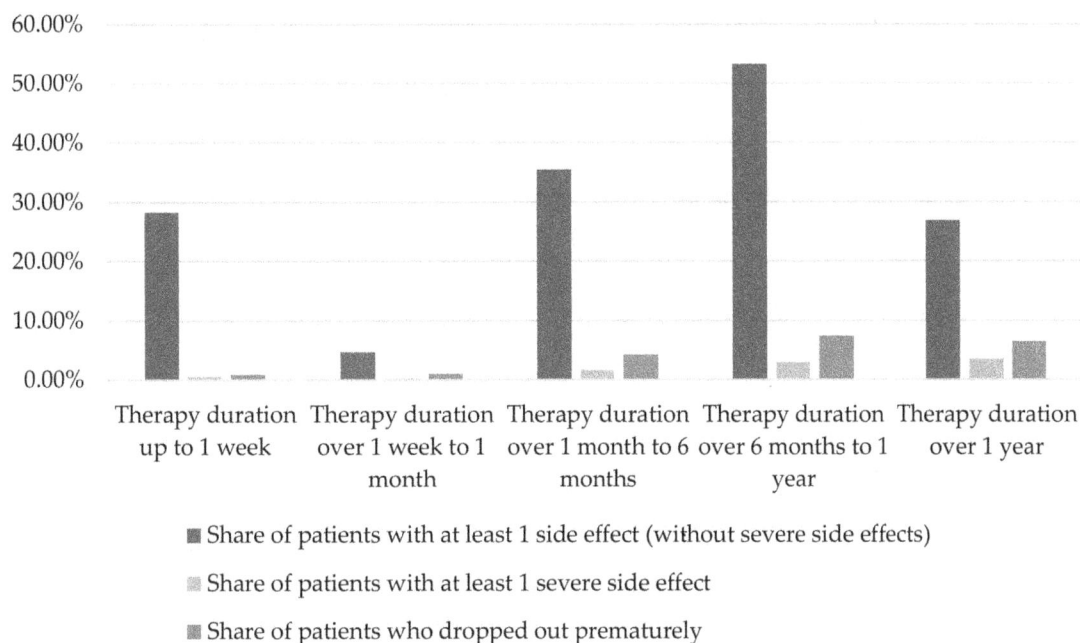

Figure 2. Occurrence of adverse events in dependence on therapy duration (n (therapy duration up to one week) = 332; n (therapy duration over one week to one month) = 6525; n (therapy duration over one month to six months) = 3170; n (therapy duration over six months to one year) = 1297; n (therapy duration over one year) = 917; per therapy period differentiation between patients with at least one side effect (column 1), patients with at least one severe side effect (column 2), patients who dropped out of the study prematurely (column 3)) [2,8–15,17–52].

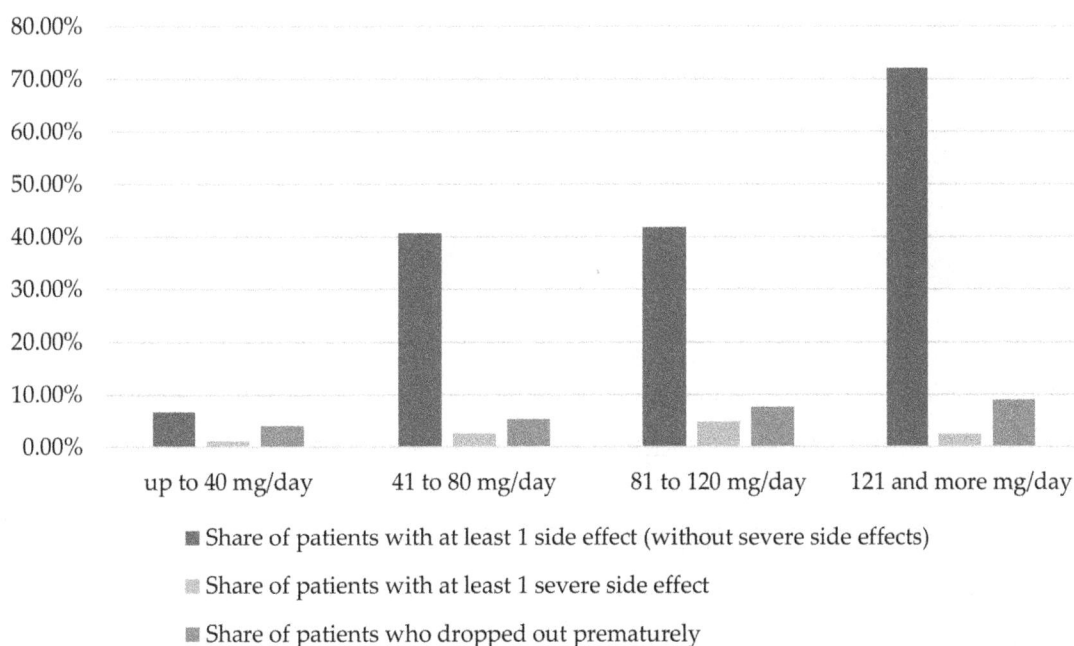

Figure 3. Occurrence of adverse events in dependence on febuxostat dosage (n (up to 40 mg/day) = 1803; n (41 to 80 mg/day) = 2361; n (81 to 120 mg/day) = 673; n (121 and more mg/day) = 200; for each dose group differentiation between: patients with at least one side effect (column 1), patients with at least one severe side effect (column 2), patients who dropped out prematurely (column 3); daily dose used in mg/day for each dose group: up to 40 mg/day: 10, 20, 30, 40; 41 to 80 mg/day: 50, 60, 70, 80; 81 to 120 mg/day: 90, 120; 121 mg/day and more: 160, 180, 240) [8,9,11–13,15,17–27,29,31,33–36,38,41,42,45,48–54].

A quantification of the interaction between the duration of therapy and the dose was not possible based on the information provided in the original studies.

2.1.2. Renal Function

The share of patients with impaired renal function, who experienced at least one side effect (without severe side effects) was a maximum of 14.3% and thus lower than for patients with normal renal function (27.4%) (see Figure 4). The maximum febuxostat dose for patients with impairment in renal function was at 80 mg/day, lower than for patients with normal renal function (maximum 240 mg/day).

2.1.3. Liver Function

The metabolisation of febuxostat in the body largely takes place in the liver [50]. In the study by Khosravan et al., the subjects were allocated into three groups based on the individual hepatic function as determined by Child-Pugh [50]. In patients with moderately impaired liver function, the share of patients with at least one side effect (without severe side effects) was 75% and therefore three times as high as in the patient group with normal liver function (25%) [50] (see Table 1). The daily dose of febuxostat in all groups was 80 mg [50]. The most frequently reported side effects (without severe side effects) were headache, abdominal pain, and diarrhea, as well as a change in the frequency of micturition [50]. It was not necessary to adjust the febuxostat dose in any of the cases [50]. No severe side effects occurred in any of the groups [50].

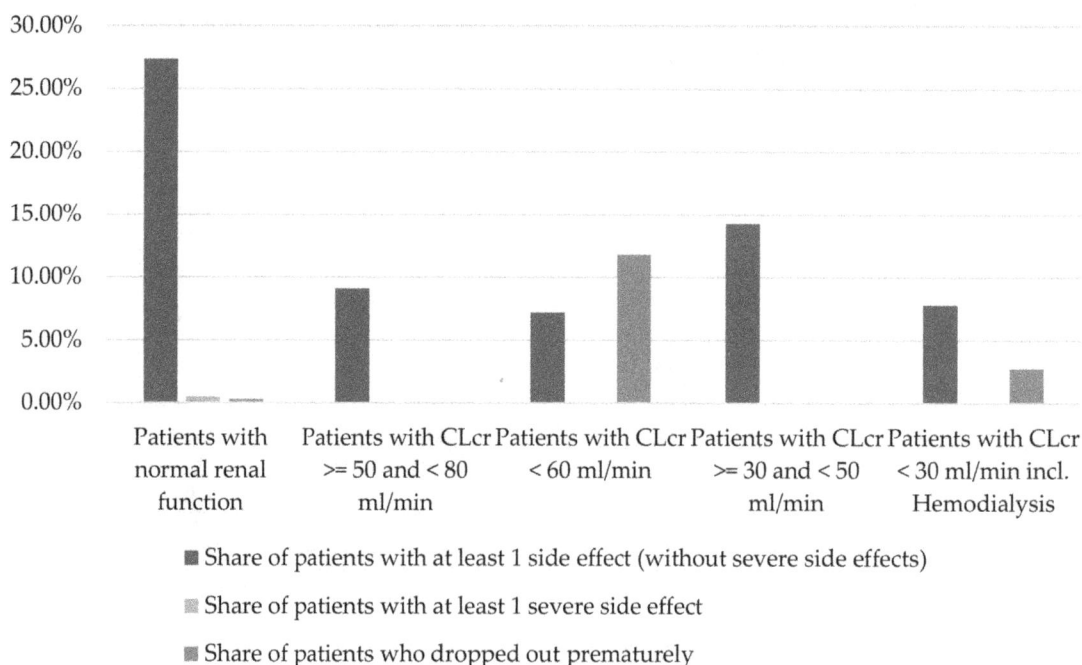

Figure 4. Occurrence of adverse events depending on renal function (n (patients with normal renal function) = 1812; n (patients with CLcr >= 50 and <80 mL/min) = 11; n (patients with CLcr <60 mL/min) = 610; n (patients with CLcr >=30 and <50 mL/min) = 35; n (patients with CLcr <30 mL/min incl. hemodialysis) = 399; per patient group (sorted by renal function, left starting with the best) differentiation between patients with at least one side effect (column 1), patients with at least one severe side effect (column 2), patients who dropped out prematurely (column 3)) [12–14,17–20,22,24–26,29,31,34,35,37,38,41,44–46,48–52,55].

Table 1. Adverse events in patients depending on liver function (number of patients examined per group (column 1); liver function of patient group (column 2); patients with at least one side effect (column 3); patients with at least one severe side effect (column 4); publications reviewed (column 5); differentiation between side effect and severe side effect in accordance with the publications, no standard definition).

Number of Patients with Febuxostat Therapy	Liver Function	Number of Patients with at Least One Side Effect (Share in %)	Number of Patients with at Least One Severe Side Effect (Share in %)	Source
12	Normal	3 (25.0)	0	
8	Mildly limited	5 (63.0)	0	[50]
8	Moderately limited	6 (75.0)	0	

2.1.4. Diabetes mellitus type 2

The occurrence of adverse events during treatment with febuxostat in patients with and without diabetes mellitus type 2 is comparable based on the publications reviewed (see Figure 5) [39,56].

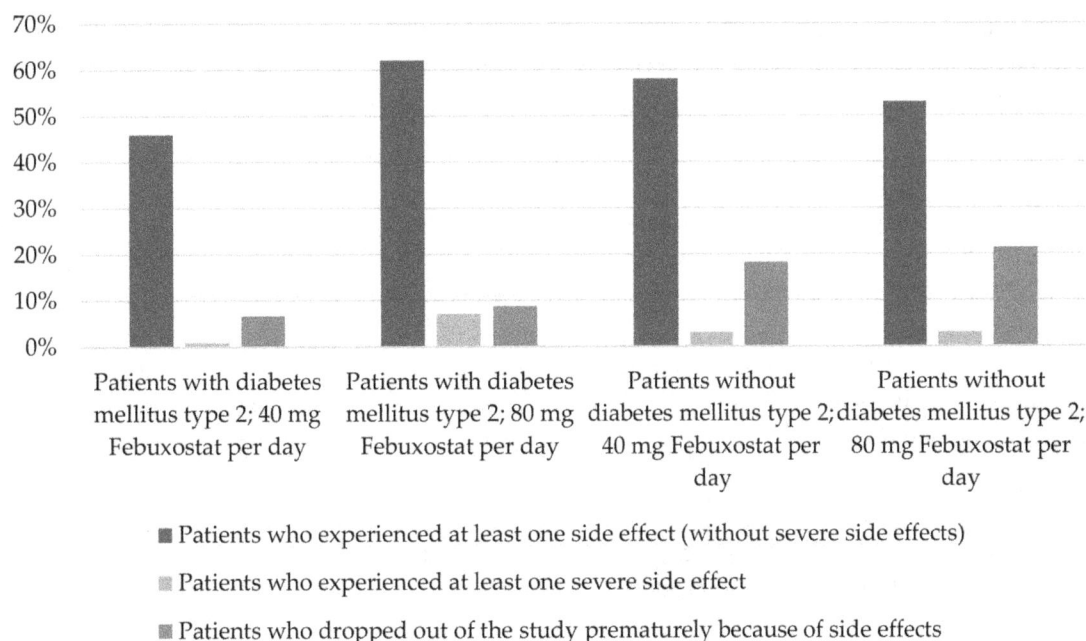

■ Patients who experienced at least one side effect (without severe side effects)

▨ Patients who experienced at least one severe side effect

■ Patients who dropped out of the study prematurely because of side effects

Figure 5. Occurrence of adverse events in patients with and without diabetes mellitus type 2 (n (Study population) = 1462; classification of patients by patients with and without diabetes mellitus type 2 as well as respective febuxostat dose (40 or 80 mg/day); in each case, illustration of patients who experienced at least one side effect (column 1), patients who experienced at least one severe side effect (column 2), patients who dropped out of the study prematurely (column 3)) [56].

In Ito et al. [39], at least one side effect (without severe side effects) occurred among 13.5% of the diabetes patients treated with febuxostat. Among patients without diabetes mellitus type 2 the share was 20% [39].

Becker et al. [56] showed that the urate lowering efficiency of febuxostat (reducing the serum urate level below 6 mg/dL) is dose dependent in both patients with and without renal insufficiency. Febuxostat at a daily dose of 80 mg was more efficient than 40 mg at any level of renal insufficiency (see Figure 6). This holds true for both diabetic and non-diabetic patients [56].

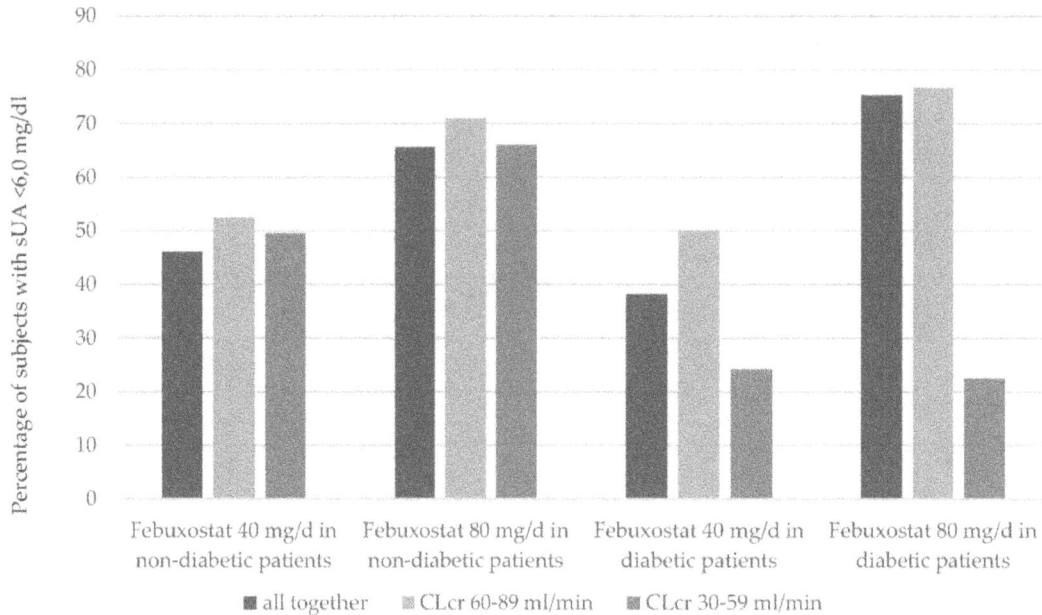

Figure 6. Comparing diabetic and non-diabetic patients and the urate lowering efficiency of febuxostat (patients with achievement of serum urate level < 6.0 mg/dL in percent) at a daily dose of febuxostat of 40 mg/day respectively 80 mg/day with regard to the renal function level (sUA: serum urate level) [56].

2.1.5. Age Dependency

Studies indicated an increase in adverse events in patients over 65 years of age [21,57]. The share of patients who experienced at least one side effect (without severe side effects) and one severe side effect was twice as high in the group of patients over the age of 65 (58.3% and 6.3%) than in the group of patients under 65 years (29.2% and 2.5%) [57]. The number of comorbidities in the study population of the patients under 65 years was in part only half as high as in the group of patients over 65 [57]. In the younger group every patient took an average of 3.8 medications versus 7.1 medications in the older patient group [57].

2.1.6. Pre-existing Allopurinol Intolerance

Based on the reviewed publications, the risk of a skin reaction (exanthem, pruritus) is higher by a factor of 3.6 under therapy with febuxostat in patients with a pre-existing allopurinol intolerance [28].

2.1.7. Combination of Febuxostat with NSAIDs

Non-steroidal anti-inflammatory drugs (NSAIDs) are frequently used to treat acute attacks of gout. The incidence of side effects was investigated during simultaneous therapy with febuxostat together with Indometacin or Naproxen (see Table 2) [52].

Table 2. Side effects during therapy with febuxostat and NSAID (applied NSAID (column 1); number of patients who were administered the NSAID (column 2); patients with at least one side effect during therapy with febuxostat (column 3), febuxostat together with NSAID (column 4); NSAID (column 5); publications reviewed (column 6)).

NSAID	Number of Patients Examined	Number of Patients with at Least One Side Effect (Share in % a Study Population)			Source
		Febuxostat	Febuxostat + NSAID	NSAID	
Indometacin	27	2 (8.0)	6 (22.0)	7 (27.0)	[52]
Naproxen	26	7 (28.0)	9 (35.0)	7 (26.0)	

Based on the publications reviewed regarding the side effect profile, Indometacin and Naproxen can be prescribed parallel to a therapy with febuxostat to the extent that there is no contraindication for NSAID therapy in a given case [52].

2.1.8. Combination of Febuxostat with Hydrochlorothiazide

In the therapy of febuxostat together with hydrochlorothiazide, 43% of the patients developed at least one side effect [12]. This share was 41% when the only treatment given was febuxostat [12]. Severe side effects did not occur [12]. The combined therapy of febuxostat and hydrochlorothiazide was well tolerated [12]. No dose adjustment is required for the simultaneous administration of febuxostat and hydrochlorothiazide [12].

2.1.9. Combination of Febuxostat with Uricosuric Drugs

Lesinurad (approved in Europe) and Arhalofenat (not yet approved in Europe) are drugs that increase the excretion of uric acid in the urine and are used to treat hyperuricemia and gout [58,59]. In 21 patients treated with febuxostat (40 or 80 mg/day) together with Lesinurad (400 to 600 mg/day), a total of 27 side effects and no severe side effects occurred [58]. During the combined use of febuxostat (40 and 80 mg/day) and Arhalofenat (600 or 80 mg/day) in 32 patients, 23 patients (72%) experienced at least one side effect and no severe side effects [59].

2.1.10. Combination of Febuxostat with Azathioprine

Two cases of a pancytopenia or eosinophilia have been published to date in response to a possible interaction between febuxostat and azathioprine [55,60]. Both authors consider an interaction of these two medications as the probable source of the symptoms [55,60]. Patients experienced, among other adverse reactions, nausea and vomiting, watery diarrhea with weight loss, as well as pancytopenia [55]; other manifestations included fever and a case of eosinophilia [60].

2.1.11. Combination of Febuxostat with Theophylline

The coadministration of febuxostat together with theophylline does not affect the pharmacokinetics of theophylline [24]. Theophylline was well tolerated when administered together with febuxostat (80 mg/day) without dose adjustment of febuxostat [24].

2.2. Findings of the Case Reports

Research revealed 14 published case reports on side effects of febuxostat. An evaluation of the cases according to a causality scale like the Naranjo score was not possible as the information given in the case reports was not detailed enough to do so.

2.2.1. Skin Reactions and DRESS Syndrome

The occurrence of hypersensitive skin reactions in conjunction with febuxostat therapy is described for 6 patients. The symptoms described range from itching and erythema [61] to "granulomatous eruption" [62] and "eruptive maculae" [63] to a potentially lethal DRESS syndrome [64–66]. DRESS syndrome is a special variant of hypersensitivity reaction (DRESS: drug reaction with eosinophilia and systemic symptoms) [64]. It is described in conjunction with febuxostat therapy in three case reports [64–66]. In two of the three patients reported with DRESS syndrome, an intolerance for allopurinol had occurred in the past [65,66]; this event had probably also occurred once in the past with the third patient during allopurinol treatment [64]. Skin reactions occurred in the past during therapy with allopurinol in a total of five of six patients (83.5%) with hypersensitive skin reactions. All described patients recovered. No patient died, see [61–66].

2.2.2. Rhabdomyolysis

Three cases of rhabdomyolysis have been described [67–69]. One of the patients had a history of a hypersensitive reaction to allopurinol [68]. Two of the patients had impaired renal function with a eGFR of 45 mL/min [67] and 35 ± 7 mL/min [68]. The authors saw a correlation with the development of rhabdomyolysis and the co-administration of a statin together with colchicine [67] or a fibrate [68] parallel to a therapy with febuxostat. In the third case, no conclusions were drawn to the causality of rhabdomyolysis [69]. There is no indication that febuxostat could be the sole cause for the occurrence of a dreaded rhabdomyolysis.

2.2.3. Agranulocytosis

In one paper, two cases of agranulocytosis in the context of treatment with febuxostat are described [70]. Both patients had chronic renal insufficiency [70]. In this context, a correlation with the therapy with febuxostat was neither proven nor excluded [70].

2.2.4. Glomerulonephritis

Izzedine et al. [71] describe the case of a 63-year-old man who developed acute kidney failure with nephrotic syndrome after five months of therapy with febuxostat at an unknown dosage [71]. An ANCA-positive Pauci-immune glomerulonephritis was diagnosed, the cause of which the authors viewed as the therapy with febuxostat [71].

2.2.5. Acute Liver Disease

Bohm et al. [72] described the case of a 34-year-old patient who developed itching, nausea, abdominal pain, fatigue, and jaundice during febuxostat therapy [72]. The authors suspect the therapy with febuxostat to be the cause for the development of this acute liver disease [72]. The authors made no statements regarding an association with febuxostat or any other causal or predisposing factors.

3. Discussion

According to the findings of the present evaluation, febuxostat is well tolerated. There are no major differences between the risk profile for allopurinol and febuxostat in regard to the occurrence of side effects [73]. However, the risk of cardiovascular death was higher under febuxostat therapy compared to allopurinol in patients with gout, whereas the overall mortality was similar [16]. In Seth et al. [74], it was demonstrated that the probability of side effects occurring was 1.12 times higher with allopurinol therapy than with febuxostat [74]. Severe side effects occurred 1.11 times more frequently when allopurinol was administered compared to febuxostat [74]. In another paper, the probability of side effects due to the administration of febuxostat was only 0.94 times as high compared to allopurinol [75]. An effect of febuxostat on arterial blood pressure as an adverse event was not reported. There is indication, that febuxostat lowers blood pressure in patients with normal renal function [76]. An influence on adverse events under febuxostat therapy in the context of the use of alcohol was not reported. With regard to cardiovascular events during febuxostat therapy, further studies need to be conducted to evaluate the effect of febuxostat on cardiovascular events and death.

In the present review of the literature, it was determined that an increase in the occurrence of side effects (without severe side effects) with febuxostat is not to be expected until the daily dose exceeds 120 mg/day. At a dose of 80 and 120 mg of febuxostat per day, the probability of side effects occurring is comparatively lower (relative risk: 0.90 and 0.93) than for therapy with allopurinol (100–300 mg/day) [77]. In the paper by Li et al. [77] it was shown that febuxostat has the lowest risk of side effects compared to allopurinol and other drugs that lower uric acid levels [77].

3.1. Renal Function

Based on the available publications, for patients with renal function disorders and extending to those requiring dialysis treatment, therapy is possible at a daily dose of 80 mg of febuxostat without an increase in the occurrence of adverse events.

Allopurinol and its active metabolite oxypurinol are excreted exclusively renally [29]. They can accumulate in patients with renal insufficiency [29]. The excretion of febuxostat is only 50% renal [29]. Its plasma levels (pharmacokinetic) in patients with renal insufficiency up to hemodialysis are stable [29]. In patients with impaired renal function, the allopurinol dose must be reduced [78]. This may result in a decline in the body's ability to reduce uric acid levels [79]. In addition, renal insufficiency increases the risk of a hypersensitivity reaction to allopurinol [79]. Consequently, a consistent dose reduction is recommended depending on creatinine clearance for allopurinol [79]. According to the findings of the present paper, a dose reduction of febuxostat is not required for patients with impaired renal function or those requiring hemodialysis. Patients with renal insufficiency must be extremely closely monitored under allopurinol therapy with careful dose adjustments. There are always cases in which this is not or not sufficiently practicable.

Bove et al. showed that, in patients with renal dysfunction, the safety profile of febuxostat compared to allopurinol was better regarding relative risk (RR) of adverse events [80]. A study with kidney transplant patients showed that the use of febuxostat in those patients was safe [81]. Using febuxostat, close monitoring of patients with renal insufficiency is not required.

Both allopurinol and febuxostat can be considered in CKD patients. Beside the risk profiles of both drugs in patients with renal insufficiency, cost and availability of intensive monitoring may also help make the decision of which to choose.

3.2. Liver Function

The present evaluation revealed an increase in the incidence of adverse events with increasing impairment of liver function. The probability of the occurrence of side effects in patients with pre-existing impairment of liver function is also higher during therapy with allopurinol [82]. This applies specifically to "generalized [...] hypersensitivity reactions" [82]. In patients with impaired liver function, a daily dose of 80 mg febuxostat should not be exceeded according to the findings of the present evaluation. This is consistent with the current product information on febuxostat: "The recommended dose for patients with mild liver function impairment [. . .] is 80 mg" of febuxostat in the treatment of gout [83].

3.3. Diabetes Mellitus Type 2

Therapy with febuxostat was tolerated equally well by patients with and without type 2 diabetes mellitus. There was no increase in the incidence of adverse events for patients with or without type 2 diabetes mellitus undergoing therapy with allopurinol [56]. A dose adjustment is required neither for febuxostat nor for allopurinol.

3.4. Age Dependence

Patients over 65 years of age developed more adverse events compared to the group of patients under 65 [21,57]. Regarding adverse events, the factors age, morbidity and medication must be considered together. From the findings of the present paper, there is no need for a general dose reduction for older patients [21,57]. It is more important that changes in the side effect profile are monitored for all patients with several secondary disorders and corresponding drug therapy. This is in particular also true for the therapy with allopurinol. Interactions must be watched for specifically in the event of combined therapy of allopurinol with "Mercaptopurine, Azathioprine, Mycophenolatmofetil, cyclosporin, aluminum hydroxide, Theophylline [or] Warfarin" [84]. Patients treated with one of these drugs should not undergo therapy designed to lower uric acid levels with allopurinol, but preferably be treated with febuxostat.

3.5. Pre-Existing Allopurinol Intolerance

Patients with a pre-existing allopurinol intolerance are more likely to develop intolerance reactions to febuxostat [28]. Patients with allopurinol intolerance require special medical attention. Patients who exhibit symptoms of a hypersensitivity reaction during therapy with febuxostat should end therapy immediately [28,61,62,64–66]. Nevertheless, "hypersensitivity to allopurinol is not a contraindication to febuxostat" [85].

3.6. Combination of Febuxostat with NSAIDs

Combining febuxostat with NSAID does not result in a significant increase in adverse events based on the present evaluation [52]. This combination is an alternative to the combination of allopurinol with an NSAID with regard to side effects.

3.7. Combination of Febuxostat with Hydrochlorothiazide

It was shown that the combined therapy with febuxostat and hydrochlorothiazide is well tolerated without a dose adjustment [12]. In a therapy with allopurinol, a simultaneous therapy with a thiazide escalates the risk of a hypersensitivity reaction [86]. Based on the publications analyzed, a therapy with febuxostat to reduce uric acid levels should be introduced for patients treated with hydrochlorothiazide. No adjustment of the febuxostat dose is necessary.

3.8. Combination of Febuxostat with Uricosuric Drugs

No severe side effects occurred during the combined therapy of febuxostat together with Lesinurad or Arhalofenat [58,59]. The question of side effects during the co-administration of Lesinurad and allopurinol is the subject of current research (see [87,88]). Before a final assessment of the tolerability of febuxostat in combination with Lesinurad or Arhalofenat can be made, the findings of additional studies must be waited for. Whether the combination of these new uricosuric agents with one of the available xanthine oxidase inhibitors has advantages for the patient cannot be inferred from the available literature.

3.9. Combination of Febuxostat with Azathioprine

In two publications [55,60], the authors report pancytopenia and eosinophilia when febuxostat and azathioprine are administered together which they consider a possible interaction of the two substances. In the scope of allopurinol therapy, the interaction with azathioprine is a known complication [89]. Severe side effects can occur [90]. To reduce this risk, the allopurinol dose should be reduced when combined with azathioprine. In addition, within the scope of allopurinol therapy, an increased risk of bone marrow suppression with a potential agranulocytosis is known through drug interaction with azathioprine [84]. Consequently, these complications and interactions should also be considered in febuxostat therapy if corresponding symptoms occur and immediate action taken, that is, the patient should discontinue taking the drug. Given an existing therapy with azathioprine, a therapy designed to lower uric acid levels, preferably with febuxostat, should follow.

3.10. Skin Reactions and DRESS Syndrome

In the present analysis, a pre-existing allopurinol intolerance was identified as a risk factor for the development of an intolerance to febuxostat [61,62,64–66]. Under therapy with allopurinol, up to 0.4% develop a DRESS syndrome [78]. For allopurinol, the greatest risk factor for the occurrence of a hypersensitivity reaction is an impairment in renal function [78]. Another risk factor is therapy of asymptomatic hyperuricemia with allopurinol [78]. A comparable correlation was not described for febuxostat.

3.11. Rhabdomyolysis

In the paper by Kang et al. [67], the authors hypothesize that the combination of febuxostat, colchicine, and rosuvastatin may have led to an increase in the plasma levels of one or more of these drugs and may thus have caused rhabdomyolysis [67]. The risk of developing rhabdomyolysis following co-administration of colchicine together with a statin is described in various case histories ([91–96]). The simultaneous existence of impaired renal function also raises the risk for rhabdomyolysis under such combination therapy [91–93,96]. The occurrence of rhabdomyolysis is also described in the combination of colchicine with fibrates [97]. With regard to patient safety, the symptoms of this side effect must expressly be watched for, and the patient must be informed if—in addition to febuxostat—a therapy with a statin, colchicine or a fibrate is intended. In this situation, regular control of the creatine kinase is to be recommended to be able to catch rhabdomyolysis at an early state. Liu et al. presented a study with 1332 patients with chronic kidney disease [98]. Forty-one patients developed a myopathy [98]. "Febuxostat was the culprit agent [...] in only two patients [...]" [98]. Further studies are required to identify the pathophysiologic relation between febuxostat and myopathy.

3.12. Agranulocytosis

In the paper by Kobayashi et al. [70], a correlation with febuxostat therapy could neither be proven nor excluded. Consequently, it is not possible to definitively state whether febuxostat can cause agranulocytosis based on the present evaluation. Further studies must be waited for.

3.13. Glomerulonephritis

One case of an ANCA-positive Pauci-immune glomerulonephritis has been published in which the authors see the cause in therapy with febuxostat [71]. The exact pathophysiological correlation remains unclarified.

3.14. Acute Liver Disease

A connection between therapy with febuxostat and an underlying acute liver disease is suspected [72]. The present evaluation has shown that changes in liver values are also one of the side effects of therapy with febuxostat. This side effect was also the main reason reported for participants dropping out of the studies prematurely considered in the present review (see studies in Table A1).

The risk of liver damage due to allopurinol is known. In a paper by Singer and Wallace, 72 patients are cited as having developed a hypersensitivity reaction to allopurinol [99]. Acute liver cell damage was diagnosed in 37 patients (51.3%) [99].

In the event of corresponding symptoms or changes in laboratory values during therapy with febuxostat, the prescribing physician should consider the risk of an acute liver disease and closely monitor therapy control.

4. Materials and Methods

Publications on the side effects and/or interactions of febuxostat were sought in the databases PubMed and Google scholar (last query on 20 March 2018) as well as in the list of references in located papers. The search terms used were: febuxostat, adverse effects, adverse events, side effects, interaction, safety. Original clinical studies, concerned with the treatment of patients with hyperuricemia and gout with febuxostat, were considered for this review in the case of presenting the number of patients with adverse events. Forty-eight original papers with 12,323 patients, six secondary analyses in these papers, as well as 14 case reports of 15 patients were systematically evaluated. The papers were evaluated for events in conjunction with therapy with febuxostat. These included side effects, severe side effects, dropping out of the study prematurely, as well as the death of a study participant. The total number of side effects that occurred is the sum of mild side effects (referred to as "side effect") and severe side effects (referred to as "severe side effect").

The rating by mild (e.g., headache, diarrhea, nausea) and severe side effect (e.g., hypersensitivity reactions, major changes in liver values, cardiovascular events) is based on the authors' rating in their respective publication. The classification is not based on a standard definition.

Events which were not evaluated as being connected to febuxostat in the respective publications were not included in this paper's evaluation. The comparison to allopurinol was made based on reviews addressing the side effects or interactions of allopurinol.

5. Conclusions

In the interest of preventing hypersensitivity reactions, such as skin reactions or DRESS syndrome, allopurinol should be carefully used and the therapy should be closely monitored in patients with impairment of renal or liver function. Febuxostat should be considered for therapy. Higher CV death rates during febuxostat therapy must also be taken into consideration, although there is no difference in the overall death rate between patients being treated with febuxostat and those with allopurinol. No across-the-board dose adjustment for febuxostat is needed for older patients. Existing concomitant medications must be considered in all age groups. Therapy with allopurinol is contraindicated for patients with a previously known intolerance for allopurinol. In these cases, febuxostat can still be used to treat hyperuricemia and gout whereby the risk of intolerances is elevated. This must be watched in daily clinical practice. In the majority of the published case reports, no correlation of side effects was shown to therapy with febuxostat.

The present analysis has shown that febuxostat is well tolerated and a modern and safe alternative to allopurinol therapy. It can be expected that these findings indicate that the agent febuxostat will continue to become more important in daily clinical practice. This will also have a positive impact on the quality of care and therapeutic safety of patients with hyperuricemia and gout.

Author Contributions: A.J. was responsible for the development of the concept as well as for the elaboration and the writing of the review. U.G. gave scientific advice. The results published are part of the dissertation by Andreas Jordan on adverse events and interactions of febuxostat (Ludwig Maximilians Universtity of Munich, Germany).

Appendix A

Table A1. Adverse events in the original works (number of patients examined per study (column 1); patients with at least one side effect (column 2); patients with at least one severe side effect (column 3); patients who dropped out of the study prematurely (column 4); patients who died (column 5); publications reviewed (column 6); differentiation between side effect and severe side effect according to the respective publication, no standard definition).

Number of Patients with Febuxostat Therapy	Number of Patients with at Least One Side Effect (Share in %)	Number of Patients with at Least One Severe Side Effect (Share in %)	Number of Patients to Drop out Prematurely (Share in %)	Number of Patients Who Died (Share in %)	Source
154	60 (38.9)	0	9 (5.8)	0	[26]
15	1 (6.7)	0	0	0	[23]
507	123 (24.3)	32 (6.3)	39 (7.7)	0	[8]
115	14 (12.2)	3 (2.6)	5 (4.3)	0	[49]
32	10 (31.3)	0	0	0	[22]
28	14 (50.0)	0	0	0	[50]
118	57 (48.3)	0	10 (8.5)	0	[51]

Table A1. *Cont.*

Number of Patients with Febuxostat Therapy	Number of Patients with at Least One Side Effect (Share in %)	Number of Patients with at Least One Severe Side Effect (Share in %)	Number of Patients to Drop out Prematurely (Share in %)	Number of Patients Who Died (Share in %)	Source
51	9 (17.6)	0	0	0	[52]
92	26 (28.3)	2 (2.2)	3 (3.3)	0	[20]
48	21 (43.8)	0	0	0	[21]
670	462 (69.0)	25 (3.7)	61 (9.1)	0	[9]
116	106 (91.0)	0	13 (11.2)	0	[10]
1513	839 (55.5)	47 (3.1)	110 (7.3)	0	[11]
34	14 (41.2)	0	0	0	[12]
13	1 (7.7)	1 (7.7)	0	0	[32]
6	3 (50.0)	0	0	0	[18]
29	3 (10.3)	0	0	0	[17]
20	8 (40.0)	0	0	0	[45]
122	10 (8.2)	0	0	0	[46]
171	63 (36.8)	0	6 (3.5)	0	[47]
161	39 (24.2)	1 (0.6)	0	0	[48]
69	11 (15.9)	0	1 (1.5)	0	[13]
39	12 (30.8)	0	0	0	[25]
12	2 (16.7)	0	0	0	[24]
33	20 (60.6)	0	2 (6.1)	0	[36]
17	5 (29.4)	0	0	0	[37]
100	1 (1.0)	0	2 (2.0)	0	[27]
344	113 (32.8)	0	21 (6.1)	0	[41]
38	1 (2.6)	0	0	0	[53]
82	10 (12.2)	0	0	0	[33]
70	5 (7.1)	0	4 (5.7) (included in pat. with ≥ 1 side effect)	0	[14]
26	0	0	0	0	[43]
5948	152 (2.6)	15 (0.25)	36 (0.6)	0	[2]
22	0	1 (4.5)	0	0	[42]
151	6 (4.0)	0	0	0	[34]
36	0	0	0	0	[19]
51	5 (9.8)	0	0	0	[29]
45	2 (4.4)	0	0	0	[38]
336	91 (27.1)	1 (0.3)	6 (1.8)	0	[35]
89	33 (37.1)	0	0	0	[30]
101	4 (4.0)	0	0	0	[28]
160	27 (16.9)	0	5 (3.1)	0	[39]
294	18 (6.1)	0	7 (2.4)	0	[44]
83	0	0	6 (7.2)	0	[40]
64	53 (82.8)	13 (20.3)	8 (12.5)	1 (1.6)	[15]
54	8 (14.8)	2 (3.7)	0	0	[31]
12,279	**2462 (20.1)**	**143 (1.2)**	**354 (2.9)**	**1 (0.008)**	**TOTAL**

Appendix B

Table A2. Adverse events in the secondary analyses (number of patients examined per study (column 1); patients with at least one side effect (column 2); patients with at least one severe side effect (column 3); patients who dropped out of the study prematurely (column 4); patients who died (column 5); publications reviewed (column 6); differentiation between side effect and severe side effect according to the respective publication, no standard definition).

Number of Patients with Febuxostat Therapy	Number of Patients with at Least One Side Effect (Share in %)	Number of Patients with at Least One Severe Side Effect (Share in %)	Number of Patients to Drop Out Prematurely (Share in %)	Number of Patients Who Died (Share in %)	Source
1513	ND	49 (3.2)	ND	2 (0.7)	[57]
116	106 (91.0)	21 (18.0)	13 (11.2)	0	[100]
137	100 (71.9)	9 (6.5)	ND	1 (0.7)	[101]
243	145 (59.7)	17 (7.0)	34 (14.0)	0	[102]
1399	770 (55.0)	44 (3.2)	0	0	[103]
1462	812 (55.5)	47 (3.2)	ND	0	[56]
4870	**1933 (39.7)**	**187 (3.8)**	**47 (1.0)**	**3 (0.06)**	**Total**

References

1. Tausche, A.-K.; Jansen, T.L.; Schroder, H.-E.; Bornstein, S.R.; Aringer, M.; Muller-Ladner, U. Gout—Current diagnosis and treatment. *Deutsches Ärzteblatt Int.* **2009**, *106*, 549–555. [CrossRef]

2. Tausche, A.-K.; Reuss-Borst, M.; Koch, U. Urate lowering therapy with febuxostat in daily practice—A multicentre, open-label, prospective observational study. *Int. J. Rheumatol.* **2014**, *2014*, 123105. [CrossRef] [PubMed]

3. Edwards, N.L. Febuxostat: A new treatment for hyperuricaemia in gout. *Rheumatology* **2009**, *48* (Suppl. 2), ii15–ii19. [CrossRef] [PubMed]

4. Spiekermann, S. Electron spin resonance characterization of vascular xanthine and NAD(P)H oxidase activity in patients with coronary artery disease: Relation to endothelium-dependent vasodilation. *Circulation* **2003**, *107*, 1383–1389. [CrossRef] [PubMed]

5. White, C.R.; Darley-Usmar, V.; Berrington, W.R.; McAdams, M.; Gore, J.Z.; Thompson, J.A.; Parks, D.A.; Tarpey, M.M.; Freeman, B.A. Circulating plasma xanthine oxidase contributes to vascular dysfunction in hypercholesterolemic rabbits. *Proc. Natl. Acad. Sci. USA* **1996**, *93*, 8745–8749. [CrossRef] [PubMed]

6. Cardillo, C.; Kilcoyne, C.M.; Cannon, R.O., 3rd; Quyyumi, A.A.; Panza, J.A. Xanthine oxidase inhibition with oxypurinol improves endothelial vasodilator function in hypercholesterolemic but not in hypertensive patients. *Hypertension* **1997**, *30 Pt 1*, 57–63. [CrossRef] [PubMed]

7. Tausche, A.-K.; Christoph, M.; Forkmann, M.; Richter, U.; Kopprasch, S.; Bielitz, C.; Aringer, M.; Wunderlich, C. As compared to allopurinol, urate-lowering therapy with febuxostat has superior effects on oxidative stress and pulse wave velocity in patients with severe chronic tophaceous gout. *Rheumatol. Int.* **2014**, *34*, 101–109. [CrossRef] [PubMed]

8. Becker, M.A.; Schumacher, H.R., Jr.; Wortmann, R.L.; MacDonald, P.A.; Eustace, D.; Palo, W.A.; Streit, J.; Joseph-Ridge, N. Febuxostat compared with allopurinol in patients with hyperuricemia and gout. *N. Engl. J. Med.* **2005**, *353*, 2450–2461. [CrossRef] [PubMed]

9. Schumacher, H.R.; Becker, M.A.; Wortmann, R.L.; MacDonald, P.A.; Hunt, B.; Streit, J.; Lademacher, C.; Joseph-Ridge, N. Effects of febuxostat versus allopurinol and placebo in reducing serum urate in subjects with hyperuricemia and gout: A 28-week, phase III, randomized, double-blind, parallel-group trial. *Arthritis Rheum.* **2008**, *59*, 1540–1548. [CrossRef] [PubMed]

10. Schumacher, H.R.; Becker, M.A.; Lloyd, E.; MacDonald, P.A.; Lademacher, C. Febuxostat in the treatment of gout: 5-yr findings of the FOCUS efficacy and safety study. *Rheumatology* **2009**, *48*, 188–194. [CrossRef] [PubMed]

11. Becker, M.A.; Schumacher, H.R.; Espinoza, L.R.; Wells, A.F.; MacDonald, P.; Lloyd, E.; Lademacher, C. The urate-lowering efficacy and safety of febuxostat in the treatment of the hyperuricemia of gout: The CONFIRMS trial. *Arthritis Res. Ther.* **2010**, *12*, R63. [CrossRef] [PubMed]

12. Grabowski, B.; Khosravan, R.; Wu, J.-T.; Vernillet, L.; Lademacher, C. Effect of hydrochlorothiazide on the pharmacokinetics and pharmacodynamics of febuxostat, a non-purine selective inhibitor of xanthine oxidase. *Br. J. Clin. Pharmacol.* **2010**, *70*, 57–64. [CrossRef] [PubMed]

13. Kamatani, N.; Fujimori, S.; Hada, T.; Hosoya, T.; Kohri, K.; Nakamura, T.; Ueda, T.; Yamamoto, T.; Yamanaka, H.; Matsuzawa, Y. Placebo-controlled, double-blind study of the non-purine-selective xanthine oxidase inhibitor Febuxostat (TMX-67) in patients with hyperuricemia including those with gout in Japan: Phase 3 clinical study. *J. Clin. Rheumatol.* **2011**, *17* (Suppl. 2), S19–S26. [CrossRef] [PubMed]

14. Shibagaki, Y.; Ohno, I.; Hosoya, T.; Kimura, K. Safety, efficacy and renal effect of febuxostat in patients with moderate-to-severe kidney dysfunction. *Hypertens. Res. Off. J. Jpn. Soc. Hypertens.* **2014**, *37*, 919–925. [CrossRef] [PubMed]

15. Saag, K.G.; Whelton, A.; Becker, M.A.; MacDonald, P.; Hunt, B.; Gunawardhana, L. Impact of febuxostat on renal function in gout patients with moderate-to-severe renal impairment. *Arthritis Rheumatol.* **2016**, *68*, 2035–2043. [CrossRef] [PubMed]

16. White, W.B.; Saag, K.G.; Becker, M.A.; Borer, J.S.; Gorelick, P.B.; Whelton, A.; Hunt, B.; Castillo, M. Cardiovascular Safety of Febuxostat or Allopurinol in Patients with Gout. *N. Engl. J. Med.* **2018**. [CrossRef] [PubMed]

17. Hosoya, T.; Ohno, I. A repeated oral administration study of febuxostat (TMX-67), a non-purine-selective

inhibitor of xanthine oxidase, in patients with impaired renal function in Japan: Pharmacokinetic and pharmacodynamic study. *J. Clin. Rheumatol.* **2011**, *17* (Suppl. 2), S27–S34. [CrossRef] [PubMed]

18. Grabowski, B.A.; Khosravan, R.; Vernillet, L.; Mulford, D.J. Metabolism and excretion of 14C febuxostat, a novel nonpurine selective inhibitor of xanthine oxidase, in healthy male subjects. *J. Clin. Pharmacol.* **2011**, *51*, 189–201. [CrossRef] [PubMed]

19. Zhang, M.; Di, X.; Xu, L.; Xu, J.; Yang, Y.; Jiang, N.; Song, L.; Xu, X. Pharmacokinetics and pharmacodynamics of febuxostat under fasting conditions in healthy individuals. *Exp. Ther. Med.* **2014**, *7*, 393–396. [CrossRef] [PubMed]

20. Khosravan, R.; Grabowski, B.; Wu, J.-T.; Joseph-Ridge, N.; Vernillet, L. Effect of food or antacid on pharmacokinetics and pharmacodynamics of febuxostat in healthy subjects. *Br. J. Clin. Pharmacol.* **2008**, *65*, 355–363. [CrossRef] [PubMed]

21. Khosravan, R.; Kukulka, M.J.; Wu, J.-T.; Joseph-Ridge, N.; Vernillet, L. The effect of age and gender on pharmacokinetics, pharmacodynamics, and safety of febuxostat, a novel nonpurine selective inhibitor of xanthine oxidase. *J. Clin. Pharmacol.* **2008**, *48*, 1014–1024. [CrossRef] [PubMed]

22. Mayer, M.D.; Khosravan, R.; Vernillet, L.; Wu, J.-T.; Joseph-Ridge, N.; Mulford, D.J. Pharmacokinetics and pharmacodynamics of febuxostat, a new non-purine selective inhibitor of xanthine oxidase in subjects with renal impairment. *Am. J. Ther.* **2005**, *12*, 22–34. [CrossRef] [PubMed]

23. Hoshide, S.; Takahashi, Y.; Ishikawa, T.; Kubo, J.; Tsuchimoto, M.; Komoriya, K.; Ohno, I.; Hosoya, T. PK/PD and safety of a single dose of TMX-67 (febuxostat) in subjects with mild and moderate renal impairment. *Nucleosides Nucleotides Nucleic Acids* **2004**, *23*, 1117–1118. [CrossRef] [PubMed]

24. Tsai, M.; Wu, J.-T.; Gunawardhana, L.; Naik, H. The effects of xanthine oxidase inhibition by febuxostat on the pharmacokinetics of theophylline. *Int. J. Clin. Pharmacol. Ther.* **2012**, *50*, 331–337. [CrossRef] [PubMed]

25. Naik, H.; Wu, J.-T.; Palmer, R.; McLean, L. The effects of febuxostat on the pharmacokinetic parameters of rosiglitazone, a CYP2C8 substrate. *Br. J. Clin. Pharmacol.* **2012**, *74*, 327–335. [CrossRef] [PubMed]

26. Becker, M.A.; Kisicki, J.; Khosravan, R.; Wu, J.; Mulford, D.; Hunt, B.; MacDonald, P.; Joseph-Ridge, N. Febuxostat (TMX-67), a novel, non-purine, selective inhibitor of xanthine oxidase, is safe and decreases serum urate in healthy volunteers. *Nucleosides Nucleotides Nucleic Acids* **2004**, *23*, 1111–1116. [CrossRef] [PubMed]

27. Hiramitsu, S.; Ishiguro, Y.; Matsuyama, H.; Yamada, K.; Kato, K.; Noba, M.; Uemura, A.; Matsubara, Y.; Yoshida, S.; Kani, A.; et al. Febuxostat (Feburic tablet) in the management of hyperuricemia in a general practice cohort of Japanese patients with a high prevalence of cardiovascular problems. *Clin. Exp. Hypertens.* **2014**, *36*, 433–440. [CrossRef] [PubMed]

28. Bardin, T.; Chales, G.; Pascart, T.; Flipo, R.-M.; Korng Ea, H.; Roujeau, J.-C.; Delayen, A.; Clerson, P. Risk of cutaneous adverse events with febuxostat treatment in patients with skin reaction to allopurinol. A retrospective, hospital-based study of 101 patients with consecutive allopurinol and febuxostat treatment. *Jt. Bone Spine* **2016**, *83*, 314–317. [CrossRef] [PubMed]

29. Hira, D.; Chisaki, Y.; Noda, S.; Araki, H.; Uzu, T.; Maegawa, H.; Yano, Y.; Morita, S.-Y.; Terada, T. Population pharmacokinetics and therapeutic efficacy of febuxostat in patients with severe renal impairment. *Pharmacology* **2015**, *96*, 90–98. [CrossRef] [PubMed]

30. Yamamoto, T.; Hidaka, Y.; Inaba, M.; Ishimura, E.; Ooyama, H.; Kakuta, H.; Moriwaki, Y.; Higami, K.; Ohtawara, A.; Hosoya, T.; et al. Effects of febuxostat on serum urate level in Japanese hyperuricemia patients. *Mod. Rheumatol.* **2015**, *25*, 779–783. [CrossRef] [PubMed]

31. Yu, K.-H.; Lai, J.-H.; Hsu, P.-N.; Chen, D.-Y.; Chen, C.-J.; Lin, H.-Y. Safety and efficacy of oral febuxostat for treatment of HLA-B*5801-negative gout: A randomized, open-label, multicentre, allopurinol-controlled study. *Scand. J. Rheumatol.* **2016**, *45*, 304–311. [CrossRef] [PubMed]

32. Chohan, S. Safety and efficacy of febuxostat treatment in subjects with gout and severe allopurinol adverse reactions. *J. Rheumatol.* **2011**, *38*, 1957–1959. [CrossRef] [PubMed]

33. Mizuno, T.; Hayashi, T.; Hikosaka, S.; Shimabukuro, Y.; Murase, M.; Takahashi, K.; Hayashi, H.; Yuzawa, Y.; Nagamatsu, T.; Yamada, S. Efficacy and safety of febuxostat in elderly female patients. *Clin. Interv. Aging* **2014**, *9*, 1489–1493. [CrossRef] [PubMed]

34. Wang, Y.S.; Ng, S.P.; Kuo, L.H.; Chien, S.Y. The effectiveness and safety of febuxostat: An experience in medical center in Taiwan. *Value Health* **2014**, *17*, A776. [CrossRef] [PubMed]

35. Xu, S.; Liu, X.; Ming, J.; Chen, S.; Wang, Y.; Liu, X.; Liu, H.; Peng, Y.; Wang, J.; Lin, J.; et al. A phase 3, multicenter, randomized, allopurinol-controlled study assessing the safety and efficacy of oral febuxostat in Chinese gout patients with hyperuricemia. *Int. J. Rheum. Dis.* **2015**, *18*, 669–678. [CrossRef] [PubMed]

36. Goldfarb, D.S.; MacDonald, P.A.; Gunawardhana, L.; Chefo, S.; McLean, L. Randomized controlled trial of febuxostat versus allopurinol or placebo in individuals with higher urinary uric acid excretion and calcium stones. *Clin. J. Am. Soc. Nephrol.* **2013**, *8*, 1960–1967. [CrossRef] [PubMed]

37. Akimoto, T.; Morishita, Y.; Ito, C.; Iimura, O.; Tsunematsu, S.; Watanabe, Y.; Kusano, E.; Nagata, D. Febuxostat for hyperuricemia in patients with advanced chronic kidney disease. *Drug Target Insights* **2014**, *8*, 39–43. [CrossRef] [PubMed]

38. Sircar, D.; Chatterjee, S.; Waikhom, R.; Golay, V.; Raychaudhury, A.; Chatterjee, S.; Pandey, R. Efficacy of febuxostat for slowing the GFR decline in patients with CKD and asymptomatic hyperuricemia: A 6-month, double-blind, randomized, placebo-controlled trial. *Am. J. Kidney Dis.* **2015**, *66*, 945–950. [CrossRef] [PubMed]

39. Ito, H.; Antoku, S.; Abe, M.; Omoto, T.; Shinozaki, M.; Nishio, S.; Mifune, M.; Togane, M.; Nakata, M.; Yamashita, T. Comparison of the renoprotective effect of febuxostat for the treatment of hyperuricemia between patients with and without type 2 diabetes mellitus: A retrospective observational study. *Intern. Med.* **2016**, *55*, 3247–3256. [CrossRef] [PubMed]

40. Quilis, N.; Andres, M.; Gil, S.; Ranieri, L.; Vela, P.; Pascual, E. Febuxostat for patients with gout and severe chronic kidney disease: Which is the appropriate dosage? Comment on the article by Saag et al. *Arthritis Rheumatol.* **2016**, *68*, 2563–2564. [CrossRef] [PubMed]

41. Huang, X.; Du, H.; Gu, J.; Zhao, D.; Jiang, L.; Li, X.; Zuo, X.; Liu, Y.; Li, Z.; Li, X.; et al. An allopurinol-controlled, multicenter, randomized, double-blind, parallel between-group, comparative study of febuxostat in Chinese patients with gout and hyperuricemia. *Int. J. Rheum. Dis.* **2014**, *17*, 679–686. [CrossRef] [PubMed]

42. Tojimbara, T.; Nakajima, I.; Yashima, J.; Fuchinoue, S.; Teraoka, S. Efficacy and safety of febuxostat, a novel nonpurine selective inhibitor of xanthine oxidase for the treatment of hyperuricemia in kidney transplant recipients. *Transplant. Proc.* **2014**, *46*, 511–513. [CrossRef] [PubMed]

43. Sofue, T.; Inui, M.; Hara, T.; Nishijima, Y.; Moriwaki, K.; Hayashida, Y.; Ueda, N.; Nishiyama, A.; Kakehi, Y.; Kohno, M. Efficacy and safety of febuxostat in the treatment of hyperuricemia in stable kidney transplant recipients. *Drug Des. Dev. Ther.* **2014**, *8*, 245–253. [CrossRef] [PubMed]

44. Lim, D.-H.; Oh, J.S.; Ahn, S.M.; Hong, S.; Kim, Y.-G.; Lee, C.-K.; Choi, S.W.; Yoo, B. Febuxostat in hyperuricemic patients with advanced CKD. *Am. J. Kidney Dis.* **2016**, *68*, 819–821. [CrossRef] [PubMed]

45. Kamatani, N.; Fujimori, S.; Hada, T.; Hosoya, T.; Kohri, K.; Nakamura, T.; Ueda, T.; Yamamoto, T.; Yamanaka, H.; Matsuzawa, Y. An allopurinol-controlled, multicenter, randomized, open-label, parallel between-group, comparative study of febuxostat (TMX-67), a non-purine-selective inhibitor of xanthine oxidase, in patients with hyperuricemia including those with gout in Japan: Phase 2 exploratory clinical study. *J. Clin. Rheumatol.* **2011**, *17* (Suppl. 2), S44–S49. [CrossRef] [PubMed]

46. Kamatani, N.; Fujimori, S.; Hada, T.; Hosoya, T.; Kohri, K.; Nakamura, T.; Ueda, T.; Yamamoto, T.; Yamanaka, H.; Matsuzawa, Y. An allopurinol-controlled, randomized, double-dummy, double-blind, parallel between-group, comparative study of febuxostat (TMX-67), a non-purine-selective inhibitor of xanthine oxidase, in patients with hyperuricemia including those with gout in Japan: Phase 3 clinical study. *J. Clin. Rheumatol.* **2011**, *17* (Suppl. 2), S13–S18. [CrossRef] [PubMed]

47. Kamatani, N.; Fujimori, S.; Hada, T.; Hosoya, T.; Kohri, K.; Nakamura, T.; Ueda, T.; Yamamoto, T.; Yamanaka, H.; Matsuzawa, Y. Multicenter, open-label study of long-term administration of febuxostat (TMX-67) in Japanese patients with hyperuricemia including gout. *J. Clin. Rheumatol.* **2011**, *17* (Suppl. 2), S50–S56. [CrossRef] [PubMed]

48. Kamatani, N.; Fujimori, S.; Hada, T.; Hosoya, T.; Kohri, K.; Nakamura, T.; Ueda, T.; Yamamoto, T.; Yamanaka, H.; Matsuzawa, Y. Placebo-controlled double-blind dose-response study of the non-purine-selective xanthine oxidase inhibitor febuxostat (TMX-67) in patients with hyperuricemia (including gout patients) in japan: Late phase 2 clinical study. *J. Clin. Rheumatol.* **2011**, *17* (Suppl. 2), S35–S43. [CrossRef] [PubMed]

49. Becker, M.A.; Schumacher, H.R., Jr.; Wortmann, R.L.; MacDonald, P.A.; Palo, W.A.; Eustace, D.; Vernillet, L.; Joseph-Ridge, N. Febuxostat, a novel nonpurine selective inhibitor of xanthine oxidase: A twenty-eight-day,

multicenter, phase II, randomized, double-blind, placebo-controlled, dose-response clinical trial examining safety and efficacy in patients with gout. *Arthritis Rheum.* **2005**, *52*, 916–923. [CrossRef] [PubMed]

50. Khosravan, R.; Grabowski, B.A.; Mayer, M.D.; Wu, J.-T.; Joseph-Ridge, N.; Vernillet, L. The effect of mild and moderate hepatic impairment on pharmacokinetics, pharmacodynamics, and safety of febuxostat, a novel nonpurine selective inhibitor of xanthine oxidase. *J. Clin. Pharmacol.* **2006**, *46*, 88–102. [CrossRef] [PubMed]

51. Khosravan, R.; Grabowski, B.A.; Wu, J.-T.; Joseph-Ridge, N.; Vernillet, L. Pharmacokinetics, pharmacodynamics and safety of febuxostat, a non-purine selective inhibitor of xanthine oxidase, in a dose escalation study in healthy subjects. *Clin. Pharmacokinet.* **2006**, *45*, 821–841. [CrossRef] [PubMed]

52. Khosravan, R.; Wu, J.-T.; Joseph-Ridge, N.; Vernillet, L. Pharmacokinetic interactions of concomitant administration of febuxostat and NSAIDs. *J. Clin. Pharmacol.* **2006**, *46*, 855–866. [CrossRef] [PubMed]

53. Maie, K.; Yokoyama, Y.; Kurita, N.; Minohara, H.; Yanagimoto, S.; Hasegawa, Y.; Homma, M.; Chiba, S. Hypouricemic effect and safety of febuxostat used for prevention of tumor lysis syndrome. *SpringerPlus* **2014**, *3*, 501. [CrossRef] [PubMed]

54. Becker, M.A.; Schumacher, H.R.; MacDonald, P.A.; Lloyd, E.; Lademacher, C. Clinical efficacy and safety of successful longterm urate lowering with febuxostat or allopurinol in subjects with gout. *J. Rheumatol.* **2009**, *36*, 1273–1282. [CrossRef] [PubMed]

55. Kaczmorski, S.; Doares, W.; Winfrey, S.; Al-Geizawi, S.; Farney, A.; Rogers, J.; Stratta, R. Gout and transplantation: New treatment option–Same old drug interaction. *Transplantation* **2011**, *92*, e13–e14. [CrossRef] [PubMed]

56. Becker, M.A.; MacDonald, P.A.; Hunt, B.J.; Jackson, R.L. Diabetes and gout: Efficacy and safety of febuxostat and allopurinol. *Diabetes Obes. Metab.* **2013**, *15*, 1049–1055. [CrossRef] [PubMed]

57. Becker, M.A.; MacDonald, P.A.; Hunt, B.; Gunawardhana, L. Treating hyperuricemia of gout: Safety and efficacy of febuxostat and allopurinol in older versus younger subjects. *Nucleosides Nucleotides Nucleic Acids* **2011**, *30*, 1011–1017. [CrossRef] [PubMed]

58. Fleischmann, R.; Kerr, B.; Yeh, L.-T.; Suster, M.; Shen, Z.; Polvent, E.; Hingorani, V.; Quart, B.; Manhard, K.; Miner, J.N.; et al. Pharmacodynamic, pharmacokinetic and tolerability evaluation of concomitant administration of lesinurad and febuxostat in gout patients with hyperuricaemia. *Rheumatology* **2014**, *53*, 2167–2174. [CrossRef] [PubMed]

59. Steinberg, A.S.; Vince, B.D.; Choi, Y.-J.; Martin, R.L.; McWherter, C.A.; Boudes, P.F. The pharmacodynamics, pharmacokinetics, and safety of arhalofenate in combination with febuxostat when treating hyperuricemia associated with gout. *J. Rheumatol.* **2016**. [CrossRef] [PubMed]

60. Dore, M.; Frenette, A.J.; Mansour, A.-M.; Troyanov, Y.; Begin, J. Febuxostat as a novel option to optimize thiopurines' metabolism in patients with inadequate metabolite levels. *Ann. Pharmacother.* **2014**, *48*, 648–651. [CrossRef] [PubMed]

61. Abeles, A.M. Febuxostat hypersensitivity. *J. Rheumatol.* **2012**, *39*, 659. [CrossRef] [PubMed]

62. Laura, A.; Luca, P.; Luisa, P.A. Interstitial granulomatous drug reaction due to febuxostat. *Indian J. Dermatol. Venereol. Leprol.* **2014**, *80*, 182–184. [CrossRef] [PubMed]

63. Oda, T.; Sawada, Y.; Ohmori, S.; Omoto, D.; Haruyama, S.; Yoshioka, M.; Nishio, D.; Nakamura, M. Fixed drug eruption-like macules caused by febuxostat. *Eur. J. Dermatol.* **2016**, *26*, 412–413. [CrossRef] [PubMed]

64. Chou, H.-Y.; Chen, C.-B.; Cheng, C.-Y.; Chen, Y.-A.; Ng, C.Y.; Kuo, K.-L.; Chen, W.-L.; Chen, C.-H. Febuxostat-associated drug reaction with eosinophilia and systemic symptoms (DRESS). *J. Clin. Pharm. Ther.* **2015**, *40*, 689–692. [CrossRef] [PubMed]

65. Paschou, E.; Gavriilaki, E.; Papaioannou, G.; Tsompanakou, A.; Kalaitzoglou, A.; Sabanis, N. Febuxostat hypersensitivity: Another cause of DRESS syndrome in chronic kidney disease? *Eur. Ann. Allergy Clin. Immunol.* **2016**, *48*, 251–255. [PubMed]

66. Lien, Y.-H.H.; Logan, J.L. Cross-reactions between allopurinol and febuxostat. *Am. J. Med.* **2017**, *130*, e67–e68. [CrossRef] [PubMed]

67. Kang, Y.; Kim, M.J.; Jang, H.N.; Bae, E.J.; Yun, S.; Cho, H.S.; Chang, S.-H.; Park, D.J. Rhabdomyolysis associated with initiation of febuxostat therapy for hyperuricaemia in a patient with chronic kidney disease. *J. Clin. Pharm. Ther.* **2014**, *39*, 328–330. [CrossRef] [PubMed]

68. Ghosh, D.; McGann, P.M.; Furlong, T.J.; Day, R.O. Febuxostat-associated rhabdomyolysis in chronic renal failure. *Med. J. Aust.* **2015**, *203*, 107–108. [CrossRef] [PubMed]

69. Chahine, G.; Saleh, K.; Ghorra, C.; Khoury, N.; Khalife, N.; Fayad, F. Febuxostat-associated eosinophilic polymyositis in marginal zone lymphoma. *Jt. Bone Spine* **2016**. [CrossRef] [PubMed]

70. Kobayashi, S.; Ogura, M.; Hosoya, T. Acute neutropenia associated with initiation of febuxostat therapy for hyperuricaemia in patients with chronic kidney disease. *J. Clin. Pharm. Ther.* **2013**, *38*, 258–261. [CrossRef] [PubMed]

71. Izzedine, H.; Boulanger, H.; Gueutin, V.; Rouvier, P.; Deray, G. ANCA-positive pauci-immune glomerulonephritis and febuxostat treatment. *Clin. Kidney J.* **2012**, *5*, 486. [CrossRef] [PubMed]

72. Bohm, M.; Vuppalanchi, R.; Chalasani, N. Febuxostat-induced acute liver injury. *Hepatology* **2016**, *63*, 1047–1049. [CrossRef] [PubMed]

73. Castrejon, I.; Toledano, E.; Rosario, M.P.; Loza, E.; Perez-Ruiz, F.; Carmona, L. Safety of allopurinol compared with other urate-lowering drugs in patients with gout: A systematic review and meta-analysis. *Rheumatol. Int.* **2015**, *35*, 1127–1137. [CrossRef] [PubMed]

74. Seth, R.; Kydd, A.S.R.; Buchbinder, R.; Bombardier, C.; Edwards, C.J. Allopurinol for chronic gout. *Cochrane Database Syst. Rev.* **2014**, *10*, CD006077. [CrossRef] [PubMed]

75. Faruque, L.I.; Ehteshami-Afshar, A.; Wiebe, N.; Tjosvold, L.; Homik, J.; Tonelli, M. A systematic review and meta-analysis on the safety and efficacy of febuxostat versus allopurinol in chronic gout. *Semin. Arthritis Rheum.* **2013**, *43*, 367–375. [CrossRef] [PubMed]

76. Gunawardhana, L.; McLean, L.; Punzi, H.A.; Hunt, B.; Palmer, R.N.; Whelton, A.; Feig, D.I. Effect of Febuxostat on Ambulatory Blood Pressure in Subjects With Hyperuricemia and Hypertension: A Phase 2 Randomized Placebo-Controlled Study. *J. Am. Heart Assoc.* **2017**, *6*. [CrossRef] [PubMed]

77. Li, S.; Yang, H.; Guo, Y.; Wei, F.; Yang, X.; Li, D.; Li, M.; Xu, W.; Li, W.; Sun, L.; et al. Comparative efficacy and safety of urate-lowering therapy for the treatment of hyperuricemia: A systematic review and network meta-analysis. *Sci. Rep.* **2016**, *6*, 33082. [CrossRef] [PubMed]

78. Markel, A. Allopurinol-induced DRESS syndrome. *Isr. Med. Assoc. J.* **2005**, *7*, 656–660. [PubMed]

79. Dalbeth, N.; Stamp, L. Allopurinol dosing in renal impairment: Walking the tightrope between adequate urate lowering and adverse events. *Semin. Dial.* **2007**, *20*, 391–395. [CrossRef] [PubMed]

80. Bove, M.; Cicero, A.F.G.; Veronesi, M.; Borghi, C. An evidence-based review on urate-lowering treatments: Implications for optimal treatment of chronic hyperuricemia. *Vasc. Health Risk Manag.* **2017**, *13*, 23–28. [CrossRef] [PubMed]

81. Baek, C.H.; Kim, H.; Yang, W.S.; Han, D.J.; Park, S.-K. Efficacy and Safety of Febuxostat in Kidney Transplant Patients. *Exp. Clin. Transplant.* **2017**. [CrossRef] [PubMed]

82. Ratiopharm GmbH. Fachinformation zu "Allopurinol-ratiopharm 100/300 mg Tabletten". 2016. Available online: http://www.ratiopharm.de/index.php?eID=dumpFile&t=f&f=70732&g=-1&r=1894%2C1894&token=38cd525615b9b72e43152a6306fbb025793a5c41 (accessed on 5 March 2017).

83. Berlin-Chemie, A.G. Fachinformation Adenuric. 2017. Available online: http://www.fachinfo.de/pdf/012335 (accessed on 18 March 2017).

84. Pea, F. Pharmacology of drugs for hyperuricemia. Mechanisms, kinetics and interactions. *Contrib. Nephrol.* **2005**, *147*, 35–46. [CrossRef] [PubMed]

85. Waller, A.; Jordan, K.M. Use of febuxostat in the management of gout in the United Kingdom. *Ther. Adv. Musculoskelet. Dis.* **2017**, *9*, 55–64. [CrossRef] [PubMed]

86. Chao, J.; Terkeltaub, R. A critical reappraisal of allopurinol dosing, safety, and efficacy for hyperuricemia in gout. *Curr. Rheumatol. Rep.* **2009**, *11*, 135–140. [CrossRef] [PubMed]

87. Perez-Ruiz, F.; Sundy, J.S.; Miner, J.N.; Cravets, M.; Storgard, C. Lesinurad in combination with allopurinol: Results of a phase 2, randomised, double-blind study in patients with gout with an inadequate response to allopurinol. *Ann. Rheum. Dis.* **2016**, *75*, 1074–1080. [CrossRef] [PubMed]

88. Bardin, T.; Keenan, R.T.; Khanna, P.P.; Kopicko, J.; Fung, M.; Bhakta, N.; Adler, S.; Storgard, C.; Baumgartner, S.; So, A. Lesinurad in combination with allopurinol: A randomised, double-blind, placebo-controlled study in patients with gout with inadequate response to standard of care (the multinational CLEAR 2 study). *Ann. Rheum. Dis.* **2016**. [CrossRef] [PubMed]

89. Stamp, L.K.; Jordan, S. The challenges of gout management in the elderly. *Drugs Aging* **2011**, *28*, 591–603. [CrossRef] [PubMed]

90. Gearry, R.B.; Day, A.S.; Barclay, M.L.; Leong, R.W.L.; Sparrow, M.P. Azathioprine and allopurinol: A two-edged interaction. *J. Gastroenterol. Hepatol.* **2010**, *25*, 653–655. [CrossRef] [PubMed]

91. Hsu, W.-C.; Chen, W.-H.; Chang, M.-T.; Chiu, H.-C. Colchicine-induced acute myopathy in a patient with concomitant use of simvastatin. *Clin. Neuropharmacol.* **2002**, *25*, 266–268. [CrossRef] [PubMed]

92. Baker, S.K.; Goodwin, S.; Sur, M.; Tarnopolsky, M.A. Cytoskeletal myotoxicity from simvastatin and colchicine. *Muscle Nerve* **2004**, *30*, 799–802. [CrossRef] [PubMed]

93. Alayli, G.; Cengiz, K.; Canturk, F.; Durmus, D.; Akyol, Y.; Menekse, E.B. Acute myopathy in a patient with concomitant use of pravastatin and colchicine. *Ann. Pharmacother.* **2005**, *39*, 1358–1361. [CrossRef] [PubMed]

94. Atasoyu, E.M.; Evrenkaya, T.R.; Solmazgul, E. Possible colchicine rhabdomyolysis in a fluvastatin-treated patient. *Ann. Pharmacother.* **2005**, *39*, 1368–1369. [CrossRef] [PubMed]

95. Tufan, A.; Dede, D.S.; Cavus, S.; Altintas, N.D.; Iskit, A.B.; Topeli, A. Rhabdomyolysis in a patient treated with colchicine and atorvastatin. *Ann. Pharmacother.* **2006**, *40*, 1466–1469. [CrossRef] [PubMed]

96. Sarullo, F.M.; Americo, L.; Di Franco, A.; Di Pasquale, P. Rhabdomyolysis induced by co-administration of fluvastatin and colchicine. *Monaldi Arch. Chest Dis.* **2010**, *74*, 147–149. [CrossRef] [PubMed]

97. Leung, Y.Y.; Yao Hui, L.L.; Kraus, V.B. Colchicine—Update on mechanisms of action and therapeutic uses. *Semin. Arthritis Rheum.* **2015**, *45*, 341–350. [CrossRef] [PubMed]

98. Liu, C.-T.; Chen, C.-Y.; Hsu, C.-Y.; Huang, P.-H.; Lin, F.-Y.; Chen, J.-W.; Lin, S.-J. Risk of Febuxostat-Associated Myopathy in Patients with CKD. *Clin. J. Am. Soc. Nephrol.* **2017**, *12*, 744–750. [CrossRef] [PubMed]

99. Singer, J.Z.; Wallace, S.L. The allopurinol hypersensitivity syndrome. Unnecessary morbidity and mortality. *Arthritis Rheum.* **1986**, *29*, 82–87. [CrossRef] [PubMed]

100. Whelton, A.; MacDonald, P.A.; Zhao, L.; Hunt, B.; Gunawardhana, L. Renal function in gout: Long-term treatment effects of febuxostat. *J. Clin. Rheumatol.* **2011**, *17*, 7–13. [CrossRef] [PubMed]

101. Chohan, S.; Becker, M.A.; MacDonald, P.A.; Chefo, S.; Jackson, R.L. Women with gout: Efficacy and safety of urate-lowering with febuxostat and allopurinol. *Arthritis Care Res. (Hoboken)* **2012**, *64*, 256–261. [CrossRef] [PubMed]

102. Jackson, R.L.; Hunt, B.; MacDonald, P.A. The efficacy and safety of febuxostat for urate lowering in gout patients >= 65 years of age. *BMC Geriatr.* **2012**, *12*, 11. [CrossRef] [PubMed]

103. Wells, A.F.; MacDonald, P.A.; Chefo, S.; Jackson, R.L. African American patients with gout: Efficacy and safety of febuxostat vs allopurinol. *BMC Musculoskelet. Disord.* **2012**, *13*, 15. [CrossRef] [PubMed]

9

Design, Synthesis, In Vitro, and Initial In Vivo Evaluation of Heterobivalent Peptidic Ligands Targeting Both NPY(Y$_1$)- and GRP-Receptors— An Improvement for Breast Cancer Imaging?

Alicia Vall-Sagarra [1], Shanna Litau [1,2], Clemens Decristoforo [3] (ID), Björn Wängler [2], Ralf Schirrmacher [4] (ID), Gert Fricker [5] and Carmen Wängler [1,*]

[1]   Biomedical Chemistry, Department of Clinical Radiology and Nuclear Medicine,
      Medical Faculty Mannheim of Heidelberg University, Theodor-Kutzer-Ufer 1-3, 68167 Mannheim, Germany;
      Alicia.Vall-Sagarra@medma.uni-heidelberg.de (A.V.-S.); Shanna.Litau@medma.uni-heidelberg.de (S.L.)

[2]   Molecular Imaging and Radiochemistry, Department of Clinical Radiology and Nuclear Medicine,
      Medical Faculty Mannheim of Heidelberg University, Theodor-Kutzer-Ufer 1-3, 68167 Mannheim, Germany;
      Bjoern.Waengler@medma.uni-heidelberg.de

[3]   Department of Nuclear Medicine, University Hospital Innsbruck, Medical University Innsbruck,
      Anichstrasse 35, 6020 Innsbruck, Austria; Clemens.Decristoforo@tirol-kliniken.at

[4]   Department of Oncology, Division Oncological Imaging, University of Alberta, 11560 University Avenue,
      Edmonton, AB T6G 1Z2, Canada; schirrma@ualberta.ca

[5]   Institute of Pharmacy and Molecular Biotechnology, University of Heidelberg, Im Neuenheimer Feld 329,
      69120 Heidelberg, Germany; gert.fricker@uni-hd.de

*   Correspondence: Carmen.Waengler@medma.uni-heidelberg.de

Abstract: Heterobivalent peptidic ligands (HBPLs), designed to address two different receptors independently, are highly promising tumor imaging agents. For example, breast cancer has been shown to concomitantly and complementarily overexpress the neuropeptide Y receptor subtype 1 (NPY(Y$_1$)R) as well as the gastrin-releasing peptide receptor (GRPR). Thus, radiolabeled HBPLs being able to bind these two receptors should exhibit an improved tumor targeting efficiency compared to monospecific ligands. We developed here such bispecific HBPLs and radiolabeled them with ^{68}Ga, achieving high radiochemical yields, purities, and molar activities. We evaluated the HBPLs and their monospecific reference peptides in vitro regarding stability and uptake into different breast cancer cell lines and found that the ^{68}Ga-HBPLs were efficiently taken up via the GRPR. We also performed in vivo PET/CT imaging and ex vivo biodistribution studies in T-47D tumor-bearing mice for the most promising ^{68}Ga-HBPL and compared the results to those obtained for its scrambled analogs. The tumors could easily be visualized by the newly developed ^{68}Ga-HBPL and considerably higher tumor uptakes and tumor-to-background ratios were obtained compared to the scrambled analogs in and ex vivo. These results demonstrate the general feasibility of the approach to use bispecific radioligands for in vivo imaging of breast cancer.

Keywords: breast cancer; ^{68}Ga; GRPR; NPY(Y$_1$)R; peptide heterodimers; PET/CT imaging

1. Introduction

Radiolabeled peptides, being able to specifically bind certain receptors overexpressed on many malignancies, have become standard radiotracers for tumor-specific imaging by positron emission tomography (PET) in a clinical routine. However, these radiolabeled peptides are able to address only one target receptor type, being thus only able to visualize tumors expressing this particular receptor.

As different tumor lesions can however overexpress different receptor types and receptor expression can change upon metastasis and disease progression, a monovalent peptidic radioligand is often not able to visualize all tumor cells with the same efficiency and some lesions might be completely missed by the applied radiopeptide.

Radiolabeled heterobivalent peptide ligands (HBPLs) on the other hand—by their ability to specifically target more than one receptor type—have been proposed to be better-suited agents for tumor imaging as they enable the visualization of the tumor by different receptor types potentially overexpressed by the target cells [1,2].

HBPLs furthermore can have favorable effects for in vivo tumor imaging compared to monovalent ligands such as improved in vivo biodistribution and enhanced avidity caused by simultaneous binding if both receptors are present on the tumor cell surface. In this case, also a higher probability of rebinding is achieved for a heterobivalent binder in case of dissociation from the receptor compared to a monovalent peptide due to "forced proximity" of the second potential binder to the second target receptor.

Furthermore, by being able to target different receptor types on the tumor cell surface, an overall higher number of receptors can be addressed by a heterobivalent ligand, increasing the probability of binding and thus tumor visualization. Thus, HBPLs are also of special interest not only for the imaging of such tumors that express both receptor types concomitantly, but also for tumors exhibiting a heterogeneous target expression with varying receptor densities between different individuals or lesions and for differential target expression during disease progression. A non-uniform distribution of target receptors between lesions results—if using monomeric peptidic radioligands—in the visualization of only some of the lesions whereas others are not depicted. Applying a HBPL for imaging, such lesions can nevertheless be addressed as long as one of the target receptors is present (Figure 1).

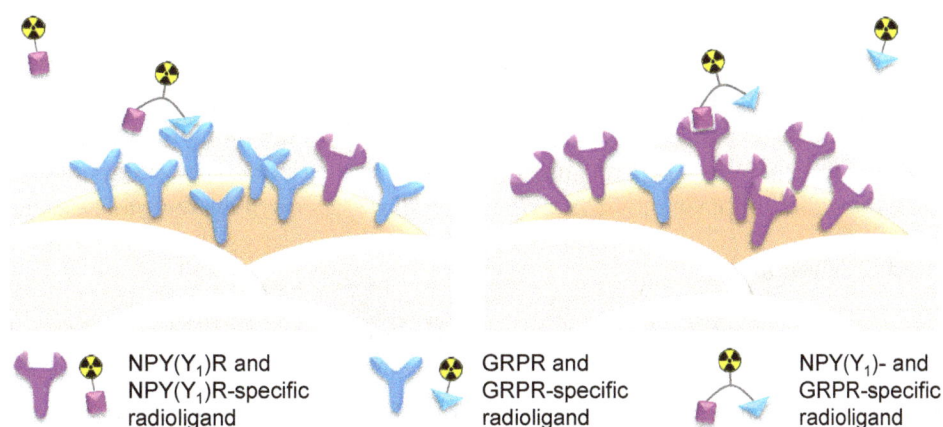

Figure 1. Schematic depiction of the functional principle of radiolabeled NPY(Y$_1$)R- and gastrin-releasing peptide receptor (GRPR)-binding heterobivalent peptidic ligands (HBPLs) for tumor imaging: Monomeric peptide radiotracers can only bind to one receptor type and thus miss tumor tissues or lesions that do not express the respective receptor due to tumor heterogeneity or disease progression whereas the use of radiolabeled HBPLs, which can bind to more than one target receptor type, results in a higher probability of target visualization.

Recently, a radiolabeled HBPL, being able to address the gastrin-releasing peptide receptor as well as integrin $\alpha_v\beta_3$ was successfully translated into the clinics for imaging of prostate cancer with PET/CT, showing a much higher tumor visualization sensitivity compared to the respective GRPR-targeting peptide monomer. This proves the clinical relevance of the heterobivalent peptide targeting concept [3].

To be able to develop a HBPL being able to more efficiently target tumor tissues than the respective peptide monomers, it is necessary to know the receptor expression profile on the target tumor type.

Regarding this point, some excellent systematical work has been carried out, determining the presence of certain receptor types and their densities on different human malignancies [2,4–6].

Human breast cancer, for example, overexpresses in about 75% of all cases the gastrin-releasing peptide receptor (GRPR) [7] and in 66–85% the neuropeptide Y receptor subtype 1 (NPY(Y_1)R) [8]. Both receptors are expressed to an insignificant amount on healthy breast tissue, thus rendering both receptor types well-suited target structures for sensitive and specific breast cancer imaging. Furthermore, Reubi and co-workers could show on 68 human breast cancer samples that 63/68 (93%) overexpressed one or both receptor types. Of these, 32 (51%) expressed both receptors concomitantly, whereas 18 (29%) expressed only the GRPR, and a further 13 (21%) expressed only the NPY(Y_1)R [5]. Thus, the combination of two peptidic ligands being able to specifically bind the NPY(Y_1)R and the GRPR to one radioligand should enable a considerably higher breast cancer visualization efficiency and sensitivity and thus give less false-negative results compared to the respective monovalent radioligands (Figure 1).

To obtain a highly potent bispecific HBPL, it is mandatory that both peptide parts of the construct are still able to bind to their respective target receptor type despite the considerable chemical modifications necessary for peptide heterodimerization. Thus, a suitable molecular design has to be found that enables the binding of both peptides to their respective target receptor.

So far, only one example of a heterobivalent NPY(Y_1)R- and GRPR-targeting ligand has been described [9,10] and for this substance, no descriptions of radiolabeling with a PET isotope, in vitro cell uptake or in vivo imaging data are available. Thus, the general feasibility of the approach has not been demonstrated so far.

Thus, the aims of this study were to: (i) Develop a synthesis strategy yielding different HBPLs varying in molecular design and consisting of a NPY(Y_1)- and a GRPR-affine peptide as well as a chelating agent (for radiolabeling with the positron-emitting radiometal nuclide ^{68}Ga); (ii) Establish the ^{68}Ga-radiolabeling and determine the $\log_D$ and in vitro stability of the resulting ^{68}Ga-HBPLs in human serum; (iii) Evaluate the uptake of the ^{68}Ga-HBPLs into human breast cancer cell lines in vitro to determine if the substances can still interact with both target receptors and are taken up by the tumor cells; (iv) Determine if the particular molecular design used has a measurable influence on tumor cell uptake; and (v) Show the general feasibility of the approach by investigating the tumor uptake of the most potent HBPL in vivo by PET/CT imaging and ex vivo biodistribution in a proof-of-concept study and determine if the tumor uptake profits from the heterodimerization of the receptor-specific peptides.

2. Results and Discussion

2.1. Synthesis of GRPR- and NPY(Y_1)R-Binding HBPLs **22–26**, *Scrambled HBPL Analogs* **24a–c**, *Blocking Agents* **3** *and* **4** *as well as Monomeric Reference Peptides* **27** *and* **28**

At first, a suitable synthesis strategy towards the GRPR- and NPY(Y_1)R-binding HBPLs was developed. The target molecular design of the substances is depicted in Figure 2 and was based on the following considerations: (i) The structure was to be based on a symmetrically branched scaffold to obtain homogenous products and the scaffold should comprise the chelator NODA-GA ((1,4,7-triazacyclononane-4,7-diyl)diacetic acid-1-glutaric acid), which is able to stably and efficiently complex ^{68}Ga [11]; (ii) The chelator should be spatially separated from the receptor-affine peptides by a short PEG linker to prevent an interference of the radiometal complex with receptor binding [12]; (iii) As we and others were able to show before for peptide di- and multimers, the distance between the peptides within the same molecule can have a significant influence on the achievable receptor interaction [13–16], thus different distances between both peptidic receptor ligands should be investigated for the target HBPLs by introducing linkers of different length; (iv) Furthermore, as it was proposed that also the rigidity of the molecules might influence cellular uptakes by a conformational stabilization of the spatial orientation of the receptor ligands, the used linker structures did not only differ in length, but also in rigidity.

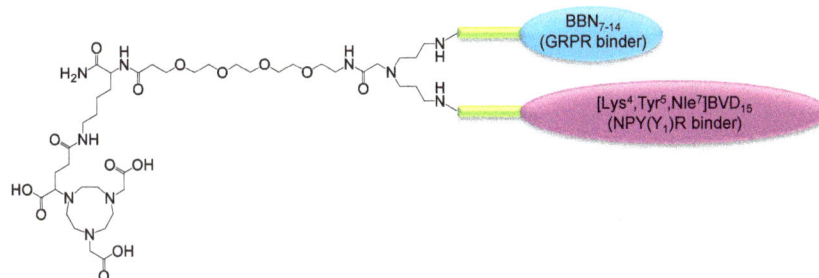

Figure 2. Schematic depiction of the general molecular design of the target HBPLs consisting of a chelating agent (NODA-GA), a short PEG_4-linker between radiometal complex and peptides, the symmetrical branching unit, the linkers of different length and rigidity (green) and the GRPR- and $NPY(Y_1)R$-binding peptides BBN_{7-14} (cyan) and $[Lys^4, Trp^5, Nle^7]BVD_{15}$ (magenta).

2.1.1. Synthesis of the Peptide Monomers 1−6

Aiming at the synthesis of GRPR-and $NPY(Y_1)R$-binding HBPLs and their following in vitro and in vivo evaluation in human breast cancer tumor cells, we first synthesized the respective peptide monomers for subsequent heterodimerization on symmetrically branched scaffolds. As GRPR-affine peptide monomer, we chose the receptor agonist PESIN (PEG_4-BBN_{7-14}), which exhibits a favorably high stability, significant tumor uptake, as well as high tumor to background ratios in vivo [17,18], and can be modified at its N-terminal end without considerably changing its receptor binding affinity [13]. As $NPY(Y_1)R$-affine peptide monomer, we chose $[Lys^4, Trp^5, Nle^7]BVD_{15}$ as this peptide was shown to exhibit good affinities to the $NPY(Y_1)R$ even when further modified in position four [9,19,20].

The peptides were to be conjugated to the symmetrically branched scaffolds by a click chemistry approach to be able to obtain the desired rather complex target HBPLs efficiently. Furthermore, the coupling products have to be stable under physiological conditions. Different click chemistry reactions fulfill these requirements; of these, we chose the oxime formation between aminooxy functionalities and aldehydes.

Both peptides were synthesized by standard solid phase peptide synthesis (SPPS) methods [13,21] by successive conjugation of the respective N_α-Fmoc-amino acids after HBTU activation to the respective rink amide resin and finally modified on resin with bis-Boc-aminooxy acetic acid, giving aminooxy-PESIN (1) and $[Lys^4(aminooxy), Trp^5, Nle^7]BVD_{15}$ (2) (Figure 3). In case of PESIN, the aminooxy functionality was introduced at the N-terminal end as the peptide can be modified in this position without considerable alterations in binding affinity. In case of $[Lys^4, Trp^5, Nle^7]BVD_{15}$, the aminooxy functionality was introduced in position 4 (N_ε amine of lysine) as modifications in this position interfere least with receptor binding.

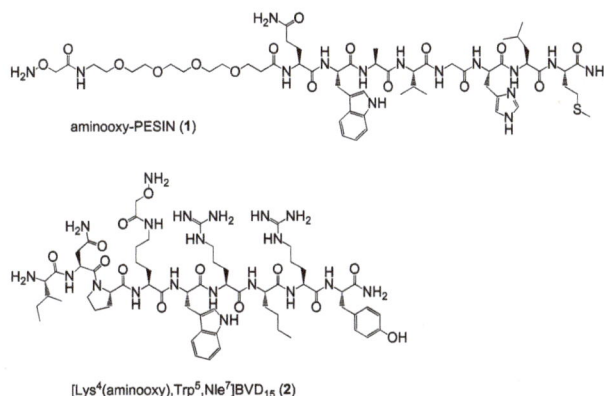

aminooxy-PESIN (1)

$[Lys^4(aminooxy), Trp^5, Nle^7]BVD_{15}$ (2)

Figure 3. Depiction of the chemical structures of aminooxy-PESIN (1) and $[Lys^4(aminooxy), Trp^5, Nle^7]BVD_{15}$ (2) used for the assembly of the HBPLs.

As the target HBPLs should be evaluated in vitro regarding their ability to be taken up by human breast cancer cell lines and the contribution of both parts of the HBPLs on tumor cell uptake should be assessed, we further synthesized the peptide monomers bombesin (3) and [Lys^4,Trp^5,Nle^7]BVD$_{15}$ (4) as blocking substances for the GRPR and the NPY(Y$_1$)R during these experiments (Figure 4).

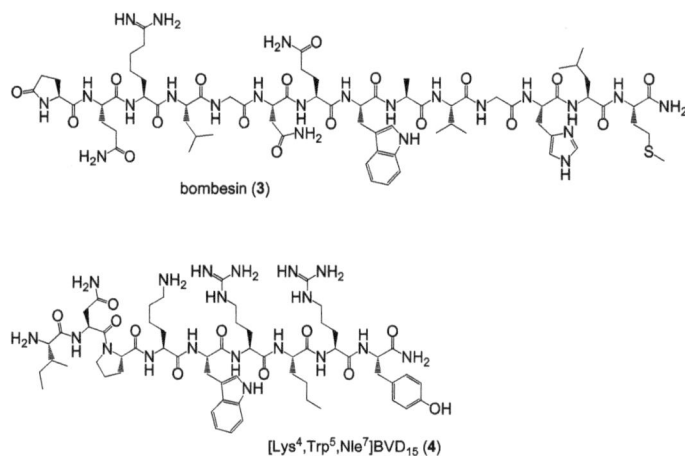

Figure 4. Depiction of the chemical structures of bombesin (3) and [Lys^4,Trp^5,Nle^7]BVD$_{15}$ (4) used as receptor blocking substances during the in vitro tumor cell uptake studies.

Regarding the in vivo evaluation of the HBPLs in tumor-bearing animals and the verification of the receptor specificity of the observed tumor uptakes and the contribution of both peptides of the HBPLs to overall tumor uptakes, two different approaches can be followed. The first one is to block the respective target receptor analogous to the in vitro assays by adding blocking substances 3 or 4 and the other one is to use scrambled HBPL analogs. To compare the in vivo tumor uptake of an HBPL to that of its scrambled analogs instead of performing blocking studies however eliminates possible difficulties that might arise from the low stability of the monomeric receptor ligands.

Thus, three different scrambled HBPL analogs were synthesized: PESIN combined with scrambled [Lys^4(aminooxy),Trp^5,Nle^7]BVD$_{15}$, scrambled PESIN combined with [Lys^4(aminooxy), Trp^5,Nle^7]BVD$_{15}$ and both peptides of the HBPL scrambled. For this purpose, the two scrambled aminooxy-modified peptide monomers aminooxy-PESIN$_{scrambled}$ (5) and [Lys^4(aminooxy),Trp^5,Nle^7] BVD$_{15,scrambled}$ (6) (Figure 5) were synthesized and analogously to 1 and 2 used during the following HBPL syntheses.

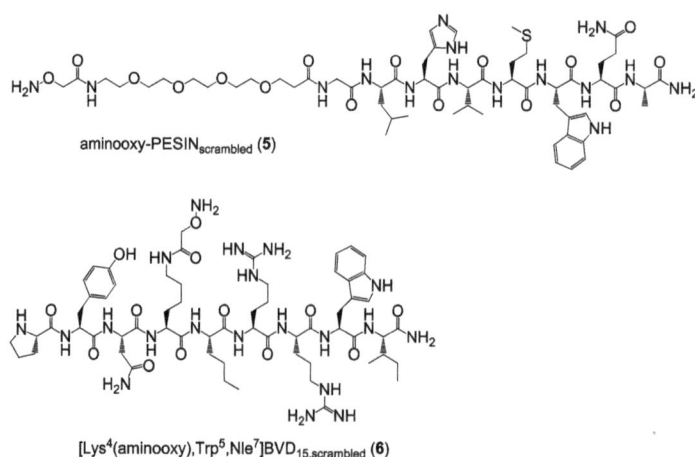

Figure 5. Depiction of the chemical structures of aminooxy-PESIN$_{scrambled}$ (5) and [Lys^4(aminooxy), Trp^5,Nle^7]BVD$_{15,scrambled}$ (6) which were used to synthesize partly or fully scrambled HBPL analogs.

2.1.2. Synthesis of the Heterobivalent Ligands **22–26**, **24a–c** and Monomeric Reference Peptides **27** and **28**

The branched *bis*-amines **7–11** and *bis*-aldehydes **12–16** (Scheme 1) were synthesized following a published procedure [22] with minor modifications (see Supplementary Materials for detailed description). In the following, these NODA-GA-modified branched *bis*-aldehyde scaffolds **12–16** were efficiently reacted with aminooxy-PESIN (**1**) and aminooxy-PESIN$_{scrambled}$ (**5**) to the monovalent intermediates **17–21** and **19a**. These were further reacted with [Lys^4(aminooxy),Trp^5,Nle^7]BVD$_{15}$ (**2**) and its scrambled analog **6** to the final heterobivalent peptidic target structures **22–26** and their partly or fully scrambled analogs **24a–c** (Scheme 1).

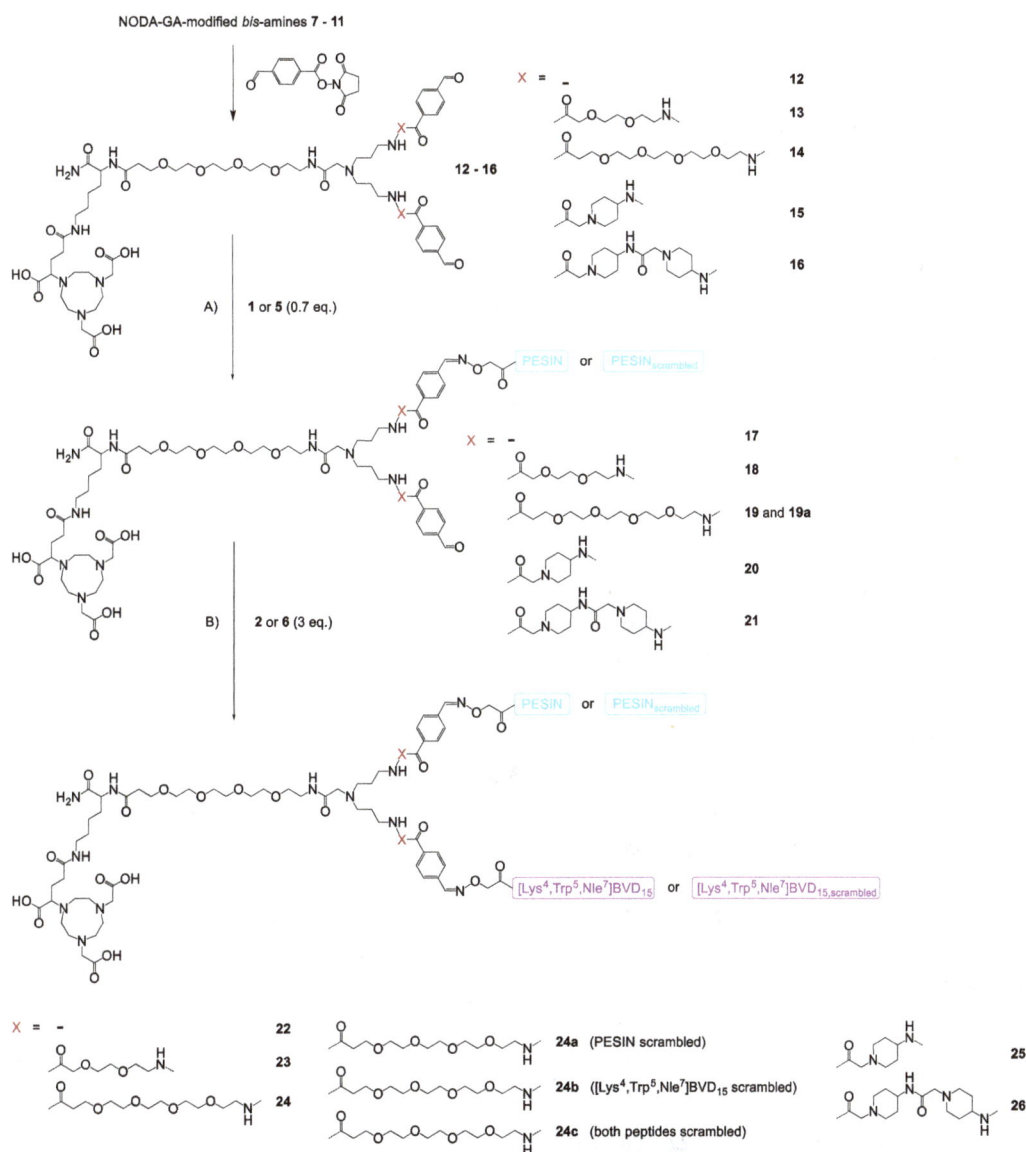

Scheme 1. Schematic depiction of the syntheses of the GRPR- and NPY(Y$_1$)R-affine HBPLs **22–26** and the scrambled analogs **24a–c**. Conditions: (**A**) **1**, H$_2$O + 0.1% TFA, phosphate buffer, pH 4.0–4.6, RT, 5 min, yields: 47% for **17**, 51% for **18**, 43% for **19**, 44% for **19a**, 58% for **20**, 55% for **21**; (**B**) **2**, H$_2$O + 0.1% TFA, phosphate buffer, pH 4.0–4.6, RT, 5 min, yields: 82% for **22**, 79% for **23**, 66% for **24**, 49% for **24a**, 63% for **24b**, 61% for **24c**, 75% for **25**, 73% for **26**.

1 as well as its scrambled analog **5** reacted efficiently within minutes with the branched *bis*-aldehydes **12–16**, giving the respective monovalent conjugation products **17–21** and **19a** in satisfactory yields of 47% to 58%. Higher yields could not be obtained as **1** and **5** had to be applied in a lower amount than the *bis*-aldehydes **12–16** to minimize the formation of the respective homobivalent PESIN-dimers, being the only observed side products in this reaction. These monovalent intermediates were in the following reacted with **2** or **6**, proceeding equally efficient than the first reaction step within minutes, giving the target HBPLs **22–26** as well as the scrambled analogs **24a–c** in good yields of 49% to 82%.

The HBPLs exhibited—depending on the linker structure used—distances between both peptidic receptor ligands of 46 (no additional linker units used), 64 (PEG_2 linkers), 78 (PEG_4 linkers), 60 (ACMP linkers), and 74 (two successive ACMP linkers) bond lengths.

Besides the target HBPLs and the scrambled analogs, also the monomeric reference compounds DOTA-PESIN (**27**) [18] and [Lys^4(DOTA),Trp^5,Nle^7]BVD$_{15}$ (**28**) [19] (Figure 6) (DOTA = (1,4,7,10-tetraazacyclododecane-1,4,7,10-tetrayl)tetraacetic acid), having been described before to be potent agents efficiently targeting the GRPR and NPY(Y$_1$)R, were synthesized in yields of 7% and 45%, respectively. These ligands, addressing only one of the target receptors types, served as monomeric reference compounds for the following in vitro evaluations.

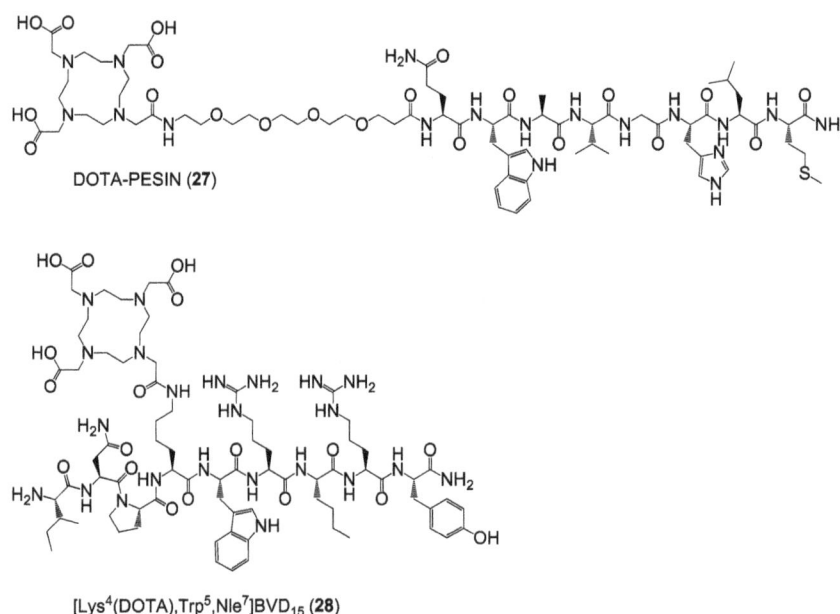

DOTA-PESIN (**27**)

[Lys^4(DOTA),Trp^5,Nle^7]BVD$_{15}$ (**28**)

Figure 6. Depiction of the structures of DOTA-PESIN (**27**) and [Lys^4(DOTA),Trp^5,Nle^7]BVD$_{15}$ (**28**), serving as mono-specific reference substances for the HBPLs in the following in vitro tumor cell uptake studies.

2.2. ^{68}Ga-Radiolabeling, log$_D$ and Stability Determination of Peptide Heterodimers [^{68}Ga]22–[^{68}Ga]26 and Monomeric Reference Peptides [^{68}Ga]27 and [^{68}Ga]28

The heterobivalent ligands **22–26** and the reference substances **27** and **28** were in the following radiolabeled with ^{68}Ga^{3+}. The ^{68}Ga^{3+} was obtained via elution of an itG or Eckert & Ziegler IGG100 ^{68}Ge/^{68}Ga generator system. After adjusting the pH of the solution to 3.5 to 4.0, the NODA-GA-comprising HBPLs **22–26** were incubated at 40–45 °C for 10 min. The DOTA-comprising reference compounds **27** and **28** were reacted at 99 °C under otherwise identical conditions. The ^{68}Ga-labeled products [^{68}Ga]22–[^{68}Ga]26, [^{68}Ga]27 and [^{68}Ga]28 were obtained in radiochemical yields and purities of 95–99% (Figure S1A) as well as non-optimized molar activities of 10–15 GBq/μmol (used for in vitro assays and obtained by using an itG generator system) or

40–46 GBq/μmol (used for in vivo evaluations, obtained by using an Eckert & Ziegler IGG100 generator system), starting from 110–150 or 420–460 MBq of $^{68}Ga^{3+}$, respectively.

Regarding a favorable in vivo biodistribution of the radioligands, the $\log_D$ of the HBPLs should be in a comparable range as that of the lead peptide monomers as we and others were able to show before that a high lipophilicity negatively influences tumor uptake, organ distribution, and unspecific background accumulation, resulting in a limited usefulness of the radiopeptides for tumor visualization [23–25]. Consequently, we determined the $\log_D$ of the developed HBPLs [^{68}Ga]22–[^{68}Ga]26 in comparison to the monomeric reference peptides [^{68}Ga]27 and [^{68}Ga]28 via the distribution coefficient of the respective radiotracer between phosphate buffer and 1-octanol. The results of these evaluations are depicted in Figure S2. The results showed a comparatively high hydrophilicity for all of the tested substances (-1.857 ± 0.054 for [^{68}Ga]27, -1.982 ± 0.162 for [^{68}Ga]28, -1.569 ± 0.111 for [^{68}Ga]22, -1.527 ± 0.109 for [^{68}Ga]23, -1.672 ± 0.086 for [^{68}Ga]24, -1.550 ± 0.114 for [^{68}Ga]25 and -1.518 ± 0.089 for [^{68}Ga]26). This indicates that the in vivo pharmacokinetics of the developed HBPLs [^{68}Ga]22–[^{68}Ga]26 should, in terms of hydrophilicity, be similar to that of the parent monomeric radiopeptides [^{68}Ga]27 and [^{68}Ga]28.

Besides lipophilicity, the stability of peptidic radioligands is an important parameter regarding their applicability for in vivo imaging. Thus, the stability of the ^{68}Ga-labeled HBPLs [^{68}Ga]22–[^{68}Ga]26 and the reference compounds [^{68}Ga]27 and [^{68}Ga]28 was determined in human serum. Typical radio-HPLC chromatograms for each substance (obtained after 90 min incubation with human serum) are depicted in Figure S1B. All of the tested compounds were stable over the testing period of 90 min, showing only a negligible degradation after this time: $3 \pm 0.2\%$ for [^{68}Ga]27, $4 \pm 0.8\%$ for [^{68}Ga]28, $2 \pm 1.6\%$ for [^{68}Ga]22, $1 \pm 0.5\%$ for [^{68}Ga]23, no observable fragmentation for [^{68}Ga]24, $2 \pm 0.3\%$ for [^{68}Ga]25 and $2 \pm 0.5\%$ for [^{68}Ga]26. From the serum stability point of view—which can however only give a rough estimation of stability under in vivo conditions [26]—all of the radioligands are applicable for in vivo tumor imaging with PET/computed tomography (CT).

2.3. In Vitro Cell Uptake Studies: Tumor Cell Uptake of [^{68}Ga]22–[^{68}Ga]26 in Comparison to the Reference Peptides [^{68}Ga]27 and [^{68}Ga]28 in Different Human Breast Cancer Cell Lines

In the following, we intended to determine if we could observe an independent binding of both peptide parts of the HBPLs to both target receptor types, being the prerequisite for improved/more likely tumor uptake (→ Figure 1). This can be achieved by tumor cell uptake studies of the radiotracers as it was shown before for radiolabeled somatostatin analogs that the in vitro cell uptake directly correlates to in vivo tumor uptakes [27], demonstrating the relevance of such in vitro tumor cell uptake studies.

The human breast cancer cell line T-47D was described to express both the GRPR [9,28] as well as the NPY(Y_1)R [29,30] (where β-estradiol in the medium increases NPY(Y_1)R-expression) and thus should be the ideal cell line to determine if both parts of the developed HBPLs bind to their respective receptor and if a synergistic effect of peptide heterodimerization on tumor cell uptake can be achieved. Of course, it would also have been feasible to use different cells lines expressing either the GRPR or the NPY(Y_1)R to demonstrate that both peptides of the HBPLs are still able to address their respective target receptor, but a cell line expressing both receptors concomitantly is far more advantageous to showcase the potential beneficial effects of heterodimerization and to determine the part each of the peptides contributes to tumor cell uptake in case of a concomitant receptor expression.

Thus, we first determined the uptake of the HBPLs [^{68}Ga]22–[^{68}Ga]26 in comparison to the peptide monomers [^{68}Ga]27 and [^{68}Ga]28 in T-47D cells. The results of the cell uptake studies of the radioligands are shown in Figure 7a (overall specific cell uptake of [^{68}Ga]22–[^{68}Ga]26, [^{68}Ga]27 and [^{68}Ga]28) and Figure 7b (uptake of [^{68}Ga]24, differentiated by overall uptake, internalization and surface binding; the results for the other tested radioligands were comparable and can be found in the Supplementary Materials in Figures S3–S7).

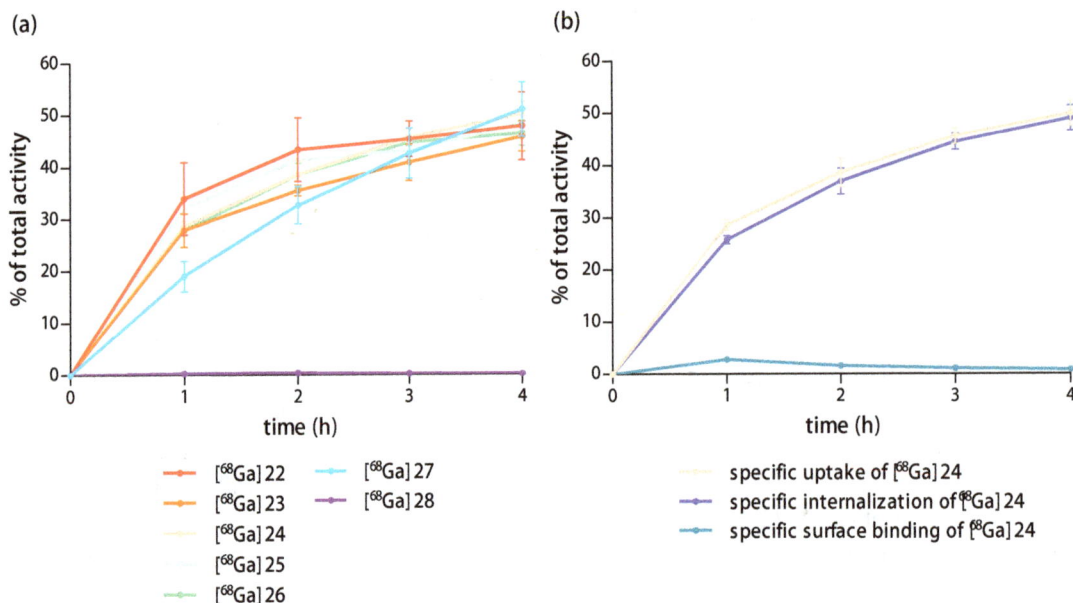

Figure 7. (a) Specific cell uptake of [^{68}Ga]**22**−[^{68}Ga]**26**, [^{68}Ga]**27** and [^{68}Ga]**28** in T-47D cells over 4 h of incubation; (b) Uptake of [^{68}Ga]**24** in the same cells, differentiated by overall uptake, internalization, and surface binding.

As expected, a high and constant specific uptake of the monovalent GRPR-specific peptide [^{68}Ga]**27** of $51.0 \pm 5.2\%$ was observed into the T-47D cells after 4 h. Also, the HBPLs [^{68}Ga]**22**−[^{68}Ga]**26** demonstrated a comparably high specific uptake into these cells of $47.8 \pm 6.5\%$, $45.8 \pm 2.9\%$, $50.1 \pm 2.4\%$, $48.2 \pm 2.8\%$ and $46.4 \pm 2.4\%$, respectively, after the same time. Interestingly, the monovalent, NPY(Y$_1$)-binding peptide [^{68}Ga]**28** showed no specific uptake ($0.2 \pm 0.03\%$). This means that the uptake of the HBPLs [^{68}Ga]**22**−[^{68}Ga]**26** into the T-47D cells is exclusively mediated by the GRPR.

These results indicate that the heterodimerization and the resulting significant chemical modification of the peptides as well as the compounds' complexity and size do not affect the GRPR-specific tumor cell uptake of the HBPLs compared to the monomeric reference [^{68}Ga]**27**. Also, the molecular design of the heterobivalent ligands comprising linkers of different length and rigidity does not seem to have a significant effect on the GRPR-mediated cellular uptake of the respective HBPL radiotracer.

In the following, we tested the uptake of the peptide monomers [^{68}Ga]**27** and [^{68}Ga]**28** in three further standard cell lines of breast cancer: BT-474, MCF-7 and MDA-MB-231 cells. Of these, the BT-474 cells were also described to express both the GRPR [31] and the NPY(Y$_1$)R [31], whereas MCF-7 cells were described to be NPY(Y$_1$)R positive [30,32] but expressing the GRPR only to a low extent [9] and MDA-MB-231 cells were described to be GRPR positive [33] but expressing the NPY(Y$_1$)R to a low extent [29,30]. The results of these experiments can be found in the Supplementary Materials (Figures S8–S10) and demonstrated contrary to the expectations only negligible uptakes of both peptide monomers in all cell lines.

As the HBPLs [^{68}Ga]**22**−[^{68}Ga]**26** and the respective monomer [^{68}Ga]**27** were however shown to be efficiently taken up by GRPR-positive T-47D cells, these results indicate that the GRPR is present to an only low amount on BT-474, MCF-7, and MDA-MB-231 cells. Concerning the missing uptake of [^{68}Ga]**28** into all tested cell lines, three explanations are possible: (i) The NPY(Y$_1$)R is present on at least some of the cells but the peptide sequence [Lys^4,Trp^5,Nle^7]BVD$_{15}$, being the NPY(Y$_1$)R-targeting sequence in monomer [^{68}Ga]**28** as well as the HBPLs [^{68}Ga]**22**−[^{68}Ga]**26**, is not able to efficiently address the NPY(Y$_1$)R; (ii) The NPY(Y$_1$)R is expressed in such low amounts that the tested radioligands cannot be efficiently taken up by the cells by this receptor; or (iii) The molar activities of the tested radioligands were too low and a significant self-blocking of the NPY(Y_1)R-mediated uptake took place, preventing the cell uptake.

In order to determine if the NPY(Y_1)R is actually present on T-47D, MCF-7 and BT-474 cells and if the molar activity of monomer [^{68}Ga]28 and the HBPLs [^{68}Ga]22–[^{68}Ga]26 prevented their cellular uptake via the NPY(Y_1)R, the cell uptake studies were repeated using commercially available ^{125}I-PYY, binding the NPY(Y_1)R [29] and exhibiting a high molar activity of 81.4 GBq/µmol. In these experiments, an about 100-fold lower amount of substance was used for the cell uptake studies compared to the ^{68}Ga-labeled ligands ([^{68}Ga]22–[^{68}Ga]26, [^{68}Ga]27 and [^{68}Ga]28: 0.37–0.40 pmol per 1.5×10^6 cells; ^{125}I-PYY: 0.003–0.005 pmol per 1.5×10^6 cells) in order to exclude the eventuality of self-blocking. In all of the three tested cell lines, the specific uptake of ^{125}I-PYY showed to be negligibly low (between 0.2 and 2.5% of the total activity applied), confirming that the target NPY(Y_1) receptor might be present on the cells but if so, then only to a very low amount, being too low to give useful results in the cell uptake studies.

Furthermore, this low receptor density prevents a successful determination of the receptor affinity of the developed radioligands. This is in contrast to other studies, using identically treated MCF-7 cells to determine NPY(Y_1)R affinities of newly developed NPY(Y_1)R-affine radioligands [9,19]. We could however not reproduce these results using MCF-7 cells of different suppliers due to the observed low expression of NPY(Y_1)R on the cells.

As it was described that MCF-7 cells can express the target NPY(Y_1)R to a much higher extent in vivo than under in vitro conditions [34], this might also be the case for the T-47D cell line, expressing besides the NPY(Y_1)R also the for our scientific question important GRPR. Thus, we in the following performed initial in vivo evaluations of HBPL [^{68}Ga]24, showing highly promising results in the preceding evaluations. Of the developed HBPLs, [^{68}Ga]24 showed the highest stability and hydrophilicity as well as a slightly higher tumor cell uptake than the other analogs in vitro and thus represents a potent representative of the developed HBPLs for a following proof-of-concept in vivo evaluation.

2.4. Proof-of-Concept: Evaluation of HBPL [^{68}Ga]24 and Its Scrambled Analogs [^{68}Ga]24a and [^{68}Ga]24b via In Vivo PET/CT Imaging in T-47D-Bearing Nude Mice and Ex Vivo Biodistribution

To investigate the in vivo pharmacokinetic properties of the most potent HBPL [^{68}Ga]24, we performed small animal PET/CT imaging studies in T-47D tumor-bearing immunodeficient mice. Likewise, also the scrambled variants of [^{68}Ga]24, [^{68}Ga]24a (PESIN$_{scrambled}$ combined with [Lys^4(aminooxy),Trp^5,Nle^7]BVD$_{15}$) and [^{68}Ga]24b (PESIN combined with [Lys^4(aminooxy),Trp^5,Nle^7]BVD$_{15,scrambled}$), were evaluated under the same conditions for comparison.

By evaluating these radioligands under the same conditions, the proportion of both peptide binders on the uptake of [^{68}Ga]24 and also the receptor-specificity of the uptake of the radioligand via both receptors should be determined. The evaluation of the partly scrambled monovalent analogs instead of the monomeric peptides, which would also have been possible, exhibits the advantage that all evaluated radioligands show a similar pharmacokinetic distribution and also a similar possible degradation pattern. Using the monovalent peptides bombesin or NPY/BVD for receptor blocking (to show the receptor specificity of both peptide parts of [^{68}Ga]24 and to determine the contribution of both peptide parts of the HBPL to overall tumor uptake) might have resulted in an incomplete blocking of the respective receptor as the GRPR-affine bombesin as well as the NPY(Y_1)R-affine peptides NPY and BVD are known for their limited in vivo stability.

For the PET/CT imaging studies, 5.5–8.0 MBq of the respective ^{68}Ga-radioligand were administered via the lateral tail vein under isoflurane anesthesia to the tumor-bearing animals. Directly after completion of the diagnostic scans, the animals were sacrificed, the organs were collected and measured in a gamma-counter. The results of these in vivo PET/CT imaging studies and the ex vivo biodistribution data are given in Figure 8 and Table S1.

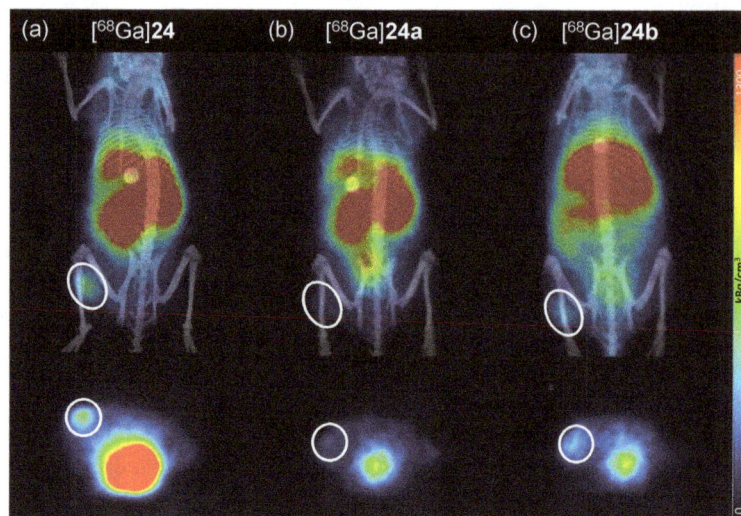

Figure 8. Representative small animal positron emission tomography/computed tomography (PET/CT) imaging results for [^{68}Ga]**24** (**a**); [^{68}Ga]**24a** (**b**) and [^{68}Ga]**24b** (**c**). The images show coronal (**upper row**) and transaxial (**lower row**) slices for all tracers at 37.5 min p.i. The same scaling was used for all images and 4 animals were examined per radioligand. The tumor is encircled in each image.

As can easily be seen from the in vivo PET/CT imaging as well as the ex vivo biodistribution data, all developed ligands showed a rather high kidney and liver uptake. Thus, further improvements in ligand design must be carried out to result in clinically relevant imaging agents for improved breast cancer visualization with PET/CT.

Compared to the bispecific ligand [^{68}Ga]**24** with which the tumor can easily be delineated via PET/CT, the scrambled analogs [^{68}Ga]**24a** and [^{68}Ga]**24b** showed a considerably less efficient tumor visualization ability (Figure 8).

This results from a lower absolute tumor uptake for [^{68}Ga]**24a** and [^{68}Ga]**24b** compared to [^{68}Ga]**24** over the course of PET imaging (Figure 9a, SUVs$_{(85min)}$ of 122.03 ± 16.27 kBq/cm^3 for [^{68}Ga]**24**, 42.95 ± 26.38 kBq/cm^3 for [^{68}Ga]**24a** and 70.29 ± 16.09 kBq/cm^3 for [^{68}Ga]**24b** were observed), which was also confirmed in the ex vivo biodistribution experiments (Figure 9b).

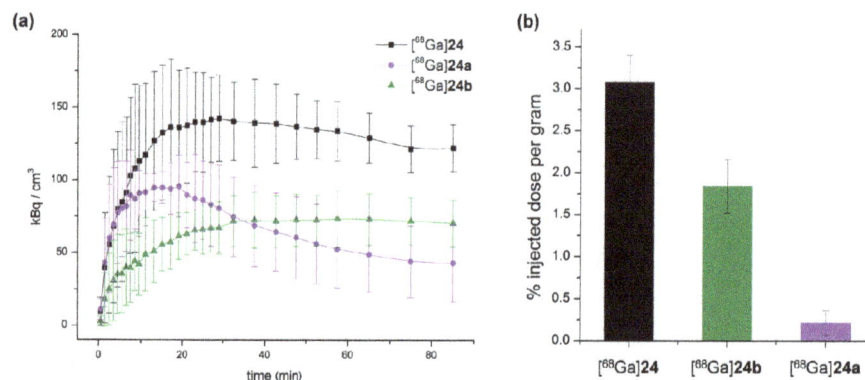

Figure 9. Absolute tumor uptakes as determined by in vivo PET imaging as well as ex vivo biodistribution experiments ($n = 4$). (**a**) Time-activity-curves are depicted, showing tumor uptakes over the course of PET imaging for [^{68}Ga]**24** (black), [^{68}Ga]**24a** (purple) and [^{68}Ga]**24b** (green); (**b**) Tumor uptakes (% injected dose per gram) are shown for [^{68}Ga]**24** (black), [^{68}Ga]**24a** (purple) and [^{68}Ga]**24b** (green) as determined by ex vivo biodistribution directly after the completed diagnostic scans.

This indicates that both parts of HBPL [^{68}Ga]**24** contributed to in vivo tumor uptake and that its uptake into the tumor was GRPR- and also NPY(Y$_1$)R-specific.

As can be observed from the time-activity-curves obtained by PET imaging (Figure 9a), those ligands comprising an intact variant of the GRPR-targeting ligand BBN$_{7-14}$ showed a stable plateau phase in tumor accumulation ([^{68}Ga]**24b**) or only a slight decrease ([^{68}Ga]**24**) whereas [^{68}Ga]**24a**, comprising a scrambled variant of BBN$_{7-14}$, shows a surge in tumor uptake followed by a decline of activity in the tumor. This might be attributable to the limited stability of BVD analogs under in vivo conditions, which has been described before [35] and might result in radioligand metabolization during imaging. If then the GRPR-binding peptide is still able to bind to its target receptor, the tumor uptake nevertheless remains largely stable due to a GRPR-mediated uptake. However, if only a scrambled variant of BBN$_{7-14}$ is present, no receptor-affine peptide binder remains for continuous radiotracer uptake into the tumor, resulting in an overall decrease in tumor accumulation.

Further, high and considerably improved tumor-to-background ratios could be achieved for [^{68}Ga]**24** (tumor-to-muscle: 11.81 ± 1.83, tumor-to-blood: 2.72 ± 0.43) compared to [^{68}Ga]**24a** (tumor-to-muscle: 1.07 ± 1.14, tumor-to-blood: 0.50 ± 0.47) and [^{68}Ga]**24b** (tumor-to-muscle: 3.83 ± 0.80, tumor-to-blood: 0.91 ± 0.24) as determined by ex vivo biodistribution at 130 min p.i. This indicates that both peptide parts of the HBPL contributed to tumor uptake and thus tumor visualization.

In summary, we were able to show here for the first time that the general concept to assemble a GRPR- and a NPY(Y$_1$)R-affine peptide to one combined radioligand is in general feasible regarding a contribution of both peptides of the HBPL to in vivo tumor uptake and thus is beneficial with regard to overall tumor uptake and tumor visualization probability compared to the monospecific agents.

3. Materials and Methods

General. All commercially available chemicals were of analytical grade and were used without further purification. Resins for solid phase-based syntheses, PyBOP (Benzotriazole-1-yl-oxy-*tris*-pyrrolidino-phosphonium hexafluorophosphate), Fmoc-protected standard amino acids as well as *bis*-Boc-aminooxy acetic acid were purchased from NovaBiochem (Darmstadt, Germany). SFB (Succinimidyl-*p*-formyl-benzoate) was synthesized according to a published procedure [36]. Fmoc-ACMP-OH (Fmoc-4-amino-1-carboxymethyl-piperidine) was obtained from Iris Biotech (Marktredwitz, Germany), respectively. Fmoc-L-Lys(Boc$_2$-Aoa)-OH, mono-Fmoc ethylene diamine hydrochloride, HBTU (*O*-(Benzotriazol-1-yl)-*N,N,N',N'*-tetramethyluronium hexafluorophosphate), Tracepur water and *N,N*-bis(*N'*-Fmoc-3-aminopropyl)-glycine potassium hemisulfate ((Fmoc-NH-Propyl)$_2$-Gly-OH) were purchased from Iris Biotech, SigmaAldrich (Schnelldorf, Germany), Carl Roth (Karlsruhe, Germany), VWR (Bruchsal, Germany) and PolyPeptide (Strasbourg, France), respectively. NODA-GA-(*t*Bu)$_3$ and DOTA-(*t*Bu)$_3$ were obtained from CheMatech (Dijon, France).

Bis-amines **7–11** and *bis*-aldehydes **12–16** were synthesized according to published procedures [22] with minor modifications of the synthesis protocols. Details of these syntheses can be found in the supplementary information.

Unless otherwise stated, the coupling reactions during solid phase-based syntheses were usually carried out in DMF for 30 min using 4 eq. of acid, 3.9 eq. of HBTU as coupling reagent and 4 eq. of DIPEA (*N,N*-Diisopropylethylamine) as base. Fmoc protecting groups were removed using 50% (*v/v*) piperidine in DMF.

For analytical and semipreparative HPLC chromatography, Dionex UltiMate 3000 systems equipped with a Chromolith Performance (RP-18e, 100-4.6 mm, Merck, Darmstadt, Germany) and a Chromolith SemiPrep (RP-18e, 100-10 mm, Merck) column were used, operated with a flow rate of 4 mL/min and H$_2$O + 0.1% TFA and MeCN + 0.1% TFA as eluents. For radio-analytical HPLC chromatography, a Dionex UltiMate 3000 system equipped with a Chromolith Performance (RP-18e, 100-4.6 mm, Merck) column and a GabiStar radioactivity detector (Raytest, Straubenhardt, Germany) or an Agilent 1200 system equipped with a Chromolith Performance (RP-18e, 100-4.6 mm, Merck) column and a GabiStar radioactivity detector (Raytest) were used and operated with a flow rate of 4 mL/min and H_2O + 0.1% TFA and MeCN + 0.1% TFA as eluents. MALDI (Matrix-Assisted Laser Desorption/Ionization) spectra were obtained with a Bruker Daltonics Microflex spectrometer (Bremen, Germany).

The human breast cancer cell lines T-47D, MDA-MB-231 and MCF-7 were purchased from SigmaAldrich (Schnelldorf, Germany), whereas the cell line BT-474 was obtained from the Leibniz-Institute DSMZ (Braunschweig, Germany). Dulbecco's Modified Eagle Medium (DMEM), RPMI-1640 medium, 200 mM L-glutamine, 0.05% trypsin/EDTA and 0.25% trypsin/EDTA were purchased from Life Technologies. Fetal calf serum (FCS) was obtained from GE Healthcare Life Sciences and phosphate buffered saline (PBS) as well as β-estradiol were purchased from Sigma Aldrich. Bovine serum albumin (BSA) was purchased from CarlRoth (Karlsruhe, Germany).

The human ^{125}I-labeled NPY(Y_1)-binding peptide [^{125}I]-Peptide-YY was obtained from PerkinElmer in a molar activity of 81.4 GBq/μmol. The γ-counter used was a 2480 WIZARD² system (PerkinElmer, Rodgau, Germany).

For the in vivo evaluations, five week old female Fox Chase SCID mice were obtained from Janvier and implanted with estradiol pellets (0.36 mg/60 days; obtained from Innovative Research of America) one week prior to tumor cell inoculation. Tumor cells were inoculated using Matrigel basal membrane matrix with reduced growth factor (obtained from VWR). For PET/CT measurements, a small animal Albira II PET/SPECT/CT system (Bruker, Eggenstein-Leopoldshafen, Germany) was used.

Synthesis of aminooxy-PESIN (1) and aminooxy-PESIN$_{scrambled}$ (5). The peptides were synthesized on solid support by standard Fmoc solid-phase peptide synthesis using a commercially available standard Rink amide MBHA resin, HBTU as coupling reagent, standard N_α-Fmoc-amino acids, N_ω-Fmoc-PEG$_4$-OH and *bis*-Boc-aminooxy acetic acid. All amino acids (apart from *bis*-Boc-aminooxy acetic acid which was reacted for 60 min) were coupled within 30 min. The crude aminooxy-modified peptides were cleaved from the solid support using a mixture of TFA:TIS:H_2O of 95:2.5:2.5 (*v/v*) for 60 min, suspended in diethyl ether and purified by semipreparative HPLC.

1 was purified using a gradient of 15–30% MeCN + 0.1% TFA in 8 min (R_t = 6.35 min) and isolated as white solid after lyophilization in yields of 27% (85.0 mg; 67.4 μmol). MALDI-MS (*m/z*) using 2,5-dihydroxybenzoic acid as matrix substance for [M + H⁺]⁺ (calculated): 1260.23 (1260.46); [M + Na⁺]⁺ (calculated): 1282.21 (1282.62); [M + K⁺]⁺ (calculated): 1298.16 (1298.60). MALDI-MS (*m/z*) using α-cyano-4-hydroxycinnamic acid as matrix substance for [M + H⁺]⁺ (calculated): 1260.63 (1260.46); [M + Na⁺]⁺ (calculated): 1282.56 (1282.62); [M + K⁺]⁺ (calculated): 1298.54 (1298.60).

5 was purified using a gradient of 10–60% MeCN + 0.1% TFA in 8 min (R_t = 5.42 min) and isolated as white solid after lyophilization in yields of 22% (28.1 mg, 22.2 μmol). MALDI-MS (*m/z*) using α-cyano-4-hydroxycinnamic acid as matrix substance for [M + H⁺]⁺ (calculated): 1260.81 (1260.46); [M + Na⁺]⁺ (calculated): 1282.84 (1282.62); [M + K⁺]⁺ (calculated): 1298.78 (1298.60).

Synthesis of [Lys⁴(aminooxy),Trp⁵,Nle⁷]BVD15 (2) and [Lys⁴(aminooxy),Trp⁵,Nle⁷]BVD15$_{scrambled}$ (6). The peptides were synthesized on solid support by standard Fmoc solid-phase peptide synthesis using a commercially available Rink amide MBHA resin, HBTU as coupling reagent, standard N_α-Fmoc-amino acids and N_α-Fmoc-L-Lys(Boc$_2$-Aoa)-OH. The crude aminooxy-modified peptides were cleaved from the solid support using a mixture of TFA:TIS:H_2O of 95:2.5:2.5 (*v/v*) for 90 min, suspended in diethyl ether and purified by semipreparative HPLC.

2 was purified using a gradient of 10–60% MeCN + 0.1% TFA in 8 min (R_t = 3.71 min) and isolated as white solid after lyophilization in yields of 35% (114.2 mg; 86.7 μmol). MALDI-MS (*m/z*) using 2,5-dihydroxybenzoic acid as matrix substance for [M + H⁺]⁺ (calculated): 1317.02 (1317.54); [M + Na⁺]⁺ (calculated): 1339.13 (1339.74); [M + K⁺]⁺ (calculated): 1355.03 (1355.71). MALDI-MS (*m/z*) using α-cyano-4-hydroxycinnamic acid as matrix substance for [M + H⁺]⁺ (calculated): 1317.89 (1317.54); [M + Na⁺]⁺ (calculated): 1339.89 (1339.74); [M + K⁺]⁺ (calculated): 1355.86 (1355.71).

6 was purified using a gradient of 10–50% MeCN + 0.1% TFA in 8 min (R_t = 4.31 min) and isolated as white solid after lyophilization in yields of 20% (26.0 mg; 19.7 μmol). MALDI-MS (*m/z*) using α-cyano-4-hydroxycinnamic acid as matrix substance for $[M + H^+]^+$ (calculated): 1317.37 (1317.54); $[M + Na^+]^+$ (calculated): 1339.38 (1339.74).

Synthesis of bombesin (3). The peptide was synthesized on solid support by standard Fmoc solid-phase peptide synthesis using a commercially available standard Rink amide resin, HBTU as coupling reagent and standard N_α-Fmoc-amino acids. All amino acids were coupled within 35 min. The crude peptide was cleaved from the solid support using a mixture of TFA:TIS:H_2O of 95:2.5:2.5 (v/v) for 90 min, suspended in diethyl ether and purified by semipreparative HPLC using a gradient of 15–60% MeCN + 0.1% TFA in 5.5 min (R_t = 3.40 min) and isolated as white solid after lyophilization in yields of 22% (35.2 mg, 21.6 μmol). MALDI-MS (m/z) using α-cyano-4-hydroxycinnamic acid as matrix substance for $[M + H^+]^+$ (calculated): 1618.56 (1618.82); $[M + Na^+]^+$ (calculated): 1640.55 (1640.81); $[M + K^+]^+$ (calculated): 1656.57 (1656.78).

Synthesis of [Lys[4],Trp[5],Nle[7]]BVD15 (4). The peptide was synthesized on solid support by standard Fmoc solid-phase peptide synthesis using a commercially available standard Rink amide resin, HBTU as coupling reagent and standard N_α-Fmoc-amino acids. All amino acids were coupled within 30 min. The crude peptide was cleaved from the solid support using a mixture of TFA:TIS:H_2O of 95:2.5:2.5 (v/v) for 120 min, suspended in diethyl ether and purified by semipreparative HPLC using a gradient of 10–60% MeCN + 0.1% TFA in 5.5 min (R_t = 3.05 min) and isolated as white solid after lyophilization in yields of 40% (49.2 mg; 39.5 μmol). MALDI-MS (m/z) using α-cyano-4-hydroxycinnamic acid as matrix substance for $[M + H^+]^+$ (calculated): 1244.63 (1244.73); $[M + Na^+]^+$ (calculated): 1266.65 (1266.72); $[M + K^+]^+$ (calculated): 1282.60 (1282.69).

General synthesis of NODA-GA-PESIN-aldehydes (17−21) and NODA-GA-PESIN$_{scrambled}$-aldehyde (19a). To a solution of the respective branched NODA-GA-*bis*-aldehyde (**12−16**) in H_2O + 0.1% TFA (250−500 μL) was added a solution of aminooxy-PESIN (**1**) or aminooxy-PESIN$_{scrambled}$ (**5**) (0.7 eq.) in H_2O + 0.1% TFA (250−500 μL). The pH of the solutions was adjusted to 4.0–4.6 by addition of phosphate buffer (0.1 M, pH 7.2, ~150 μL) and the reaction progress was monitored by analytical HPLC. The reactions were found to be finished within 5 min and the products were purified by semipreparative HPLC. The products were isolated as white solids after lyophilization. Gradients used for HPLC purification and synthesis yields for each compound are given below.

17: gradient: 20–45% MeCN + 0.1% TFA in 5 min (R_t = 4.45 min), yield: 47%. MALDI-MS (m/z) using α-cyano-4-hydroxycinnamic acid as matrix substance for $[M + H^+]^+$ (calculated): 2427.33 (2427.22); $[M + Na^+]^+$ (calculated): 2449.30 (2449.21); $[M + K^+]^+$ (calculated): 2465.49 (2465.18). MALDI-MS (m/z) using 2,5-dihydroxybenzoic acid as matrix substance for $[M + H^+]^+$ (calculated): 2426.69 (2427.22); $[M + Na^+]^+$ (calculated): 2448.99 (2449.21); $[M + K^+]^+$ (calculated): 2464.93 (2465.18). MALDI-MS (m/z) using sinapic acid as matrix substance for $[M + H^+]^+$ (calculated): 2427.38 (2427.22); $[M + Na^+]^+$ (calculated): 2449.25 (2449.21).

18: gradient: 25–45% MeCN + 0.1% TFA in 5 min (R_t = 3.76 min), yield: 51%. MALDI-MS (m/z) using α-cyano-4-hydroxycinnamic acid as matrix substance for $[M + H^+]^+$ (calculated): 2717.48 (2717.37); $[M + Na^+]^+$ (calculated): 2739.21 (2739.36); $[M + K^+]^+$ (calculated): 2755.49 (2755.33). MALDI-MS (m/z) using 2,5-dihydroxybenzoic acid as matrix substance for $[M + H^+]^+$ (calculated): 2717.18 (2717.37); $[M + Na^+]^+$ (calculated): 2739.60 (2739.36); $[M + K^+]^+$ (calculated): 2755.13 (2755.33).

19: gradient: 25–45% MeCN + 0.1% TFA in 5 min (R_t = 4.26 min), yield: 43%. MALDI-MS (m/z) using α-cyano-4-hydroxycinnamic acid as matrix substance for $[M + H^+]^+$ (calculated): 2921.63 (2921.50); $[M + Na^+]^+$ (calculated): 2943.64 (2943.49); $[M + K^+]^+$ (calculated): 2959.46 (2959.47). MALDI-MS (m/z) using 2,5-dihydroxybenzoic acid as matrix substance for $[M + H^+]^+$ (calculated): 2921.63 (2921.50); $[M + Na^+]^+$ (calculated): 2943.34 (2943.49); $[M + K^+]^+$ (calculated): 2959.57 (2959.47).

19a (PESIN scrambled): gradient: 25–45% MeCN + 0.1% TFA in 5.5 min (R_t = 4.18 min), yield: 44%. MALDI-MS (m/z) using α-cyano-4-hydroxycinnamic acid as matrix substance for $[M + H^+]^+$ (calculated): 2921.59 (2921.50); $[M + Na^+]^+$ (calculated): 2943.56 (2943.49); $[M + K^+]^+$ (calculated): 2959.52 (2959.47).

20: gradient: 20–45% MeCN + 0.1% TFA in 5 min (R_t = 3.93 min), yield: 58%. MALDI-MS (m/z) using α-cyano-4-hydroxycinnamic acid as matrix substance for $[M + H^+]^+$ (calculated): 2707.24 (2707.41); $[M + Na^+]^+$ (calculated): 2729.30 (2729.40); $[M + K^+]^+$ (calculated): 2745.58 (2745.37). MALDI-MS (m/z) using 2,5-dihydroxybenzoic acid as matrix substance for $[M + H^+]^+$ (calculated): 2706.98 (2707.41); $[M + Na^+]^+$ (calculated): 2728.88 (2729.40); $[M + K^+]^+$ (calculated): 2744.78 (2745.37).

21: gradient: 25–45% MeCN + 0.1% TFA in 5 min (R_t = 2.85 min), yield: 55%. MALDI-MS (m/z) using α-cyano-4-hydroxycinnamic acid as matrix substance for $[M + H^+]^+$ (calculated): 2987.39 (2987.60); $[M + Na^+]^+$ (calculated): 3009.40 (3009.59); $[M + K^+]^+$ (calculated): 3025.80 (3025.56). MALDI-MS (m/z) using 2,5-dihydroxybenzoic acid as matrix substance for $[M + H^+]^+$ (calculated): 2987.03 (2987.60). MALDI-MS (m/z) using sinapic acid as matrix substance for $[M + H^+]^+$ (calculated): 2987.81 (2987.60).

General synthesis of heterobivalent ligands 22−26 and scrambled analogs 24a–c. To a solution of the respective NODA-GA-PESIN-aldehyde (**17−21** or **19a**) in H_2O + 0.1% TFA (250−500 μL) was added a solution of **2** or **6** (3 eq.) in H_2O + 0.1% TFA (250−500 μL). The pH of the solutions was adjusted to 4.0–4.6 by addition of phosphate buffer (0.1 M, pH 7.2, ~150 μL) and the reaction progress was monitored by analytical HPLC. The reactions were found to be finished within 5 min and the products were purified by semipreparative HPLC. The products were isolated as white solids after lyophilization. Gradients used for HPLC purification and synthesis yields for each compound are given below.

22: gradient: 25–50% MeCN + 0.1% TFA in 5 min (R_t = 3.19 min), yield: 82%. MALDI-MS (m/z) using α-cyano-4-hydroxycinnamic acid as matrix substance for $[M + H^+]^+$ (calculated): 3728.21 (3728.29); $[M + Na^+]^+$ (calculated): 3750.49 (3750.28). MALDI-MS (m/z) using 2,5-dihydroxybenzoic acid as matrix substance for $[M + H^+]^+$ (calculated): 3728.71 (3728.29); $[M + Na^+]^+$ (calculated): 3750.76 (3750.28).

23: gradient: 25–45% MeCN + 0.1% TFA in 5 min (R_t = 3.65 min), yield: 79%. MALDI-MS (m/z) using α-cyano-4-hydroxycinnamic acid as matrix substance for $[M + H^+]^+$ (calculated): 4018.99 (4018.61); $[M + Na^+]^+$ (calculated): 4040.69 (4040.60). MALDI-MS (m/z) using 2,5-dihydroxybenzoic acid as matrix substance for $[M + H^+]^+$ (calculated): 4018.95 (4018.61); $[M + Na^+]^+$ (calculated): 4040.02 (4040.60).

24: gradient: 25–45% MeCN + 0.1% TFA in 6 min (R_t = 3.86 min), yield: 66%. MALDI-MS (m/z) using α-cyano-4-hydroxycinnamic acid as matrix substance for $[M + H^+]^+$ (calculated): 4222.98 (4222.87). MALDI-MS (m/z) using 2,5-dihydroxybenzoic acid as matrix substance for $[M + H^+]^+$ (calculated): 4222.48 (4222.87); $[M + Na^+]^+$ (calculated): 4244.96 (4244.86); $[M + K^+]^+$ (calculated): 4260.51 (4260.97). MALDI-MS (m/z) using sinapic acid as matrix substance for $[M + H^+]^+$ (calculated): 4222.87 (4222.87).

24a (PESIN scrambled): gradient: 25–45% MeCN + 0.1% TFA in 6 min (R_t = 3.55 min), yield: 49%. MALDI-MS (m/z) using α-cyano-4-hydroxycinnamic acid as matrix substance for $[M + H^+]^+$ (calculated): 4222.54 (4222.87). MALDI-MS (m/z) using 2,5-dihydroxybenzoic acid as matrix substance for $[M + H^+]^+$ (calculated): 4222.17 (4222.87); $[M + Na^+]^+$ (calculated): 4244.94 (4244.86).

24b ([Lys^4,Trp^5,Nle^7]BVD$_{15}$ scrambled): gradient: 25–40% MeCN + 0.1% TFA in 5.5 min (R_t = 4.58 min), yield: 63%. MALDI-MS (m/z) using α-cyano-4-hydroxycinnamic acid as matrix substance for $[M + H^+]^+$ (calculated): 4222.35 (4222.87). MALDI-MS (m/z) using 2,5-dihydroxybenzoic acid as matrix substance for $[M + H^+]^+$ (calculated): 4222.29 (4222.87); $[M + Na^+]^+$ (calculated): 4244.99 (4244.86); $[M + K^+]^+$ (calculated): 4260.49 (4260.97).

24c (PESIN and [Lys^4,Trp^5,Nle^7]BVD$_{15}$ scrambled): gradient: 25–45% MeCN + 0.1% TFA in 5.5 min (R_t = 4.36 min), yield: 61%. MALDI-MS (m/z) using α-cyano-4-hydroxycinnamic acid as matrix substance for $[M + H^+]^+$ (calculated): 4222.67 (4222.87); $[M + K^+]^+$ (calculated): 4260.98 (4260.97). MALDI-MS (m/z) using 2,5-dihydroxybenzoic acid as matrix substance for $[M + H^+]^+$ (calculated): 4222.48 (4222.87); $[M + Na^+]^+$ (calculated): 4244.90 (4244.86).

25: gradient: 25–50% MeCN + 0.1% TFA in 6 min (R_t = 2.76 min), yield: 75%. MALDI-MS (m/z) using α-cyano-4-hydroxycinnamic acid as matrix substance for $[M + H^+]^+$ (calculated): 4008.53 (4008.66); $[M + Na^+]^+$ (calculated): 4030.76 (4030.65); $[M + K^+]^+$ (calculated): 4046.33 (4046.76). MALDI-MS (m/z) using 2,5-dihydroxybenzoic acid as matrix substance for $[M + H^+]^+$ (calculated): 4009.12 (4008.66).

26: gradient: 25–45% MeCN + 0.1% TFA in 6 min (R_t = 2.83 min), yield: 73%. MALDI-MS (m/z) using 2,5-dihydroxybenzoic acid as matrix substance for $[M + H^+]^+$ (calculated): 4288.72 (4289.03). MALDI-MS (m/z) using sinapic acid as matrix substance for $[M + H^+]^+$ (calculated): 4289.59 (4289.03).

Synthesis of DOTA-PESIN (27). The peptide was synthesized on solid support by standard Fmoc solid-phase peptide synthesis using a commercially available standard Rink amide MBHA resin, HBTU as coupling reagent, standard N_α-Fmoc-amino acids, and N_ω-Fmoc-PEG$_4$-OH. After the conjugation of the PEG$_4$ linker to the peptide sequence, DOTA-(tBu)$_3$ was coupled within 120 min using an excess of the synthon of 2.7 eq. together with 2.6 eq. HBTU and 4 eq. DIPEA. The crude product was cleaved from the solid support using a mixture of TFA:TIS:H$_2$O of 95:2.5:2.5 (v/v) for 3 h, suspended in diethyl ether and purified by semipreparative HPLC using a gradient of 20–35% MeCN + 0.1% TFA in 8 min (R_t = 4.34 min) and isolated as white solid after lyophilization in yields of 7% (10.7 mg; 6.8 µmol). MALDI-MS (m/z) using 2,5-dihydroxybenzoic acid as matrix substance for $[M + H^+]^+$ (calculated): 1573.02 (1573.80); $[M + Na^+]^+$ (calculated): 1595.06 (1595.79); $[M + K^+]^+$ (calculated): 1610.94 (1611.76). MALDI-MS (m/z) using α-cyano-4-hydroxycinnamic acid as matrix substance for $[M + H^+]^+$ (calculated): 1573.75 (1573.80); $[M + Na^+]^+$ (calculated): 1595.85 (1595.79).

Synthesis of [Lys^4(DOTA),Trp^5,Nle^7]BVD$_{15}$ (28). The peptide was synthesized on solid support by standard Fmoc solid-phase peptide synthesis using a commercially available standard Rink amide MBHA resin, HBTU as coupling reagent, standard N_α-Fmoc-amino acids and Fmoc-Lys(Mtt)-OH. After conjugation of the last amino acid, the lysine side chain Mtt-protecting group was removed with diluted TFA (TFA:DCM 1:99 (v/v)) within 2 h and DOTA-(tBu)$_3$ was coupled in this position within 120 min using an excess of the synthon of 2.7 eq. together with 2.6 eq. HBTU and 4 eq. DIPEA. The crude DOTA-modified peptide was cleaved from the solid support using a mixture of TFA:TIS:H$_2$O of 95:2.5:2.5 (v/v) for 3 h, suspended in diethyl ether and purified by semipreparative HPLC using a gradient of 20–25% MeCN + 0.1% TFA in 8 min (R_t = 2.58 min) and isolated as white solid after lyophilization in yields of 45% (73.4 mg; 45.0 µmol). MALDI-MS (m/z) using 2,5-dihydroxybenzoic acid as matrix substance for $[M + H^+]^+$ (calculated): 1630.38 (1630.91); $[M + Na^+]^+$ (calculated): 1652.59 (1652.90); $[M + K^+]^+$ (calculated): 1668.39 (1668.87). MALDI-MS (m/z) using α-cyano-4-hydroxycinnamic acid as matrix substance for $[M + H^+]^+$ (calculated): 1630.54 (1630.91). MALDI-MS (m/z) using sinapic acid as matrix substance for $[M + H^+]^+$ (calculated): 1630.53 (1630.91).

^{68}Ga-radiolabeling of NODAGA-modified peptide heterodimers (22−26) and peptide monomers 27 and 28 for in vitro evaluations. The respective labeling precursor (10 nmol, dissolved in 10 µL of Tracepur water) was reacted with 110–150 MBq of ^{68}Ga^{3+} obtained by an itG ^{68}Ge/^{68}Ga generator system (Garching, Germany). The generator was eluted with HCl (0.05 M, 3 mL) and the eluate was trapped on a cation exchange cartridge (Macherey-Nagel, Chromafix PS-H$^+$). The ^{68}Ga^{3+} was eluted from the cartridge using a NaCl solution (5 M, 1.5 mL) and the pH was adjusted to 3.5–4.0 by addition of sodium acetate solution (1.25 M, ~50 µL). After reaction for 10 min at 45 °C (**22−26**) or 99 °C (**27 and 28**), the reaction mixtures were analyzed by analytical radio-HPLC. The radiolabeled products were found to be 95–99% pure and obtained in molar activities of 10–15 GBq/µmol (non-optimized).

^{68}Ga-radiolabeling of NODAGA-modified peptide heterodimers (24 and 24a–c) for in vivo evaluations. The respective labeling precursor (10 nmol, dissolved in 10 µL of Tracepur water) was reacted with 420–460 MBq of ^{68}Ga^{3+} obtained by fractioned elution of an Eckert & Ziegler ^{68}Ge/^{68}Ga generator system (IGG100, Eckert & Ziegler, Berlin, Germany). The generator was eluted with HCl (0.1 M, 1.4 mL) and the pH was adjusted to 3.5–4.0 by addition of sodium acetate solution (1.25 M, 90–95 µL). After reaction for 10 min at 45 °C, the reaction mixtures were analyzed by analytical radio-HPLC. The radiolabeled products were found to be 95–99% pure and obtained in molar activities of 40–46 GBq/μmol (non-optimized). The pH of the radiotracer solution was adjusted to 6.0–7.0 using HEPES buffer (2.0 M, pH 8.0, 200 μL) and used for the in vivo studies.

Determination of radiotracer lipophilicity. The heterobivalent ligands (**22–26**) as well as the monomeric reference compounds (**27** and **28**) were radiolabeled with ^{68}Ga as described before and 2 μL of the product solution (~65 pmol of the respective radioligand) were added to a mixture of phosphate buffer (0.05 M, pH 7.4, 800 μL) and 1-octanol (800 μL) and incubated for 5 min at ambient temperature under vigorous shaking. Both phases were separated by centrifugation and 100 μL of each phase were measured for radioactivity in a gamma-counter. From these data, the distribution coefficient log$D$ was calculated from the following equation: log$D_{o/w}$ = log(cpm$_o$/cpm$_w$), where: cpm$_o$ = activity in the 1-octanol phase [cpm] (cpm = counts per minute), cpm$_w$ = activity in the aqueous phase [cpm]. These experiments were performed six times independently.

Determination of the stability of the ligands in human serum. The heterobivalent ligands (**22–26**) as well as the monomeric reference compounds (**27** and **28**) were radiolabeled with ^{68}Ga as described before and 125 μL of the product solution were added to 500 μL of human serum and incubated at 37 °C. At defined time-points of 5, 15, 30, 60 and 90 min, aliquots of 75 μL of the mixture were added to 75 μL of ethanol and the precipitation of serum proteins was enhanced by ice-cooling for 2 min. After centrifugation, supernatant and precipitate were measured for radioactivity and the supernatant was analyzed by analytical radio-HPLC. These experiments were performed thrice.

Cell culture. All cell lines were grown in suitable culture medium at 37 °C in a humidified CO$_2$ (5%) atmosphere. The human breast cancer cell lines T-47D, MDA-MB-231 and MCF-7 were grown in Dulbecco's Modified Eagle Medium (DMEM), supplemented with 10% (v/v) fetal calf serum (FCS) and 1% (v/v) L-Glutamine. For a high expression of the NPY(Y$_1$) receptor on T-47D cells, the medium for this cell line was further supplemented with 0.15% (w/v) β-estradiol. The BT-474 and PC-3 cell lines were grown in RPMI-1640 medium, also supplemented with 10% (v/v) fetal calf serum (FCS) and 1% (v/v) L-Glutamine.

Internalization studies. Cells (T-47D, MDA-MB-231, MCF-7, BT-474 and PC-3, 1.5 × 10^6 cells per well) were seeded into 6-well plates and incubated overnight at 37 °C in a humidified CO$_2$ (5%) atmosphere. The next day, the medium was removed and the cells were washed twice with the respective medium without supplements (ice-cold, 1 mL) and incubated with 3.7–4.0 kBq (0.37–4.0 pmol) of the respective ^{68}Ga-radiolabeled ligand [^{68}Ga]**22**–[^{68}Ga]**26**, [^{68}Ga]**27** or [^{68}Ga]**28** (in 1.5 mL medium, containing 0.5% (w/v) BSA) for defined time-points of 1, 2, 3 or 4 h at 37 °C in a humidified CO$_2$ (5%) atmosphere. A 1000-fold excess of the respective peptide (**3** or **4**) was used for blocking to determine the non-specific cell uptake. At each time point, the medium was removed and the cells were washed twice with the respective medium without supplements (ice-cold, 1 mL). Cells were treated twice with 1 mL glycine buffer (ice-cold, 50 mM glycine, 100 mM NaCl, pH 2.8) for 5 min at room temperature, followed by 2 mL NaOH solution (1 M) for 10 min at 37 °C. The supernatants were collected and the radioactivity measured in a gamma counter. The internalized and surface bound activity was expressed as percentage of measured to total added activity. Each data point was generated thrice in triplicates.

These internalization studies were performed accordingly on T-47D, MCF-7, BT-474 and PC-3 (negative control) cells with ^{125}I-PYY (PerkinElmer, molar activity 81.4 GBq/μmol, 0.3 kBq, 0.0032 pmol). The cells were incubated for 1 h with the radioligand and additional blocking experiments were performed using a 1000-fold excess of **4**, **28** and **24**.

In vivo experiments. All animal experiments were performed in compliance with the German animal protection laws and protocols of the local committee (Regierungspräsidium Karlsruhe, approval number: 35-9185.81/G-206/15). 20, six week old female immunodeficient Fox Chase SCID (CB17/Icr-Prkdc^{scid}/IcrIcoCrl) mice with an average weight of 20 g were subcutaneously implanted with 17β-estradiol pellets (0.36 mg/60 days). 4 days later, the tumors were induced by subcutaneous inoculation of 5 × 10^6 T-47D cells into the left flank of the approval number s. After induction, the tumors were allowed to grow for 8–10 weeks and reached a diameter of about 0.5 cm.

For imaging, the animals were anaesthetized with isoflurane and injected with 5.5–8.0 MBq of the respective radioligand ([^{68}Ga]**24**, [^{68}Ga]**24a** or [^{68}Ga]**24b**) into the lateral tail vein. Dynamic PET images were acquired over 90 min and CT images were obtained within further 30 min. After the end of the diagnostic scan, the animals were sacrificed, the organs were collected and measured in a gamma-counter.

The dynamic PET images were reconstructed using the Albira Suite Reconstructor (Bruker) with an iterative dynamic reconstruction with 12 iterations using an 2D-Maximum-Likelihood Expectation-Maximization (MLEM) algorithm and a cubic image voxel size of 0.5 mm after scatter and decay correction. Data were divided into time frames from 1 to 10 min (10×1 min, 10×2 min, 6×5 min and 3×10 min) for the assessment of temporal changes in regional tracer accumulation. The CT images were obtained at 45 kVp, with currents of 0.4 mA (high dose, good resolution). Acquisitions of 400 projections were taken and a 250 μm isotropic voxel size image was reconstructed via filtered back projection. The reconstructed PET data were manually fused with the CT images using PMOD 3.6.1.1. and analyzed. Volumes of interest (VOIs) were defined for the quantification of tracer accumulation in heart, liver, kidneys, tumor, and muscle. The results for each VOI were calculated as SUV (kBq/cm^3) averaged for each time frame.

4. Conclusions

We were able to show that is chemically and radiochemically feasible to synthesize radiolabeled heterobivalent peptides consisting of a GRPR- and a NPY(Y_1)R-affine peptide on symmetrically branched scaffolds, resulting in bispecific heterobivalent peptidic PET radiotracers. The compounds demonstrated high stabilities in human serum, hydrophilicities comparable to the monomeric lead peptides and high GRPR-mediated tumor cell uptakes in vitro.

The performed in vivo imaging and ex vivo biodistribution studies indicated a contribution of both peptides of the evaluated HBPL to overall in vivo tumor uptake, showing the feasibility of the general concept to develop GRPR- and NPY(Y_1)R-bispecific PET radiotracers with regard to an improved and more sensitive tumor visualization of human breast cancer.

Nevertheless, the results also show that further work is required to obtain GRPR- and NPY(Y_1)R-bispecific imaging agents being useful for clinical application due to the high kidney and liver accumulation of the agents developed so far.

Author Contributions: Conceptualization, C.D., B.W., R.S., G.F. and C.W.; Methodology, C.W.; Investigation, A.V.-S., S.L., C.D.; Writing, A.V.-S., R.S., C.W.; Supervision, C.W.

Funding: This research was funded by German Research Foundation, grant number [WA3555/1-1], the Hella-Bühler Foundation for Cancer Research and the Medical Faculty Mannheim of Heidelberg University.

Acknowledgments: O. Prante (Erlangen, Germany) is acknowledged for the valuable discussions about NPY(Y_1)R-expression on breast cancer cell lines.

References

1.   Fischer, G.; Schirrmacher, R.; Wangler, B.; Wangler, C. Radiolabeled heterobivalent peptidic ligands: An approach with high future potential for in vivo imaging and therapy of malignant diseases. *ChemMedChem* **2013**, *8*, 883–890. [CrossRef] [PubMed]

2.   Reubi, J.C.; Maecke, H.R. Approaches to multireceptor targeting: Hybrid radioligands, radioligand cocktails, and sequential radioligand applications. *J. Nucl. Med.* **2017**, *58*, 10s–16s. [CrossRef] [PubMed]

3.   Zhang, J.J.; Niu, G.; Lang, L.X.; Li, F.; Fan, X.R.; Yang, X.F.; Yao, S.B.; Yan, W.G.; Huo, L.; Chen, L.B.; et al. Clinical translation of a dual integrin alpha(v)beta(3)- and gastrin-releasing peptide receptor-targeting pet radiotracer, ga-68-bbn-rgd. *J. Nucl. Med.* **2017**, *58*, 228–234. [CrossRef] [PubMed]

4.   Reubi, J.C.; Fleischmann, A.; Waser, B.; Rehmann, R. Concomitant vascular grp-receptor and vegf-receptor expression in human tumors: Molecular basis for dual targeting of tumoral vasculature. *Peptides* **2011**, *32*, 1457–1462. [CrossRef] [PubMed]

5.   Reubi, J.C.; Gugger, M.; Waser, B. Co-expressed peptide receptors in breast cancer as a molecular basis for in vivo multireceptor tumour targeting. *Eur. J. Nucl. Med. Mol. Imaging* **2002**, *29*, 855–862. [CrossRef] [PubMed]

6.   Reubi, J.C.; Waser, B. Concomitant expression of several peptide receptors in neuroendocrine tumours: Molecular basis for in vivo multireceptor tumour targeting. *Eur. J. Nucl. Med. Mol. Imaging* **2003**, *30*, 781–793. [CrossRef] [PubMed]

7.   Gugger, M.; Reubi, J.C. Gastrin-releasing peptide receptors in non-neoplastic and neoplastic human breast. *Am. J. Pathol.* **1999**, *155*, 2067–2076. [CrossRef]

8.   Reubi, J.C.; Gugger, M.; Waser, B.; Schaer, J.C. Y-1-mediated effect of neuropeptide y in cancer: Breast carcinomas as targets. *Cancer Res.* **2001**, *61*, 4636–4641. [PubMed]

9.   Shrivastava, A.; Wang, S.H.; Raju, N.; Gierach, I.; Ding, H.M.; Tweedle, M.F. Heterobivalent dual-target probe for targeting grp and y1 receptors on tumor cells. *Bioorg. Med. Chem. Lett.* **2013**, *23*, 687–692. [CrossRef] [PubMed]

10. Ghosh, A.; Raju, N.; Tweedle, M.; Kumar, K. In vitro mouse and human serum stability of a heterobivalent dual-target probe that has strong affinity to gastrin-releasing peptide and neuropeptide y1 receptors on tumor cells. *Cancer Biother. Radio* **2017**, *32*, 24–32. [CrossRef] [PubMed]

11. Wängler, C.; Wängler, B.; Lehner, S.; Elsner, A.; Todica, A.; Bartenstein, P.; Hacker, M.; Schirrmacher, R. A universally applicable (68)ga-labeling technique for proteins. *J. Nucl. Med.* **2011**, *52*, 586–591. [CrossRef] [PubMed]

12. Liu, Z.F.; Yan, Y.J.; Chin, F.T.; Wang, F.; Chen, X.Y. Dual integrin and gastrin-releasing peptide receptor targeted tumor imaging using f-18-labeled pegylated rgd-bombesin heterodimer f-18-fb-peg(3)-glu-rgd-bbn. *J. Med. Chem.* **2009**, *52*, 425–432. [CrossRef] [PubMed]

13. Lindner, S.; Michler, C.; Wängler, B.; Bartenstein, P.; Fischer, G.; Schirrmacher, R.; Wängler, C. Pesin multimerization improves receptor avidities and in vivo tumor targeting properties to grpr-overexpressing tumors. *Bioconjug. Chem.* **2014**, *25*, 489–500. [CrossRef] [PubMed]

14. Fischer, G.; Lindner, S.; Litau, S.; Schirrmacher, R.; Wangler, B.; Wangler, C. Next step toward optimization of grp receptor avidities: Determination of the minimal distance between bbn(7–14) units in peptide homodimers. *Bioconjug. Chem.* **2015**, *26*, 1479–1483. [CrossRef] [PubMed]

15. Josan, J.S.; Handl, H.L.; Sankaranarayanan, R.; Xu, L.P.; Lynch, R.M.; Vagner, J.; Mash, E.A.; Hruby, V.J.; Gillies, R.J. Cell-specific targeting by heterobivalent ligands. *Bioconjug. Chem.* **2011**, *22*, 1270–1278. [CrossRef] [PubMed]

16. Vagner, J.; Xu, L.P.; Handl, H.L.; Josan, J.S.; Morse, D.L.; Mash, E.A.; Gillies, R.J.; Hruby, V.J. Heterobivalent ligands crosslink multiple cell-surface receptors: The human melanocortin-4 and delta-opioid receptors. *Angew. Chem. Int. Ed.* **2008**, *47*, 1685–1688. [CrossRef] [PubMed]

17. Ananias, H.J.; de Jong, I.J.; Dierckx, R.A.; van de Wiele, C.; Helfrich, W.; Elsinga, P.H. Nuclear imaging of prostate cancer with gastrin-releasing-peptide-receptor targeted radiopharmaceuticals. *Curr. Pharm. Des.* **2008**, *14*, 3033–3047. [CrossRef] [PubMed]

18. Schroeder, R.P.J.; Muller, C.; Reneman, S.; Melis, M.L.; Breeman, W.A.P.; de Blois, E.; Bangma, C.H.; Krenning, E.P.; van Weerden, W.M.; de Jong, M. A standardised study to compare prostate cancer targeting efficacy of five radiolabelled bombesin analogues. *Eur. J. Nucl. Med. Mol. Imaging* **2010**, *37*, 1386–1396. [CrossRef] [PubMed]

19. Guerin, B.; Dumulon-Perreault, V.; Tremblay, M.C.; Ait-Mohand, S.; Fournier, P.; Dubuc, C.; Authier, S.; Benard, F. [lys(dota)(4)]bvd15, a novel and potent neuropeptide y analog designed for y-1 receptor-targeted breast tumor imaging. *Bioorg. Med. Chem. Lett.* **2010**, *20*, 950–953. [CrossRef] [PubMed]

20. Chatenet, D.; Cescato, R.; Waser, B.; Erchegyi, J.; Rivier, J.E.; Reubi, J.C. Novel dimeric dota-coupled peptidic y1-receptor antagonists for targeting of neuropeptide y receptor-expressing cancers. *EJNMMI Res.* **2011**, *1*, 21. [CrossRef] [PubMed]

21. Litau, S.; Niedermoser, S.; Vogler, N.; Roscher, M.; Schirrmacher, R.; Fricker, G.; Wangler, B.; Wangler, C. Next generation of sifalin-based tate derivatives for pet imaging of sstr-positive tumors: Influence of

molecular design on in vitro sstr binding and in vivo pharmacokinetics. *Bioconjug. Chem.* **2015**, *26*, 2350–2359. [CrossRef] [PubMed]

22. Lindner, S.; Fiedler, L.; Wängler, B.; Bartenstein, P.; Schirrmacher, R.; Wängler, C. Design, synthesis and in vitro evaluation of heterobivalent peptidic radioligands targeting both grp- and vpac1-receptors concomitantly overexpressed on various malignancies—Is the concept feasible? *Eur. J. Med. Chem.* **2018**, *155*, 84–95. [CrossRef] [PubMed]

23. Glaser, M.; Morrison, M.; Solbakken, M.; Arukwe, J.; Karlsen, H.; Wiggen, U.; Champion, S.; Kindberg, G.M.; Cuthbertson, A. Radiosynthesis and biodistribution of cyclic rgd peptides conjugated with novel [18f]fluorinated aldehyde-containing prosthetic groups. *Bioconjug. Chem.* **2008**, *19*, 951–957. [CrossRef] [PubMed]

24. Garayoa, E.G.; Schweinsberg, C.; Maes, V.; Brans, L.; Blauenstein, P.; Tourwe, D.A.; Schibli, R.; Schubiger, P.A. Influence of the molecular charge on the biodistribution of bombesin analogues labeled with the [tc-99m(co)(3)]-core. *Bioconjug. Chem.* **2008**, *19*, 2409–2416. [CrossRef] [PubMed]

25. Niedermoser, S.; Chin, J.; Wängler, C.; Kostikov, A.; Bernard-Gauthier, V.; Vogler, N.; Soucy, J.P.; McEwan, A.J.; Schirrmacher, R.; Wängler, B. In vivo evaluation of f-18-sifalin-modified tate: A potential challenge for ga-68-dotatate, the clinical gold standard for somatostatin receptor imaging with pet. *J. Nucl. Med.* **2015**, *56*, 1100–1105. [CrossRef] [PubMed]

26. Sparr, C.; Purkayastha, N.; Yoshinari, T.; Seebach, D.; Maschauer, S.; Prante, O.; Hubner, H.; Gmeiner, P.; Kolesinska, B.; Cescato, R.; et al. Syntheses, receptor bindings, in vitro and in vivo stabilities and biodistributions of dota-neurotensin(8-13) derivatives containing beta-amino acid residues—A lesson about the importance of animal experiments. *Chem. Biodivers.* **2013**, *10*, 2101–2121. [CrossRef] [PubMed]

27. Storch, D.; Behe, M.; Walter, M.A.; Chen, J.H.; Powell, P.; Mikolajczak, R.; Macke, H.R. Evaluation of [tc-99m/edda/hynic0]octreotide derivatives compared with [in-111-dota(0),tyr(3), thr(8)]octreotide and [in-111-dtpa(0)]octreotide: Does tumor or pancreas uptake correlate with the rate of internalization? *J. Nucl. Med.* **2005**, *46*, 1561–1569. [PubMed]

28. Fournier, P.; Dumulon-Perreault, V.; Ait-Mohand, S.; Tremblay, S.; Benard, F.; Lecomte, R.; Guerin, B. Novel radiolabeled peptides for breast and prostate tumor pet imaging: Cu-64/and ga-68/nota-peg-[d-tyr(6),beta ala(11),thi(13),nle(14)]bbn(6-14). *Bioconjug. Chem.* **2012**, *23*, 1687–1693. [CrossRef] [PubMed]

29. Amlal, H.; Faroqui, S.; Balasubramaniam, A.; Sheriff, S. Estrogen up-regulates neuropeptide yy1 receptor expression in a human breast cancer cell line. *Cancer Res.* **2006**, *66*, 3706–3714. [CrossRef] [PubMed]

30. Rennert, R.; Weber, L.; Richter, W. Receptor Ligand Linked Cytotoxic Molecules. WO2014040752A1, 20 March 2014.

31. Liu, Z.; Yan, Y.; Liu, S.; Wang, F.; Chen, X. (18)f, (64)cu, and (68)ga labeled rgd-bombesin heterodimeric peptides for pet imaging of breast cancer. *Bioconjug. Chem.* **2009**, *20*, 1016–1025. [CrossRef] [PubMed]

32. Memminger, M.; Keller, M.; Lopuch, M.; Pop, N.; Bernhardt, G.; von Angerer, E.; Buschauer, A. The neuropeptide y y-1 receptor: A diagnostic marker? Expression in mcf-7 breast cancer cells is down-regulated by antiestrogens in vitro and in xenografts. *PLoS ONE* **2012**, *7*, e51032. [CrossRef] [PubMed]

33. Chao, C.; Ives, K.; Hellmich, H.L.; Townsend, C.M.; Hellmich, M.R. Gastrin-releasing peptide receptor in breast cancer mediates cellular migration and interleukin-8 expression. *J. Surg. Res.* **2009**, *156*, 26–31. [CrossRef] [PubMed]

34. Keller, M.; Maschauer, S.; Brennauer, A.; Tripal, P.; Koglin, N.; Dittrich, R.; Bernhardt, G.; Kuwert, T.; Wester, H.J.; Buschauer, A.; et al. Prototypic f-18-labeled argininamide-type neuropeptide y y1r antagonists as tracers for pet imaging of mammary carcinoma. *ACS Med. Chem. Lett.* **2017**, *8*, 304–309. [CrossRef] [PubMed]

35. Ait-Mohand, S.; Dumulon-Perreault, V.; Benard, F.; Guerin, B. Design optimization of a new 64cu/nota truncated npy analog with improved stability and y1 affinity, the first step toward successful breast cancer pet imaging. *J. Nucl. Med.* **2016**, *57*, S1076.

36. Ebner, A.; Wildling, L.; Kamruzzahan, A.S.M.; Rankl, C.; Wruss, J.; Hahn, C.D.; Holzl, M.; Zhu, R.; Kienberger, F.; Blaas, D.; et al. A new, simple method for linking of antibodies to atomic force microscopy tips. *Bioconjug. Chem.* **2007**, *18*, 1176–1184. [CrossRef] [PubMed]

10

Phytochemical Study of the Ecuadorian Species *Lepechinia mutica* (Benth.) Epling and High Antifungal Activity of Carnosol against *Pyricularia oryzae*

Jorge Ramírez [1,*] , Gianluca Gilardoni [1] , Erika Ramón [1], Solveig Tosi [2] , Anna Maria Picco [2], Carlo Bicchi [3] and Giovanni Vidari [4]

[1] Departamento de Química y Ciencias Exactas, Universidad Técnica Particular de Loja (UTPL), Calle M. Champagnat s/n, 1101608 Loja, Ecuador; gianluca.gilardoni@gmail.com (G.G.); erika11116@gmail.com (E.R.)

[2] Dipartimento di Scienza della Terra e dell'Ambiente, Università degli Studi di Pavia, Via S. Epifanio 14, 27100 Pavia, Italy; solveig.tosi@unipv.it (S.T.); annamaria.picco@unipv.it (A.M.P.)

[3] Dipartimento di Scienza e Tecnologia del Farmaco, Università degli Studi di Torino, Via P. Giuria 9, 10125 Torino, Italy; carlo.bicchi@unito.it

[4] Dipartimento di Chimica, Università degli Studi di Pavia, Via T. Taramelli 10, 27100 Pavia, Italy; cistre@unipv.it

* Correspondence: jyramirez@utpl.edu.ec

Abstract: The plant *Lepechinia mutica* (Benth.) Epling (family Lamiaceae) is endemic to Ecuador. In the present study, we report some major non-volatile secondary metabolites from the leaves and the chemistry of the essential oil distilled from the flowers. The main identified compounds were carnosol, viridiflorol, ursolic acid, oleanolic acid, chrysothol, and 5-hydroxy-4′,7-dimethoxy flavone. Their structures were determined by X-ray diffraction and NMR and MS techniques. The essential oil showed a chemical composition similar to that distilled from the leaves, but with some qualitative and quantitative differences regarding several minor compounds. The main constituents (>4%) were: δ-3-carene (24.23%), eudesm-7(11)-en-4-ol (13.02%), thujopsan-2-α-ol (11.90%), β-pinene (7.96%), valerianol (5.19%), and co-eluting limonene and β-phellandrene (4.47%). The volatile fraction was also submitted to enantioselective analysis on a β-cyclodextrin column, obtaining the separation and identification of the enantiomers for α-thujene, β-pinene, sabinene, α-phellandrene, limonene and β-phellandrene. Furthermore, the anti-fungal activity of non-volatile secondary metabolites was tested in vitro, with carnosol resulting in being very active against the "blast disease" caused by the fungus *Pyricularia oryzae*.

Keywords: *Lepechinia mutica*; Lamiaceae; carnosol; secondary metabolites; essential oil; Ecuador; *Pyricularia oryzae*

1. Introduction

The family Lamiaceae comprises approximately 224 genera and more than 5600 species distributed all over the world. One of these genera is *Lepechinia* Willd., consisting of 43 species growing from Northern California, in Western USA, to Central Argentina, in South America [1–4]. The flora of Ecuador contains 21 genera of Lamiaceae, for a total number of 135 species, 33 of which are endemic. In particular, the genus *Lepechinia* Willd. includes nine species, among which four are endemic to Ecuador [2,5]. *Lepechinia* species are perennial herbs to shrubs, rarely gynodioecious or dioecious, often aromatic. Leaves are entire to toothed, often rugose; inflorescences are terminal and often axillary [2,5]. Several *Lepechinia* spp. are valued in the horticultural trade, and indigenous peoples of North and South America commonly use *Lepechinia* plants for medicinal and antiseptic purposes. Plants of this genus are used in folk medicine for the treatment of uterine tumors, stomach ailments, diabetes mellitus control and diarrhea treatment. In particular, the leaves of *L. mutica* are used to treat headache and nervous affections [1,3,6,7], whereas the *L. caulescens* extract has been patented as a cosmetic constituent [8].

Fungal infections or mycoses are common public health problems, ranging from superficial to deep infections. Superficial mycoses sometimes reach high endemic levels, especially in tropical areas where dermatophyte fungi are usually the principal infection factor [9,10]. Indeed, it is often argued that dermatophyte infections are the most common human infection in the world (not just the most common fungal infection). On the other hand, rice blast disease, caused by *Pyricularia oryzae* Cavara (anamorph of *Magnaporthe oryzae* B. Couch sp. nov.) [11], is a severe hemibiotrophic pathogen of rice (*Oryza sativa* L.). This pathogen may destroy wide extensions of rice cultures, reaching up to 50−70% of a whole regional production. It has been calculated that the amount of rice annually destroyed by *P. oryzae* could feed more than 60 million people [12,13].

This fungus can cause two symptoms: leaf blast and neck blast [14]. The leaf blast is characterized by white to gray green lesions or spots with darker borders appearing on the leaves. The old lesions are elliptical or spindle-shaped and whitish to gray with necrotic border. The neck blast is characterized by dark brown lesions on the base of the panicle neck, so that it cannot support the panicle. *P. oryzae* can infect the rice plant at various growth stages [15]. Our research group is interested in the discovery of new antidermatophyte substances from natural resources [16] and new agents against plant pathogenic fungi. The aim of this research was the isolation and identification of antifungal compounds from *L. mutica*. In order to accomplish this task, the dermatophyte *Microsporum canis* and the phytopatogen *P. oryzae* were selected as targets for the in vitro antifungal assay of our samples. Up to now, the antifungal activity of this plant has been described only for the essential oil distilled from leaves [17,18]. To the best of the authors' knowledge, the phytochemistry and the biological activity of *L. mutica* non-volatile fraction have not been described so far.

2. Results

2.1. Non-Volatile Fraction

Six known compounds were identified after the fractionation of the ethyl acetate (EtOAc) extract, obtained from leaves of *L. mutica*, namely the phenolic diterpene, carnosol (**1**), the sesquiterpene alcohol viridiflorol (**2**), the pentacyclic triterpene acids, ursolic acid (**3**) and oleanolic acid (**4**), the flavonoid 5-hydroxy-4',7-dimethoxy flavone (**5**), and the sesquiterpene alcohol chrysothol (**6**) (Figure 1). The presence of compounds **1–6** in *L. mutica* is reported here for the first time.

The structure of carnosol (**1**) was established by single crystal X-ray diffraction analysis. The crystallographic data were the same as those reported in the literature [19]: orthorhombic crystal; P21212; a = 15.762 (1), b = 13.757 (1), c = 7.7747 (7) Å, Z = 4, V = 1688.2 Å3, and R = 0.031. The structure elucidation was also supported by the comparison of the ^{1}H NMR, ^{13}C NMR, and ESI-MS data with those in the literature [20,21]. The ^{13}C NMR and DEPT spectra indicated the presence of four methyls, four methylenes, two methines, one oxymethine, six aromatic carbons, two quaternary carbons and one ester carbon [22,23]. The aromatic ring must be penta-substituted and one substituent was an isopropyl group, according to the ^{1}H NMR spectrum [20].

The aromadendrene sesquiterpene alcohol viridiflorol (**2**) was identified by comparison of the ^{1}H NMR, ^{13}C NMR, and ESI-MS data with those reported in the literature [24–27].

The pentacyclic triterpenoid acids ursolic acid (**3**) and the isomeric oleanolic acid (**4**) are widely occurring in plants in both free and glycosidic forms (saponins) [28]. They were identified by comparison of the ^{1}H NMR, ^{13}C NMR, and ESI-MS data with the literature [29–32].

5-Hydroxy-4′,7-dimethoxy flavone (**5**) was identified by comparison of the ^{1}H NMR, ^{13}C NMR, and ESI-MS data with those reported in the literature [33–35]. The ^{1}H NMR spectrum clearly indicated that compound **5** was a flavone containing a free phenolic OH group and two methoxy groups. The one-proton singlet at δ 13.60 in the ^{1}H NMR spectrum, exchangeable with D_2O and assignable to a phenolic proton bridged to the carbonyl group, suggested a free phenolic OH group in position C-5 [35].

The oxygenated sesquiterpenoid chrysothol (**6**) was identified by comparison of the ^{1}H NMR, ^{13}C NMR, and ESI-MS data with those in the literature [36–38]. The ^{1}H and ^{13}C NMR spectra in $CDCl_3$ showed signals of a guaiane sesquiterpenoid skeleton. The ^{1}H NMR spectrum displayed a broad doublet at δ 3.94 (1H, *J* = 4.0 Hz, H-6), a multiplet at δ 2.26 for two protons (H-1 and H-5), and a multiplet at δ 2.07 (1H, H-3a). Additionally, signals assignable to the two secondary methyl groups of an isopropyl unit, at δ 0.87 (6H, *J* = 7.0 Hz, H-12 and H-13), and to two tertiary methyls at δ 1.12 and 1.34 (H-14 and H-15), respectively [34,39], were found. The ^{13}C NMR and DEPT spectra data revealed 15 carbon signals assignable to four methyls, four methylenes, five methines and two quaternary carbons. Three oxygenated carbons were observed at δ 76.1 (d), 74.7 (s), and 74.6 (s) and the other 12 signals were for aliphatic carbons. All spectra data are available as supplementary material.

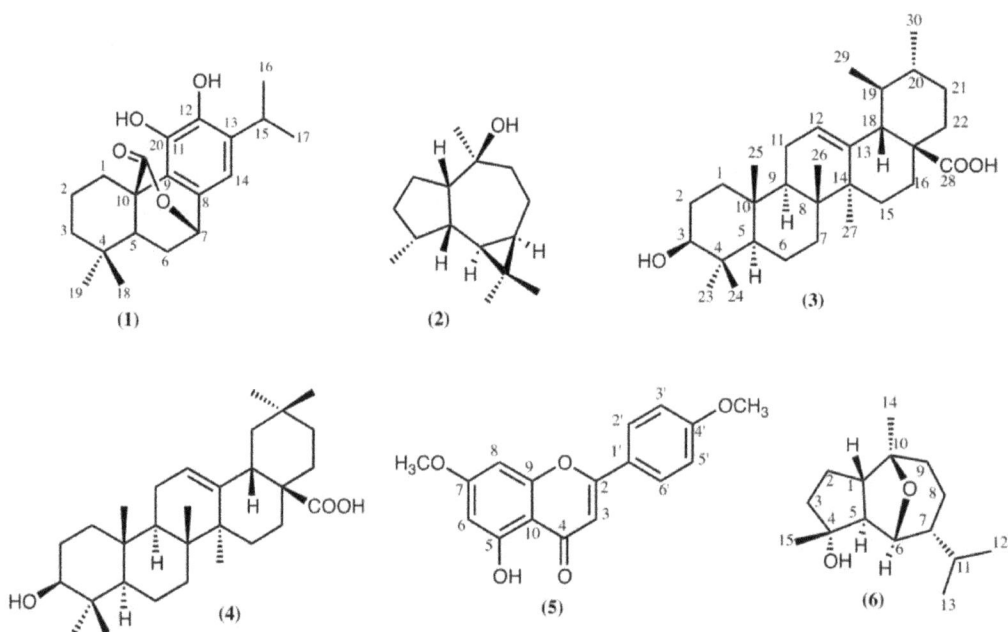

Figure 1. Compounds isolated from the leaves of *Lepechinia mutica*.

2.2. Chemical Analysis of the Volatile Fraction from Flowers

The flowers of *L. mutica* provided an essential oil in a yield of 0.317 ± 0.096% (*w/w*), referred to fresh plant material. The relative density was d^{20} = 0.8526 ± 0.0127, and the refractive index n^{20} = 1.4906 ± 0.0015. The specific rotation was $[\alpha]_D^{20}$ = −6.0 (c 0.08 in CH_2Cl_2). The qualitative and percent compositions are reported in Table 1. About 93.9% of the volatile components have been identified and most of them quantified (see Sections 4.5 and 4.6, respectively). All constituents with an abundance <0.1% were considered as trace. The significant difference between calculated and reference linear retention indices (LRIs) [40] is within the experimental error. It can be due to different analysis conditions, carried out with a more recent instrumentation.

Table 1. Chemical composition of the essential oils from flowers and leaves of *Lepechinia mutica* on a DB-5 capillary column.

Calculated LRI [a]	Reference LRI [b]	Compounds	Flowers		Leaves [17]	
			%	σ	%	σ
921	926	Tricyclene	-	-	Trace	-
924	924	Thujene <α->	Trace	-	Trace	-
931	932	Pinene <α->	2.68	0.95	1.23	0.89
946	949	Camphene	-	-	0.75	0.80
948	945	Fenchene <α->	Trace	-	-	-
971	969	Sabinene	Trace	-	0.24	0.15
974	983	Oct-3-en-1-ol	-	-	Trace	-
976	974	Pinene <β->	7.96	0.99	3.78	1.76
979	989	Hepten-2-ol <6-methyl-5->	0.32	0.12	-	-
984	979	Octanone <3->	0.16	0.17	-	-
988	988	Myrcene	1.51	0.47	0.52	0.28
998	-	Undetermined (MW 136)	0.13	0.14	-	-
1003	1003	Mentha-1(7),8-diene <p->	Trace	-	0.16	0.13
1006	1002	Phellandrene <α->	0.34	0.13	3.80	1.70
1008	1008	Carene <δ-3->	24.23	6,00	8.69	4.24
1016	1014	Terpinene <α->	Trace	-	0.11	0.07
1019	1020	Cymene <p->	1.97	0.50	0.10	0.06
1023	1022	Cymene <o->	2.04	0.52	-	-
1025	1023	Sylvestrene	-	-	0.29	0.18
1029	1024	Limonene	4.47	0.71	3.79	2.18
1029	1030	Phellandrene <β->				
1043	-	Undetermined (MW 98)	0.23	0.46	-	-
1045	1044	Ocimene <(E)-β->	0.35	0.42	-	-
1052	1054	Terpinene <γ->	Trace	-	0.23	0.12
1057	-	Undetermined (MW 136)	0.52	0.20	-	-
1065	1071	cis-Sabinene hydrate	-	-	Trace	-
1070	-	Undetermined (MW 136)	0.20	0.40	-	-
1080	1085	Mentha-2,4(8)-diene <p->	0.86	0.25	0.35	0.18
1084	1086	Terpinolene	1.78	0.40	0.60	0.33
1084	1086	trans-Linalool oxide	-	-	Trace	-
1088	1082	Cymenene <m->	1.97	0.55	-	-
1095	1102	Linalool	-	-	0.20	0.09
1108	-	Undetermined (MW 136)	3.26	0.71	-	-
1110	1109	Oct-1-en-3-yl acetate	-	-	1.37	0.60
1120	-	Undetermined (MW 136)	0.27	0.12	-	-
1124	1117	Sabina ketone <dehydro->	Trace	-	-	-
1141	1145	Camphor	-	-	Trace	-
1142	-	Undetermined (MW 136)	0.10	0.19	-	-
1165	1172	Borneol	-	-	0.25	0.05
1174	1180	4-Terpineol	-	-	0.14	0.02
1194	1186	Terpineol <α->	0.16	0.04	0.11	0.02
1283	1281	Isobornyl acetato	-	-	2.20	1.04
1284	1284	Bornyl acetate	Trace	-	-	-
1335	1328	Elemene <δ->	-	-	Trace	-
1345	1348	Cubebene <α->	0.22	0.07	0.57	0.08
1346	1342	Terpinyl acetate <α->				
1373	1373	Ylangene <α->	0.26	0.09	0.15	0.05
1374	1362	Isoledene	0.20	0.05		
1374	1367	Copaene <α->	-	-	1.46	0.23
1381	1387	Bourbonene <β->	0.20	0.05	0.47	0.25
1385	1382	Modheph-2-ene	0.21	0.05	-	-
1392	1387	Cubebene <β->	0.20	0.05	0.15	0.04
1395	1398	Cyperene	0.20	0.05	-	-

Table 1. *Cont.*

Calculated LRI [a]	Reference LRI [b]	Compounds	Flowers		Leaves [17]	
			%	σ	%	σ
1404	1400	Sibirene	0.28	0.09	-	-
1407	1409	Gurjunene <α->	0.20	0.05	1.94	0.37
1407	1418	Longifolene	-	-	0.15	0.07
1417	1411	Funebrene <2-*epi*-β->	0.57	0.19	Trace	-
1417	1412	(*E*)-Caryophyllene	-	-	4.55	2.16
1424	1431	Copaene <β->	0.20	0.05	0.50	0.08
1427	1421	Duprezianene <β->	0.21	0.06	-	-
1431	1431	Gurjunene <β->	0.21	0.05	1.47	0.78
1435	1437	Guaiene <α->	0.25	0.07	-	-
1439	1449	Aromadendrene	-	-	0.56	0.10
1443	1442	Guaiadiene <6,9->	0.20	0.05	-	-
1446	1448	Muurola-3,5-diene <*cis*->	0.21	0.06	0.45	0.36
1453	1452	Humulene <α->	0.29	0.08	1.20	0.47
1457	1452	Clovene <α-*neo*->	0.22	0.06	-	-
1459	1464	Caryophyllene <9-*epi*-(*E*)->	0.21	0.06	-	-
1461	1452	*cis*-Cadina-1(6),4-diene	-	-	0.99	1.36
1469	1465	Muurola-4(14),5-diene <*cis*->	0.22	0.06	-	-
1471	1463	Dauca-5,8-diene	-	-	0.38	0.09
1472	1469	Acoradiene <β->	0.23	0.07	-	-
1475	1466	*trans*-Cadina-1(6),4-diene	-	-	0.99	0.12
1478	1479	Amorpha-4,7(11)-diene	0.21	0.06	0.15	0.07
1482	1478	Muurolene <γ->	0.21	0.06	0.92	0.23
1486	1489	Selinene <β->	0.23	0.06	-	-
1488	1485	Himachala-1,4-diene <11-αH->	0.23	0.06	-	-
1492	1481	*cis*-b-Guaiene	-	-	0.71	0.11
1493	1486	Bicyclogermacrene				
1493	1489	*epi*-Cubebol	-	-	4.62	0.58
1493	1489	Zingiberene <α->				
1493	1492	Selinene <δ->	0.24	0.07	0.81	0.08
1496	1493	Muurola-4(14),5-diene <*trans*->	0.25	0.07	-	-
1500	1505	Cuprenene <α->	0.20	0.05	-	-
1503	1505	Farnesene <(*E,E*)-α->	0.20	0.05	0.83	0.25
1510	1500	Muurolene <α->	0.32	0.11	0.91	0.17
1513	1505	Cadinene <γ->	-	-	2.86	0.37
1514	1508	Cubebol	-	-	0.36	0.21
1516	1511	Amorphene <δ->	0.44	0.19	-	-
1521	1512	*trans*-Calamenene	-	-	0.15	0.04
1522	1511	Cadinene <δ->	-	-	6.96	0.99
1529	1528	Zonarene	0.21	0.06	-	-
1533	1523	*trans*-Cadina-1,4-diene	-	-	0.37	0.10
1534	1537	Cadinene <α->	0.21	0.06	0.39	0.12
1538	1545	Selina-3,7(11)-diene	0.20	0.05	0.14	0.04
1548	-	Undetermined (MW 204)	0.21	0.07	-	-
1555	-	Undetermined (MW 204)	0.21	0.06	-	-
1559	1556	Dauca-4(11),7-diene <*trans*->	0.20	0.05	-	-
1567	1559	Germacrene B	0.21	0.05	0.18	0.06
1574	1567	Germacrene D-4-ol	-	-	1.46	0.40
1574	-	Undetermined (MW 204)	0.25	0.04	-	-
1579	-	Undetermined (MW 204)	0.21	0.05	-	-
1582	1569	Caryophyllene oxide	-	-	0.29	0.24
1583	-	Undetermined (MW 204)	0.21	0.05	-	-
1590	1584	Globulol	-	-	5.91	2.61
1591	1586	Thujopsan-2-α-ol	11.9	1.76	-	-
1592	1592	Viridiflorol	-	-	1.29	0.45

Table 1. *Cont.*

Calculated LRI [a]	Reference LRI [b]	Compounds	Flowers		Leaves [17]	
			%	σ	%	σ
1601	1600	Guaiol	0.15	0.12	-	-
1612	-	Undetermined (MW 204)	0.22	0.06	-	-
1618	1617	1,10-di-*epi*-Cubenol	-	-	0.27	0.11
1618	1623	Junenol	-	-	1.39	0.42
1629	1622	Eudesmol <10-*epi*-γ->	0.83	0.10	0.54	0.15
1634	1630	Eudesmol <γ->	2.02	1.48	-	-
1636	1639	Acorenol <β->	-	-	0.47	0.81
1639	1632	Acorenol <α->	0.60	1.20	Trace	-
1642	1635	Cadin-4-en-7-ol <*cis*->	0.88	1.75	-	-
1649	1644	Eudesmol <β->				
1652	1644	Eudesmol <α->	-	-	4.47	1.93
1652	1646	Cadinol <α->				
1652	1656	Valerianol	5.19	0.66	-	-
1668	1658	Selin-11-en-4-α-ol	Trace	-	-	-
1688	1681	Shyobunol	-	-	10.80	5.91
1691	1700	Eudesm-7(11)-en-4-ol	13.02	4.25	-	-
		Aliphatic monoterpene hydrocarbons	48.89	-	24.54	-
		Aromatic monoterpene hydrocarbons	5.98	-	0.10	-
		Monoterpene alcohols	0.48	-	0.70	-
		Monoterpene ketones	0.16	-	Traces	-
		Aliphatic esters	-	-	3.57	-
		Aliphatic sesquiterpene hydrocarbons	9.86	-	35.98	-
		Sesquiterpene alcohols	34.59	-	27.25	-
		TOTAL	99.96	-	92.14	-

[a] According to van den Dool and Kratz [41]. [b] According to Adams [40].

2.3. Enantiomeric Analysis of the Volatile Fraction from the Flowers

The results of the GC-MS analysis on a β-cyclodextrin enantioselective column are reported in Table 2, including both the enantiomeric distribution and the enantiomeric excess (*ee*) for each enantiomeric couple. The chromatogram of the enantioselective analysis is shown in Figure 2; only the enantiomeric couples that underwent separation have been reported. It is worthy of note that most of the detected enantiomers were baseline separated.

Table 2. Enantiomeric analysis of the essential oil from flowers of *Lepechinia mutica* on a 30% 2,3-diethyl-6-*tert*-butyldimethylsilyl-β-CDX column.

Enantiomers	Retention Time (min)	LRI	Enantiomeric Distribution (%)	*ee* (%)
(+)-α-thujene	9.05	924	44.19	11.62
(−)-α-thujene	9.26	928	55.81	
(+)-β-pinene	11.12	962	1.48	97.04
(−)-β-pinene	11.51	969	98.52	
(+)-sabinene	12.55	988	46.37	7.26
(−)-sabinene	13.21	1000	53.63	
(R)-α-phellandrene	14.64	1024	7.17	85.66
(S)-α-phellandrene	14.79	1027	92.83	
(S)-limonene	16.73	1059	34.19	31.62
(R)-limonene	16.87	1062	65.81	
(−)-β-phellandrene	16.63	1058	4.34	91.32
(+)-β-phellandrene	17.14	1066	95.66	

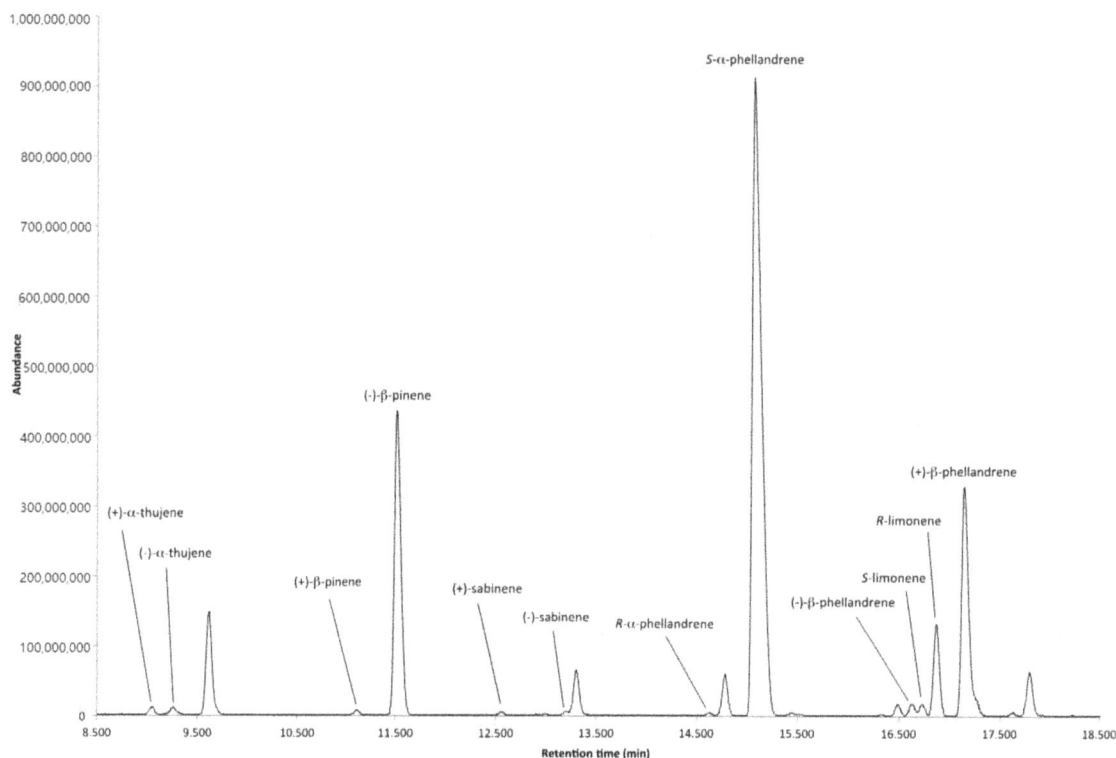

Figure 2. Chromatogram of enantiomers separated by enantioselective GC.

2.4. Biological Activity

Antifungal activities were determined for carnosol (**1**) and the results are shown in Table 3. Carnosol (**1**) showed a potent antifungal activity against the dermatophyte *Mircrosporum canis* (CBS 136538) and against *Pyricularia oryzae* (LM 120). The minimum inhibitory concentration (MIC) and minimum fungicidal concentration (MFC) values (mg/mL) determined for carnosol against *P. oryzae* are very close to those of the reference well-known pesticide flutriafol (0.01 mg/mL). Although this result does not validate a property of the plant extract, it constitutes a new biological property described for compound **1**. These results clearly show that the activity of carnosol (**1**) is similar to that of flutriafol on *Pyricularia oryzae* but not competitive to that of intraconazol on *Mircrosporum canis*. More experiments are under way in this respect.

Table 3. MIC and MFC of carnosol against *M. canis* and *P. oryzae*.

Compound	*Microsporum canis* (CBS 136538)		*Pyricularia oryzae* (LM120)	
	MIC (mg/mL)	MFC (mg/mL)	MIC (mg/mL)	MFC (mg/mL)
Carnosol (1)	0.0250 < MIC ≤ 0.0500	MFC > 0.1000	0.0125 < MIC ≤ 0.0250	0.0500 < MFC ≤ 0.1000
Flutriafol	-	-	0.0100	0.0100
Intraconazol	0.0005	-	-	-

3. Discussion

3.1. Non-Volatile Fraction

Over 71 years ago, a bitter principle was isolated from sage, *Salvia carnosa* Dougl. The natural substance, having the formula $C_{20}H_{26}O_4$, was named carnosol and noted to be a diphenolic ester, containing a hydrophenanthrene moiety, presumably identical to a compound also obtained from *S. officinalis* L. Indeed, the correct structure was eventually deduced from chemical studies mainly performed on a sample isolated from *Rosmarinus officinalis*. It was also showed that carnosol was identical with pikrosalvin (picrosalvin) isolated from *S. officinalis* L. [23,39]. Other sources of carnosol are *S. triloba* L., *Sphacele eremophila* Boiss., *S. pachyphyla*, *S. clevelandii*, and *Lepechinia hastate* [39,42]. Carnosol was also isolated, as the main diterpene constituent, from the aerial parts of *Sphacele chamaedryoides*, and it was determined to be more cytotoxic against gastric tumour cells AGS than normal fibroblasts [43]. Moreover, it showed a significant activity against the gram (+) bacteria *Staphylococcus aureus*, *Bacillus subtilis*, *Escherichia coli*, and *Candida albicans* [44].

Carnosol showed strong inhibitory effect on the EBV-EA induction and exhibited a remarkable effect on mouse skin tumor promotion in an in vivo two-stage carcinogenesis model. Carnosol has also been shown to be partly responsible for the antioxidant and anti-tumorogenesis properties of rosemary (*Rosmarinus officinalis* L.). Recently, carnosol has been proved to be efficacious in the chemoprevention and/or chemotherapy of hormone-responsive cancers [45–47].

The cytotoxicity activity of carnosol (**1**) has been determined in vitro against A-549 (human lung carcinoma), HeLa (human carcinoma of the cervix), HEp-2 (human carcinoma of the larynx), and MCF-7 (human breast adenocarcinoma) cell lines, and against a *Vero* (African green monkey kidney) cell line [46].

Viridiflorol (**2**) was previously isolated, as the major component, from the essential oils obtained from *Cistus ladaniferus* L. [27], "niaouli" (*Melaleuca viridiflora*, *M. quinquenervia*) [24,48], and the liverwort *Bazzania trilobata* L. [49]. It has also been synthesized via (-)-alloaromadendrene [26]. Viridiflorol (**2**) showed antifungal activity against *C. cucumerinum* and *P. oryzae* [26,49].

Oleanolic acid (**4**) was isolated from more than 120 plant species, as it results from a partial survey about its occurrence in plants used in folk medicine, and its biological activity. As a typical example, both oleanolic acid (**4**) and ursolic acid (**3**) are present in *Sambucus chinesis* Lindl. This plant is used in folk medicine to treat inflammatory disorders and acute hepatitis. Compounds **3** and **4** were identified as the metabolite responsible for this activity [29]. Ursolic acid is chemically and pharmacologically similar to oleanolic acid. The multiple uses of oleanolic or ursolic acid containing plants in folk medicines are due to anti-inflammatory, hepatoprotective, analgesic, cardiotonic, sedative and tonic effects, among others [29].

Ursolic acid (**3**) was identified as an active hepatoprotective component in the preparation of *Sambucus chinesis* Lindl., *Solanum incanum* L., *Tripterospermum taiwanense*, and *Eucalyptus hybrid*. In addition to its protective effects against CCl_4-induced liver injury, ursolic acid (**3**) also shows protective properties against D-galactosamine-induced liver injury in rats, and preventive effects against acetaminophen-induced cholestasis [28].

Ursolic acid (**3**) and oleanolic acid (**4**) was also isolated from *Lepechinia caulescens*. The vascular activity of ursolic acid (**3**) depended on the presence of a functional endothelium and possible NO release [29].

Flavonoid **5** was previously isolated from the aerial parts of *Sphacele chamaedryoides* [41], *Ballota inaequidens* [34], *Salvia texana* [35], *Artemisia pontica* [50], and *Combretum erythohyllum* [51]. It was also identified and quantified in *Kaempferia parviflora* and *Cistus libanotis* [52,53]. Compound **5** showed good activity against *Vibrio cholerae* and *Enterococcus faecalis*, with MIC values in the range of 25–50 μg/mL. Furthermore, it is also potentially toxic to human cells [51], and possesses high anti-allergenic activity against antigen-induced β-hexosaminidase release as a marker of degranulation in RBL-2H3 cells, with an IC_{50} of 26 μM [52].

Chrysothol (**6**) was isolated before from *Chrysothamnus viscidiflorus* (Asteraeceae) and *Fagonia boveana* [38], and showed important anti-cancer activity against human breast cancer cells [36].

3.2. Volatile Fraction

The essential oil distilled from flowers of *L. mutica* is composed of monoterpenoid and sesquiterpenoid compounds (55.6% and 44.4% respectively). The main constituents (>4%) were: δ-3-carene (24.2%), eudesm-7(11)-en-4-ol (13.0%), thujopsan-2-α-ol (11.9%), β-pinene (8.0%), valerianol

(5.2%), and co-eluting monoterpenoids limonene and β-phellandrene (4.5%). Since major constituents of the essential oil distilled from flowers are the same as the one distilled from leaves, the two chromatograms result in being qualitatively quite similar. However, quantitative analysis demonstrates that the overall composition of the two volatile fractions is actually different. In Table 1, the quantitative chemical composition of the two essential oils, expressed as percent abundance, is reported. Aliphatic monoterpens and sesquiterpens are the families showing the greatest difference, passing respectively from 24.5% to 48.9% in flowers and from 9.9% to 36.0% in leaves.

4. Materials and Methods

4.1. Instruments and Disposables

Solvents were reagent grade or HPLC grade and were purchased from Sigma-Aldrich (St. Louis, MO, USA). Low pressure preparative column chromatography was carried out on Merck LiChroprep RP-18 (Darmstadt, Germany) (25–40 μm) or Merck silica gel (230–400 mesh), in reversed and normal phase column chromatography, respectively. Medium pressure flash-chromatography was carried out on Biotage® Isolera™ Spektra equipment (Biotage AB, Uppsala, Sweden), equipped with a UV detector (205 and 254 nm) and a C-18 Cartridge (KP-18-HS), 100 g, operating with an eluent flow of 30 mL/min. TLC was performed over Merck F_{254} glass plates (RP-18) or aluminum supported silica sheets (0.25 mm), purchased from Sigma-Aldrich. Spots were detected under UV light (254 and 366 nm) and, additionally, stained by exposure to a 0.5% solution of vanillin in H_2SO_4-EtOH (4:1), followed by heating at 100 °C. The SPE columns, used for chlorophyll removal, were Discovery DSC-18 (Sigma-Aldrich) 60 mL tubes, containing 10 g of C-18 reversed phase. Optical rotations were measured on a Perkin-Elmer 241 polarimeter (Waltham, MA, USA) (concentration expressed in g/mL). Melting points were measured with a Thermo Scientific Fisher–Johns hot-plate instrument. Refractive indices were measured with an Abbe refractometer (Boeco Germany, Hamburg, Germany). LC-MS spectra were obtained with a Thermo Scientific LTQ XL Linear ION Trap mass spectrometer, equipped with an ESI source. X-ray crystallographic analysis was performed at the "Centro Grandi Strumenti (CGS)" of the University of Pavia. NMR spectra were recorded on an NMR Varian 400 MHz spectrometer or, alternatively, on Bruker 300 MHz and 200 MHz instruments. Chemical shifts (δ are given in ppm and coupling constants (J) in Hz. GC-MS and GC-FID analyses were performed with an Agilent Technologies 6890N GC, coupled to a mass spectrometry detector model 5973 *inert*, and to a flame ionization detector. In qualitative and quantitative GC analyses, a J&W DB-5 capillary column (30 m × 0.25 mm × 0.15 μm), purchased from Agilent Technologies, was used. GC enantioselective analysis was performed with a cyclodextrin-based capillary column (30% 2,3-diethyl-6-*tert*-butyldimethylsilyl-β-CDX, 25 m × 0.25 mm × 0.25 μm), purchased from Mega (Legnano, Italy).

4.2. Plant Material

The collection of *L. mutica*, authorized by the Ministry of Environment of Ecuador (MAE), with authorization no. 001-IC-FLO-DBAP-VS-DRLZCH-MA, was performed in the canton Quilanga, Loja province, Ecuador, in September 2009. The botanical specimen was identified by Dr. Bolivar Merino at the herbarium of the "Universidad Nacional de Loja". A voucher specimen, with number PPN-la-005, was deposited at the herbarium of the "Universidad Técnica Particular de Loja". After collection, leaves and flowers were separated and submitted to different processes. After drying in the dark at 35 °C, the leaves were submitted to solvent extraction. Fresh leaves and flowers were both steam distilled to obtain the essential oils. A quite complete study of the essential oil from leaves has recently been published [17].

4.3. Extraction and Purification of Non-Volatile Metabolites

The extract was obtained from 250 g of dried leaves of L. mutica, using EtOAc as the extraction solvent. The process was carried out statically, at room temperature, for three consecutive times, one hour each. After solvent evaporation, 24.1 g of the EtOAc extract were obtained (yield: 9.6%). The extract underwent subsequent removal of chlorophylls by filtration through a C-18 SPE column; elution was done with MeOH-H_2O, 9:1 v/v, followed by 100% acetone. After chlorophyll removal and solvent evaporation chlorophyll, a free EtOAc extract (13.8 g) was obtained. In addition, 1 g of this extract was fractionated by medium-pressure flash chromatography on a C-18 cartridge, containing 100 g of stationary phase, with an elution gradient from methanol/water (2:1) to 100% methanol. The eluent flow was set at 30 mL/min, giving 19 main fractions. Fraction #11 (511.5 mg) was subjected to normal phase (silica gel) column chromatography. Elution with a mixture of hexane/EtOAc (97:3) gave 38.5 mg of carnosol (1). Fraction #12 and fraction #13 (58.6 mg) were collected together and submitted to silica gel column chromatography. From the elution with a mixture of hexane/EtOAc (95:5), 10.0 mg of viridiflorol (2) was obtained. Fraction #18 (79.9 mg) was submitted to C-18 reversed phase column chromatography. Elution with a mixture of MeOH/H_2O (95:5) afforded 14.2 mg of ursolic acid (3), and 23.5 mg of oleanolic acid (4). A second amount of the EtOAc chlorophyll-free extract (11 g) was fractionated by preparative column chromatography on silica gel in order to get larger amounts of metabolites from L. mutica. Elution with an increasing polarity gradient of a hexane/EtOAc mixture afforded 16 main fractions. Fraction #11 (4.9 g) was subjected to silica gel column chromatography. Elution with an increasing polarity gradient of a hexane/EtOAc mixture gave 11.9 mg of 5-hydroxy-4',7-dimethoxy flavone (5), and 127.7 mg of carnosol (1). Collected fractions #13 and #14 (2.4 g) were submitted to silica gel column chromatography. Elution with an increasing polarity gradient of a hexane/EtOAc mixture gave 11 main fractions (F38-F49). Fraction #44 (158.3 mg) was also submitted to silica gel column chromatography. Elution with an increasing polarity gradient of a dichloromethane/EtOAc mixture afforded 77.7 mg of isolated chrysothol (6).

4.4. Distillation of the Volatile Fraction

Fresh flowers of L. mutica (5 kg) were divided into four equal amounts and steam was distilled in four stainless steel Clevenger-type apparatus for 4 h. After distillation, each organic layer was separated from the aqueous phase, dried over anhydrous sodium sulfate and weighted. For each distilled fraction, yield, relative density, refractive index and specific rotation were measured. The flowers were handled and distilled in the same way described for leaves [17].

4.5. Qualitative Analysis of the Essential Oil

The qualitative analysis of the essential oil was performed by GC-MS, injecting 1 μL of each distilled fraction, 1% (v/v) diluted in cyclohexane. The injector was kept at 220 °C, operating in split mode with a split ratio of 40:1. The carrier gas (He) was set at a constant flow of 1 mL/min. The analysis was performed in thermal gradient conditions, with the following temperature program: 60 °C for 5 min, increased to 110 °C at a rate of 5 °C/min, then to 148 °C at a rate of 2 °C/min. and to 250 °C at a rate of 20 °C/min, and then held at 250 °C for 2.4 min. The MS was operated in a SCAN mode, with a scan rate of 2 scan/s within a mass range of 40–350 m/z at 70 eV. For each chromatographic peak, the corresponding linear retention index (LRI) was calculated, according to Van den Dool and Kratz [41], with reference to a mixture of a homologous series of n-alkanes, from nonane to heptadecane. The constituents of the essential oil were identified, by comparing their LRIs and EI-MS spectra with data present in literature [40]. The identification was considered as acceptable in a range of ±13 units of LRI values, according to the injection of some standard compounds belonging to the different terpenic families.

4.6. Quantitative Analysis of the Essential Oil

The quantitative analysis of the essential oil was performed by GC-FID, with the same instrumental configuration and method of the qualitative analysis. The constituents were quantified by external calibration, using *n*-nonane as the internal standard. According to the literature [54], the response factor in FID detection is almost constant and close to value 1 within isomeric compounds, allowing the use of a single standard to quantify a family of analytes, all characterized by the same molecular formula. The same considerations are reported in reference [55]. Therefore, an isomer was used to quantify isomeric metabolites; if an isomer was not available, a structurally closely related terpene was selected. Hence, the following terpenoids (purity > 98%) were used as calibration standards: limonene for aliphatic monoterpene hydrocarbons (R^2 = 0.9962), *p*-cymene for aromatic monoterpene hydrocarbons (R^2 = 0.9986), linalool for monoterpene alcohols (R^2 = 0.9956), carvone for monoterpene ketones (R^2 = 0.9958), cedrene for sesquiterpene hydrocarbons (R^2 = 0.9998), and nerolidol for sesquiterpene alcohols (R^2 = 0.9997). All calibration curves were built on six points. Quantitative results were reported as the main values and standard deviations of three replicates for each distillation.

4.7. Enantioselective Analysis of the Essential Oil

The enantioselective analysis was performed by GC-MS, under the same conditions reported above except for the oven temperature that was set according to this program: initial temperature hold at 60 °C for 2 min, then increased to 220 °C at a rate of 2 °C/min, and then held at 220 °C for 2 min. The elution order of the separated enantiomers was determined by injection of enantiomerically pure standards, available in the laboratory of one of the authors (C.B.). LRIs were calculated as in qualitative analysis, according to Van den Dool and Kratz (see Section 4.5).

4.8. Antifungal Activity

Antifungal activities were expressed as the minimum inhibitory concentration (MIC) and minimum fungicidal concentration (MFC). MIC and MFC values were measured using a stereoscope and were determined for two strains of *Microsporum canis* (CBS 136538, from CBS-KNAW culture collection, NL), a human dermatophyte fungus, and a *Pyricularia oryzae* (LM120 strain, isolated by S.T. and A.M.P. from leaf lesions of Italian rice varieties), a plant pathogenic fungus. The compounds were dissolved in dimethylsulfoxide (DMSO), 1% *v*/*v*, in the liquid medium culture Sabouraud. The tested concentrations (expressed as mg/mL) were: 0.1000, 0.0500, 0.0250, 0.0125, and 0.0060.

The commercial well-known pesticide flutriafol, containing the antifungal compound (*R,S*)-2,4-difluoro(1H-1,2,4-triazol-1-ylmethyl)benzhydryl alcohol, was used as the positive control against *P. oryzae*, and was tested at the following concentrations: 0.2000, 0.1000, 0.0500, 0.0250, 0.0125, and 0.0060 mg/mL. Itraconazole was used as the positive control to test carnosol against *Microsporum canis*, using the ATB FUNGUS 3 strip system (BioMerieux, La Balme-les Grottes, France). The following concentrations were used (µg/mL): 4.000, 2.000, 1.000, 0.500, 0.250, and 0.125.

The activities of the reference pesticides are assumed as criteria to evaluate the carnosol (**1**) antifungal properties.

5. Conclusions

In this work, the results of the first chemical investigation on both non-volatile and volatile secondary metabolites from the leaves and flowers, respectively, of *L. mutica* are reported. Carnosol (**1**), ursolic acid (**3**), oleanolic acid (**4**), viridoflorol (**2**), chrysothol (**6**), and 5-hydroxy-4',7-dimethoxy flavone (**5**) have been isolated from the leaves. Furthermore, the chemical analysis and the enantiomeric recognition of the essential oil distilled from the flowers of *L. mutica* are described. The qualitative compositions of the essential oils from the flowers and leaves of *L. mutica* have also been compared. δ-3-Carene, eudesm-7(11)-en-4-ol, thujopsan-2-α-ol, β-pinene, valerianol, limonene, and β-phellandrene were the major components of both oils, while at least 16 minor compounds can be considered qualitatively different in the two volatile fractions.

The known phenolic diterpene lactone carnosol (**1**) was the main secondary metabolite isolated from *L. mutica*. It showed a powerful antifungal activity against the plant pathogenic fungus *P. oryzae* and an important antifungal activity against the dermatophyte fungus *Microsporum canis*.

Acknowledgments: This work has been supported by a grant (No. 20110941) from Secretaría Nacional de Educación Superior, Ciencia y Tecnología (SENESCYT) of Ecuador, during the PhD program of one of the authors (J.R.). We are grateful to Massimo Boiocchi (University of Pavia) for X-ray diffraction experiments.

Author Contributions: J.R. and E.R. realized the experimental work; J.R. and G.G. collected the plant; J.R., G.V. and G.G. realized the experimental design and interpreted experimental data; S.T. and A.M.P. realized antifungal experiments; C.B. advised on quantitative and enantioselective analysis of the essential oil. All of the authors contributed to writing the article.

References

1. Drew, B.T.; Sytsma, K.J. The South American radiation of *Lepechinia* (Lamiaceae): Phylogenetics. divergence times and evolution of dioecy. *Bot. J. Linn. Soc.* **2013**, *171*, 171–190. [CrossRef]

2. Epling, C. A Synopsis of the Tribe Lepechinieae (Labiatae). *Brittonia* **1948**, *6*, 352–364. [CrossRef]

3. Esteves, P.F.; Kuster, R.M.; Barbi, N.S.; Menezes, F.d.S. Chemical Composition and Cytotoxic Activity of *Lepechinia speciosa* (St. Hill) Epling. *Lat. Am. J. Pharm.* **2010**, *29*, 38–44.

4. Delgado, G.; Hernández, J.; Chávez, M.I.; Alvarez, L.; Gonzaga, V.; Martínez, E. Di- and triterpenpoid acids from *Lepechinia caulescens*. *Phytochemistry* **1994**, *37*, 1119–1121. [CrossRef]

5. Jorgensen, P.; León-Yánez, S. *Catalogue of the Vascular Plants of Ecuador*; Monographs in Systematic Botany; Missouri Botanical Garden: St. Louis, MO, USA, 1999; pp. 1–1182.

6. Naranjo, P.; Escaleras, R. *La Medicina Tradicional en el Ecuador: Memorias de las Primeras Jornadas Ecuatorianas de Etnomedicina Andina*, 1st ed.; Universidad Andina Simón Bolívar-Corporación Editora Nacional: Quito, Ecuador, 1995; pp. 1–192.

7. Tene, V.; Malagón, O.; Vita Finzi, P.V.; Vidari, G.; Armijos, C.; Zaragoza, T. An ethnobotanical survey of medicinal plants used in Loja and Zamora-Chinchipe, Ecuador. *J. Ethnopharmacol.* **2007**, *111*, 63–81. [CrossRef] [PubMed]

8. Pecher, V.; Leplanquais, V.; Lazou, K.; Dumas, M.C. Use of a *Lepechinia caulescens* Extract as a Cosmetic Agent and Cosmetic Composition Containing Same. U.S. Patent 2009/0304829 A1, 3 June 2009.

9. Roderick, J.H. Fungal infections. *Clin. Dermatol.* **2006**, *24*, 201–212. [CrossRef]

10. Larypoor, M.; Akhavansepahy, A.; Rahimifard, N.; Rashedi, H. Antidermatophyte activity of the essential oil of *Hypericum perforatum* of North of Iran. *J. Med. Plants* **2009**, *8*, 110–117.

11. Couch, B.C.; Kohn, L.M. A multilocus gene genealogy concordant with host preference indicates segregation of a new species, *Magnaporthe oryzae*, from *M. grisea*. *Mycologia* **2002**, *94*, 683–693. [CrossRef] [PubMed]

12. Zeigler, R.S.; Leong, S.A.; Teeng, P.S. *Rice Blast Disease*; CAB International: Wallingford, UK; International Rice Research Institute: Los Banos, Philippines, 1994; pp. 1–626.

13. Khush, G.S.; Jena, K.K. Current status and future prospects for research on blast resistance in rice (*Oryza sativa* L.). In *Advances in Genetics, Genomics and Control of Rice Blast Disease*; Wang, X., Valent, B., Eds.; Springer: Dordrecht, the Netherlands, 2009; pp. 1–10.

14. Suriani, N.; Suprapta, D.; Sudana, I.; Temaja, I.G. Antingungal Activity of Piper caninum against Pyricularia oryzae Cav. The Cause of Rice Blast Disease on Rice. *J. Biol. Agric. Healthc.* **2015**, *5*, 72–78.

15. Yolanda, K. *Penyakit Blas Pada Padi*; BPTP Bangka Balitung, Balitbang Pertanian RI: Pangkalpinang, Indonesia, 2013.

16. Ramirez, J.; Cartuche, L.; Morocho, V.; Aguilar, S.; Malagon, O. Antifungal activity of raw extract and flavanons isolated from *Piper ecuadorense* from Ecuador. *Braz. J. Pharm.* **2013**, *23*, 370–373. [CrossRef]

17. Ramírez, J.Y.; Gilardoni, G.; Jácome, M.J.; Montesinos, J.V.; Rodolfi, M.; Guglielminetti, M.L.; Cagliero, C.; Bicchi, C.; Vidari, G. Chemical composition, enantiomeric analysis, AEDA sensorial evaluation and antifungal

activity of the essential oil from the Ecuadorian plant *Lepechinia mutica* Benth (Lamiaceae). *Chem. Biodivers* **2017**, *14*, e1700292. [CrossRef] [PubMed]

18.   Malagón, O.G.; Vila, R.; Iglesias, J.; Zaragoza, T.; Cañigueral, S. Composition of the essential oils of four medicinal plants from Ecuador. *Flavour Fragr. J.* **2003**, *18*, 527–531. [CrossRef]

19.   Gajhede, M.; Anthoni, U.; Nielsen, P.H.; Pedersen, E.J.; Christophersen, C. Carnosol. Crystal structure. absolute configuration. and spectroscopic properties of a diterpene. *J. Crystallogr. Spectrosc. Res.* **1990**, *20*, 165–171. [CrossRef]

20.   Abdelhalim, A.; Chebib, M.; Aburjai, T.; Johnston, G.R.; Hanrahan, J.R. GABAa Receptor Modulation by Compounds Isolated from *Salvia triloba* L. *Adv. Biol. Chem.* **2014**, *4*, 148–159. [CrossRef]

21.   Dimayuga, R.; Garcia, S.; Nielsen, P.H.; Christophersen, C. Traditional medicine of Baja California sur (Mexico) III. Carnosol. A diterpene antibiotic from *Lepechinia hastata*. *J. Ethnopharmacol.* **1991**, *31*, 43–48. [PubMed]

22.   Inatani, R.; Fuwa, H.; Seto, H.; Nakatani, N. Structure of a new antioxidative phenolic diterpene isolated from rosemary (*Rosmarinus officinalis* L.). *Agric. Biol. Chem.* **1982**, *46*, 1661–1666. [CrossRef]

23.   Brieskorn, C.; Fuchs, A.; Bredenberg, J.B.; McChesney, J.D.; Wenkert, E. The structure of carnosol. *J. Org. Chem.* **1964**, *29*, 2293–2298. [CrossRef]

24.   Bombarda, I.; Raharivelomanana, P.; Ramanoelina, P.R.; Faure, R.; Bianchini, J.P.; Gaydou, E.M. Spectrometric identifications of sesquiterpene alcohols from niaouli (*Melaleuca quinquenervia*) essential oil. *Anal. Chim. Acta* **2001**, *447*, 113–123. [CrossRef]

25.   Faure, R.; Ramanoelina, A.; Rakatonirainy, O.; Jean-Pierre, B.; Gaydou, E.M. Two-Dimensional Nuclear Magnetic Resonance of Sesquiterpenes. 4*-Application to Complete Assignment of ^{1}H and ^{13}C NMR Spectra of Some Aromadendrane Derivatives. *Magn. Reson. Chem.* **1991**, *29*, 969–971. [CrossRef]

26.   Gijsen, H.; Wijnberg, J.; Stork, G.; De Groot, A. The Synthesis of Mono- and Dihydroxy Aromadendrane Sesquiterpenes. Starting from Natural (+)-Armomadendrene-III. *Tetrahedron* **1992**, *48*, 2465–2476. [CrossRef]

27.   Mariotti, J.P.; Tomi, F.; Casanova, J.; Costa, J.; Bernardini, A.F. Composition of the essential oil of *Cistus ladaniferus* L. cultivated in Corsica (France). *Flavour Fragr. J.* **1997**, *12*, 147–151. [CrossRef]

28.   Liu, J. Pharmacology of oleanolic acid and ursolic acid. *J. Ethnopharmacol.* **1995**, *49*, 57–68. [CrossRef]

29.   Aguirre-Crespo, F.; Vergara-Galicia, J.; Villalobos-Molina, R.; López-Guerrero, J.J.; Navarrete-Vázquez, G.; Estrada-Soto, S. Ursolic acid mediates the vasorelaxant activity of *Lepechinia caulescens* via NO release in isolated rat thoracic aorta. *Life Sci.* **2006**, *79*, 1062–1068. [CrossRef] [PubMed]

30.   Hill, R.A.; Connolly, J.D. Triterpenoids. *Nat. Prod. Rep.* **2011**, *28*, 1087–1117. [CrossRef] [PubMed]

31.   Mahato, S.; Kundu, A. ^{13}C NMR spectra of pentacyclic Triterpenoids—A compilation and some salient features. *Phytochemistry* **1994**, *37*, 1517–1575. [CrossRef]

32.   Seebacher, W.; Simic, N.; Weis, R.; Saf, R.; Kunert, O. Complete assignments of ^{1}H and ^{13}C NMR resonances of oleanolic acid, 18α-oleanolic acid, ursolic acid and their 11-oxo derivatives. *Magn. Reson. Chem.* **2003**, *41*, 636–638. [CrossRef]

33.   Sutthanut, K.; Sripanidkulchai, B.; Yenjai, C.; Jay, M. Simultaneous identification and quantitation of 11 flavonoid constituents in *Kaempferia parviflora* by gas chromatography. *J. Chromatogr. A* **2007**, *1143*, 227–233. [CrossRef] [PubMed]

34.   Citoglu, G.; Sever, B.; Antus, S.; Baitz-Gacs, E.; Altanlar, N. Antifungal Diterpenoids and Flavonoids from *Ballota inaequidens*. *Pharm. Biol.* **2004**, *42*, 659–663. [CrossRef]

35.   Gonzalez, A.G.; Aguiar, Z.E.; Luis, G.; Ravelo, A.G.; Vázquez, J.; Domínguez, X.A. Flavonoids from *Salvia texana*. *Phytochemistry* **1989**, *28*, 2871–2872. [CrossRef]

36.   Ahmed, A.A.; Hegazy, M.F.; Hassan, N.M.; Wojcinska, M.; Karchesy, J.; Pare, P.W.; Mabry, T.J. Constituents of *Chrysothamnus viscidiflorus*. *Phytochemistry* **2006**, *67*, 1547–1553. [CrossRef] [PubMed]

37.   El-Askary, H.I. Terpenoids from *Cleome droserifolia* (Forssk.) Del. *Molecules* **2005**, *10*, 971–977. [CrossRef] [PubMed]

38.   Gedara, S.R.; Abdel-halim, O.B.; El-Sharkawy, S.H.; Salama, O.M.; Shier, T.W.; Halim, A.F. New Erythroxane-Type Diterpenoids from *Fagonia boveana* (Hadidi) Hadidi & Graf. *Z. Naturforsch C* **2003**, *58*, 23–32. [PubMed]

39.   Moghaddam, F.; Farimani, M.; Amin, G. Carnosol from *Salvia eremophila* Boiss. *DARU* **2000**, *8*, 45–46. [CrossRef]

40. Adams, R.P. *Identification of Essential Oil Components by Gas Chromatography/Mass Spectrometry*, 4th ed.; Allured Publishing Corporation: Carol Stream, IL, USA, 2009.

41. Van Den Dool, H.; Kratz, P.D. A Generalization of the Retention Index System Including Linear Temperature Programmed Gas-Liquid Partition Chromatography. *J. Chromatogr.* **1963**, *11*, 463–471. [CrossRef]

42. Birtić, S.; Dussort, P.; Pierre, F.X.; Bily, A.C.; Roller, M. Carnosic acid. *Phytochemistry* **2015**, *115*, 9–19. [CrossRef] [PubMed]

43. Areche, C.; Schmeda-Hirschmann, G.; Theoduloz, C.; Rodríguez, J.A. Gastroprotective effect and cytotoxicity of abietane diterpenes from the Chilean Lamiaceae *Sphacele chamaedryoides* (Balbis) Briq. *J. Pharm. Pharmacol.* **2009**, *61*, 1689–1697. [CrossRef] [PubMed]

44. Almada, G.; Virgen, M. Minimum antimicrobial inhibitory concentration of carnosol and of the ethanol extract from *Lepichinia hastata* (Lamiaceae). *Phytomedicine* **1998**, *5*, 301–305. [CrossRef]

45. Guerrero, I.; Andrés, L.; León, L.; Machín, R.; Padrón, J.M.; Luis, J.; Delgadillo, J. Abietane Diterpenoids from *Salvia pachyphylla* and *S. clevelandii* with Cytotoxic Activity against Human Cancer Cell Lines. *J. Nat. Prod.* **2006**, *69*, 1803–1805. [CrossRef] [PubMed]

46. Marrero, J.G.; Moujir, L.; Andrés, L.S.; Montaño, N.P.; Araujo, L.; Luis, J.G. Semisynthesis and biological evaluation of abietane-type diterpenes. Revision of the structure of rosmaquinone. *J. Nat. Prod.* **2009**, *72*, 1385–1389. [CrossRef] [PubMed]

47. Núñez, M.J.; Reyes, C.P.; Jiménez, I.A.; Hayashi, H.; Tokuda, H.; Bazzocchi, I.L. Ent-Rosane and abietane diterpenoids as cancer chemopreventive agents. *Phytochemistry* **2011**, *72*, 385–390. [CrossRef] [PubMed]

48. Ireland, B.F.; Hibbert, D.B.; Goldsack, R.J.; Doran, J.C.; Brophy, J.J. Chemical variation in the leaf essential oil of *Melaleuca quinquenervia* (Cav.) S.T. Blake. *Biochem. Syst. Ecol.* **2002**, *30*, 457–470. [CrossRef]

49. Scher, J.M.; Speakman, J.B.; Zapp, J.; Becker, H. Bioactivity guided isolation of antifungal compounds from the liverwort *Bazzania trilobata* (L.) S.F. Gray. *Phytochemistry* **2004**, *65*, 2583–2588. [CrossRef] [PubMed]

50. Talzhanov, N.A.; Sadyrbekov, D.T.; Smagulova, F.M.; Mukanov, R.M.; Raldugin, V.A.; Shakirov, M.M.; Tkachev, A.V.; Atazhanova, G.A.; Tuleuov, B.I.; Adekenov, S.M. Components of *Artemisia pontica*. *Chem. Nat. Compd.* **2005**, *41*, 143–145. [CrossRef]

51. Martini, N.D.; Katerere, D.R.P.; Eloff, J.N. Biological activity of five antibacterial flavonoids from *Combretum erythrophyllum* (Combretaceae). *J. Ethnopharmacol.* **2004**, *93*, 207–212. [CrossRef] [PubMed]

52. Tewtrakul, S.; Subhadhirasakul, S.; Kummee, S. Anti-allergic activity of compounds from *Kaempferia parviflora*. *J. Ethnopharmacol.* **2008**, *116*, 191–193. [CrossRef] [PubMed]

53. Venditti, A.; Bianco, A.; Bruno, M.; Jemia, M.; Ben Jemia, M.; Nicoletti, M. Phytochemical study of *Cistus libanotis*. *Nat. Prod. Res.* **2015**, *29*, 189–192. [CrossRef] [PubMed]

54. De Saint Laumer, J.Y.; Cicchetti, E.; Merle, P.; Egger, J.; Chaintreau, A. Quantification in Gas Chromatography: Prediction of Flame Ionization Detector Response Factors from Combustion Enthalpies and Molecular Structures. *Anal. Chem.* **2010**, *82*, 6457–6462. [CrossRef] [PubMed]

55. Costa, R.; d'Acampora Zellner, B.; Crupi, M.L.; De Fina, M.R.; Valentino, M.R.; Dugo, P.; Dugo, G.; Mondello, L. GC-MS, GC-O and enantio-GC investigation of the essential oil of *Tarchonanthus camphoratus* L. *Flavour Fragr. J.* **2008**, *23*, 40–48. [CrossRef]

11

In Silico Study, Synthesis, and Cytotoxic Activities of Porphyrin Derivatives

Fransiska Kurniawan [1], Youhei Miura [2], Rahmana Emran Kartasasmita [1], Abdul Mutalib [3], Naoki Yoshioka [2] (ID) and Daryono Hadi Tjahjono [1,*] (ID)

[1] School of Pharmacy, Bandung Institute of Technology, Jalan Ganesha 10, Bandung 40132, Indonesia; fransiskakurniawan@yahoo.com (F.K.); kartasasmita@fa.itb.ac.id (R.E.K.)

[2] Department of Applied Chemistry, Faculty of Science and Technology, Keio University, 3-14-1 Hiyoshi, Kohoku-ku, Yokohama 223-8522, Japan; y-miura@applc.keio.ac.jp (Y.M.); yoshioka@applc.keio.ac.jp (N.Y.)

[3] Center for Radioisotope and Radiopharmaceutical Technology, National Nuclear Energy Agency (BATAN), Serpong, Tangerang 15310, Indonesia; mutalib@batan.go.id

* Correspondence: daryonohadi@fa.itb.ac.id

Abstract: Five known porphyrins, 5,10,15,20-*tetrakis*(p-tolyl)porphyrin (TTP), 5,10,15,20-*tetrakis* (p-bromophenyl)porphyrin (TBrPP), 5,10,15,20-*tetrakis*(p-aminophenyl)porphyrin (TAPP), 5,10,15-*tris*(tolyl)-20-mono(p-nitrophenyl)porphyrin (TrTMNP), 5,10,15-*tris*(tolyl)-20-mono(p-aminophenyl) porphyrin (TrTMAP), and three novel porphyrin derivatives, 5,15-di-[*bis*(3,4-ethylcarboxymethylenoxy) phenyl]-10,20-di(p-tolyl)porphyrin (DBECPDTP), 5,10-di-[*bis*(3,4-ethylcarboxymethylenoxy)phenyl]-15, 20-di-(methylpyrazole-4-yl)porphyrin (cDBECPDPzP), 5,15-di-[*bis*(3,4-ethylcarboxymethylenoxy) phenyl]-10,20-di-(methylpyrazole-4-yl)porphyrin (DBECPDPzP), were used to study their interaction with protein targets (in silico study), and were synthesized. Their cytotoxic activities against cancer cell lines were tested using 3-(4,5-dimetiltiazol-2-il)-2,5-difeniltetrazolium bromide (MTT) assay. The interaction of porphyrin derivatives with carbonic anhydrase IX (CAIX) and REV-ERBβ proteins were studied by molecular docking and molecular dynamic simulation. In silico study results reveal that DBECPDPzP and TrTMNP showed the highest binding interaction with REV- ERBβ and CAIX, respectively, and both complexes of DBECPDPzP-REV-ERBβ and TrTMNP-CAIX showed good and comparable stability during molecular dynamic simulation. The studied porphyrins have selective growth inhibition activities against tested cancer cells and are categorized as marginally active compounds based on their IC_{50}.

Keywords: porphyrin derivative; molecular dynamics; synthesis; cytotoxicity; cancer cell lines

1. Introduction

Cancer is a disease related to abnormal growth of cells. The primary cause of death in cancer cases is due to the cancer cells growing into the surrounding tissues and spreading (metastasis) to distant organs [1]. Based on the National Centre for Health Statistics, it was predicted that, in the USA, about 1,688,780 new cancer cases will appear in 2017 [2]. Early detection and treatment of cancer in early stages can increase the chance for curing the cancer and decrease the number of deaths significantly [3].

Several proteins that become important targets in cancer therapy are the ErbB receptor [4,5], HER-2/Neu [4], EGFR [4], tyrosin kinase [4], and carbonic anhydrase [6]. The description with respect to nine isozymes of carbonic anhydrase (CA I through IX) has been reported and it is known that CAs performs a variety of biological functions [6–10]. CA isozymes I through VII are expressed in normal tissue with various intensity and may be expressed in the malignant cell lines derived from the CA-expressing cells, but show no evidence for their direct relationships [6]. Carbonic anhydrase IX

(CAIX) is an exception due to its expression, which is associated with tumorigenesis [6]. CAIX cannot be found in non-tumorigenic hybrid cells, but it is expressed in tumorigenic clones [11,12]. This enzyme was initially found in the surface of the HeLa cell line and its potential role to be a biomarker of cervical neoplasms has been investigated [13]. Another potential target for developing anticancer agents is REV-ERB, which is a protein in the nuclear receptor group containing most of the transcription factors. REV-ERB consists of REV-ERBα and REV-ERBβ, which regulate several physiological processes, including the circadian rhythm and metabolism [5]. Disruption of circadian rhythmicity is associated with the development of breast cancer based on epidemiological data [14–18] and the World Health Organization has classified shift-work associated with a disrupted circadian rhythm as a probable carcinogen [18,19]. Between these two types of REV-ERB, the REV-ERBβ is overexpressed in the cancer cell and its transcription is more than 95% from the total mRNA of REV-ERB [5].

The main treatment of cancer is surgery to remove the cancer cells from the normal tissue. However, this method only effective for the local cancer and it will be very difficult to handle metastatic cancer. Other methods are radiation therapy and chemotherapy. Each method can only kill a fraction of the cancer cells, thus, both methods are complementary [20]. A recent method applied to treat cancer is immune-based therapy (immunotherapy). This method can prevent the development of many cancers, but is not effective for all cancer-types [21].

Previous study showed that porphyrin derivatives bearing five-member rings of pyrazolium as *meso*-substituents have been successfully synthesized and it is known that they have strong interaction with DNA [22,23]. The porphyrin containing two carboxylate groups as *meso*-substituent, such as 3,4-*bis*(carboxymethyleneoxy)phenyl (3,4-BCP), has also been synthesized and reported to be used as a radiopharmaceutical ligand due to its selectivity to the melanoma and hepatoma cancer [24–26]. Furthermore, porphyrin molecules are known to have higher inhibition activity to cancer cells than to normal cells [27,28]. Thus, porphyrin derivatives bearing a combination of methyl pyrazole and 3,4-BCP as a *meso*-subtituent shows potential to be designed and developed as anticancer agent candidates.

The purpose of the present research was to design and synthesize novel porphyrin derivatives with methyl pyrazole and 3,4-BCP as a *meso*-subtituent, as well as their in silico study to obtain information on their interaction with CAIX and nuclear receptor REV-ERBβ which are associated with the cancer cells, and their cytotoxic effect on cancer cell lines. Five known porphyrins with more simple structure were also studied as comparison. The study was started with an in silico study to design and predict the interaction between porphyrin derivatives and the protein targets. The designed porphyrins were then synthesized and tested for their cytotoxicity against HeLa, WIDR, T47D, HepG2, and MCF-7 cancer cell lines. In addition, a comparison of the cytotoxic selectivity of porphyrin derivatives to cancer cells and normal cells was also evaluated by cytotoxicity testing against the Vero cell line.

2. Results

2.1. In Silico Study

All porphyrin derivatives were docked into carbonic anhydrase IX (PDB ID: 5FL6) and REV-ERBβ (PDB ID: 4N73) as targets. Table 1 shows the results of the docking simulation of the porphyrin derivatives.

As summarized in Table 1, it showed that complexes 5FL6-TrTMNP and 4N73-DBECPDPzP have the largest negative binding energy and, hence, these complexes were predicted to have good binding interaction. Molecular dynamic simulation was performed for these two complexes for further study to provide structural, dynamic, and energetic information on their interaction. The stability of the complexes were then analyzed by the RMSD parameter (Figure 1).

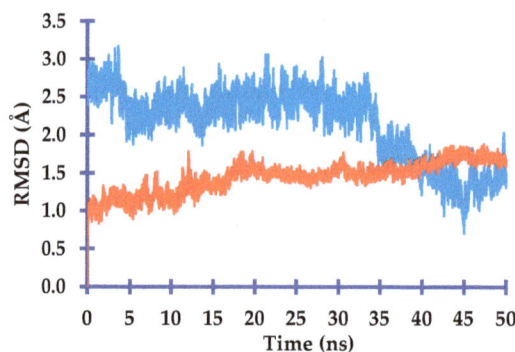

Figure 1. Plot of the RMSD value of the 5FL6-TrTMNP complex (red) and the 4N73-DBECPDPzP complex (blue) during the molecular dynamic simulation.

Table 1. Binding energy of porphyrin to protein targets.

Porphyrin Ligand	Binding Energy (kJ/mol)	
	5FL6	**4N73**
TTP	−26.82	−22.84
TBrPP	−29.00	−16.11
TAPP	−21.30	179.37
TrTMNP	−30.08	−15.69
TrTMAP	−28.66	−23.81
cDBECPDPzP	−22.34	36.15
DBECPDPzP	−16.90	−29.75
DBECPDTP	−18.87	224.26

The trajectory of both complexes were visualized to observe the position of the ligand and also to analyze their interaction. The visualization of their trajectory are shown in Figure 2 (for 5FL6-TrTMNP) and Figure 3 (for 4N73-DBECPDPzP).

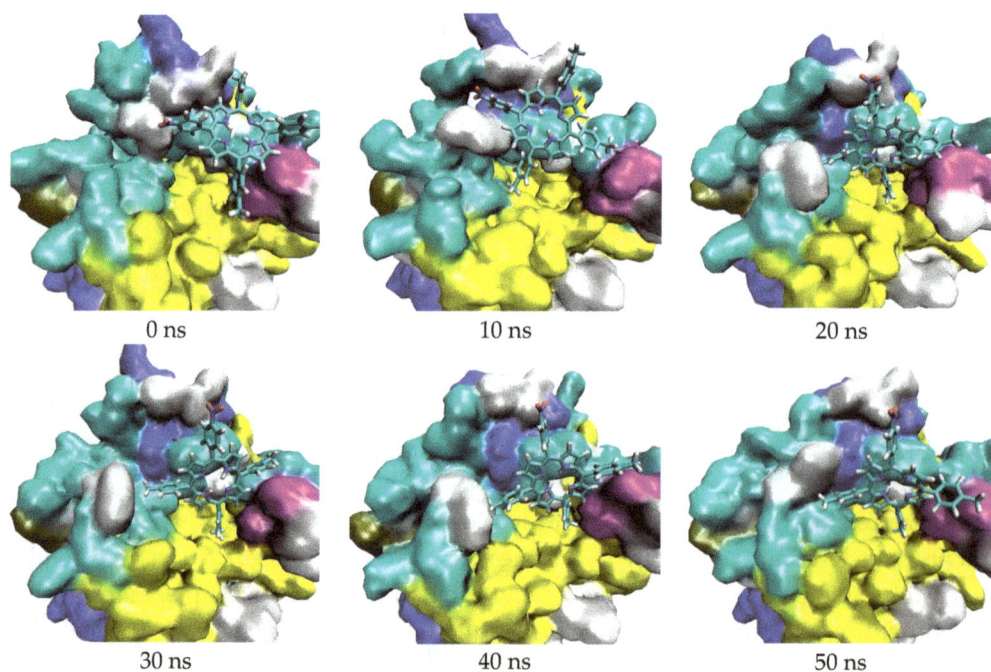

0 ns 10 ns 20 ns

30 ns 40 ns 50 ns

Figure 2. Trajectory of TrTMNP against 5FL6.

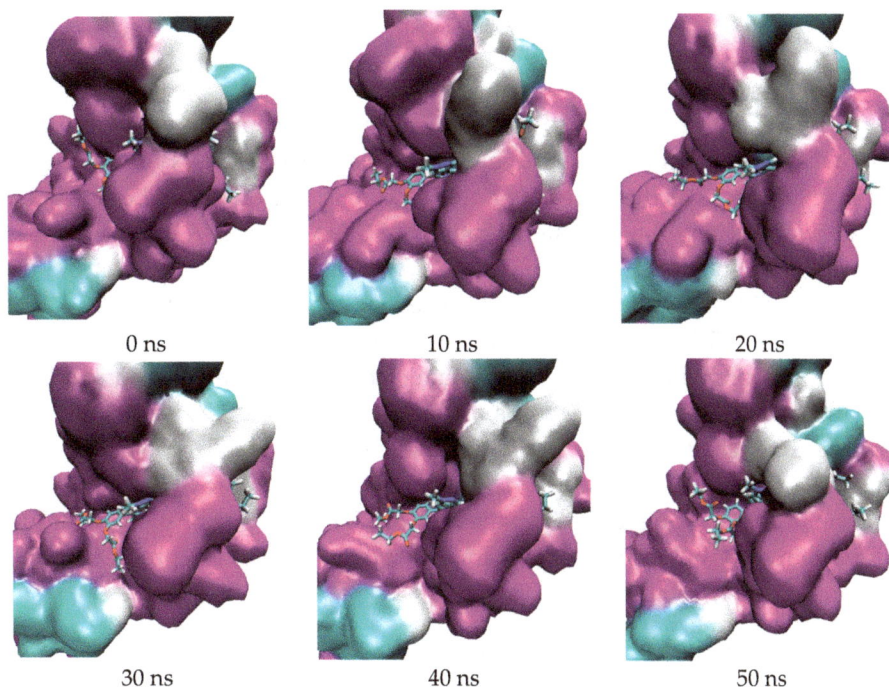

Figure 3. Trajectory of DBECPDPzP against 4N73.

After running the molecular dynamic simulation, the calculations of MM/PBSA were conducted to predict the value of ΔG_{Bind} (binding free energy), the contribution of each energy to the total calculated of binding free energy, and to evaluate the relative stability of each complex [29,30]. The results of MM/PBSA calculation for 5FL6-TrTMNP and 4N73-DBECPDPzP complexes is summarized in the Table 2.

Table 2. The binding free energies and their corresponding components of porphyrin bound to related protein targets.

Complex	ΔE_{vdw} (kJ/mol)	ΔE_{ele} (kJ/mol)	ΔG_{PB} (kJ/mol)	ΔG_{NP} (kJ/mol)	ΔG_{Bind} (kJ/mol)
5FL6-TrTMNP	−53.49	−9.39	53.51	−6.13	−15.50
4N73-DBECPDPzP	−477.91	−42.45	282.05	−38.15	−276.46

Note: ΔE_{vdw} = van der Waals contribution, ΔE_{ele} = electrostatic contribution, ΔG_{PB} = polar contribution of desolvation, ΔG_{NP} = non-polar contribution of desolvation.

2.2. Cytotoxicity Test

All of the porphyrin derivatives were evaluated for their cytotoxicity activities against several cancer cell lines and Vero cell line as a representative of normal cells. Table 3 shows the result of cytotoxicity test for porphyrin derivatives.

Table 3. Cytotoxicity (IC_{50}) of porphyrin derivatives against cell lines.

Porphyrins	IC_{50} (µM) ± SD					
	HeLa	WIDR	HepG2	T47D	MCF-7	Vero
TTP	714.6 ± 1.1	969.8 ± 1.2	1120.0 ± 1.3	1241.0 ± 1.2	1305.0 ± 1.3	15,612.0 ± 1.6
TBrPP	595.6 ± 1.3	772.7 ± 1.3	882.7 ± 1.3	443.9 ± 1.1	870.6 ± 1.3	1176.0 ± 1.1
TAPP	1007.0 ± 1.1	205.1 ± 1.2	36.0 ± 1.2	332.6 ± 1.2	262.2 ± 1.3	2264.0 ± 1.2
TrTMNP	226.1 ± 1.1	897.5 ± 1.1	146.6 ± 1.2	5372.0 ± 1.4	505.2 ± 1.2	10,079.0 ± 1.2
TrTMAP	593.1 ± 1.2	835.4 ± 1.3	106.7 ± 1.3	1099.0 ± 1.3	328.4 ± 1.4	4784.0 ± 1.2
cDBECPDPzP	1083.0 ± 1.2	28.9 ± 1.1	28.6 ± 1.2	164.5 ± 1.2	47.9 ± 1.1	548.8 ± 1.2
DBECPDPzP	941.9 ± 1.2	34.1 ± 1.1	31.7 ± 1.2	177.8 ± 1.2	64.2 ± 1.1	363.4 ± 1.1
DBECPDTP	201.7 ± 1.3	33.5 ± 1.1	37.2 ± 1.1	166.7 ± 1.3	42.1 ± 1.1	372.2 ± 1.1

3. Discussion

3.1. In Silico Study

Each porphyrin derivative was docked to both targets and the complex having the largest negative binding energy was used to run molecular dynamic simulation and MM/PBSA calculation. Data in Table 1 shows that TrTMNP has the largest negative binding energy to the 5FL6 (CAIX target). All of the porphyrin derivatives have similar interaction to the CAIX (indicated by similar binding energy value). In general, the interaction of porphyrin with CAIX was dominated by electrostatic interaction with Arg129, Asp131, Glu132, and hydrophobic interaction with Arg64, Leu199, Arg62, Arg129, Pro22, and Ala23. Interaction of 5FL6-TrTMNP (Figure 4) consists of three hydrogen bonds (with Trp9), one electrostatic interaction (with Asp131), two π-σ interaction (with Asp131 and Pro203), three π-alkyl interactions (with Val20, Pro22, and Ala23), and three alkyl-alkyl interactions (with Pro22, Ala23, and Pro57). The docking result in Table 1 shows that DBECPDPzP has the lowest binding energy to the 5FL6. Visualization of the docking pose of TrTMNP and DBECPDPzP to 5FL6 (Figure 5) reveals that the position of the porphyrin ring shifted. In the case of DBECPDPzP, the shifting of the porphyrin core made different hydrophobic interactions and this phenomenon was predicted as the cause for increasing the binding energy value.

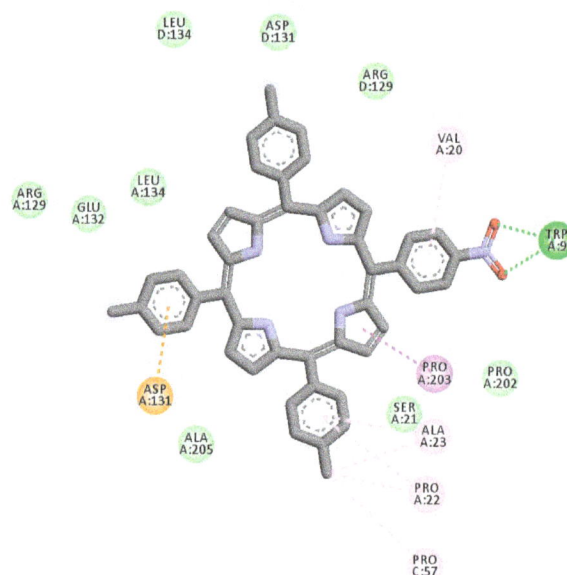

Figure 4. 2D interaction between TrTMNP and CAIX.

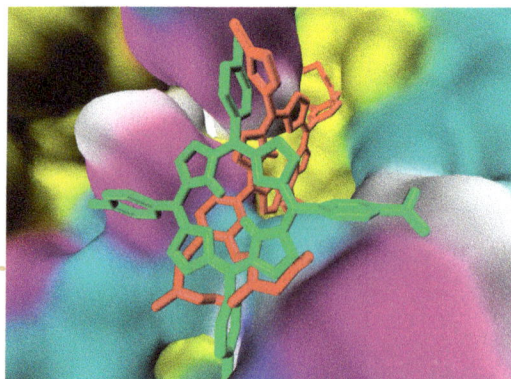

Figure 5. Overlay the docking pose of TrTMNP (green) and DBECPDPzP (red) in the binding site of 5FL6.

The interaction between porphyrin derivatives and REV-ERBβ were dominated by hydrophobic interaction. Some of the porphyrin derivatives also show hydrogen bonds with the protein which contributes to stabilizing the complexes. Table 1 show that TAPP, cDBECPDPzP, and DBECPDTP have positive values of binding energy. Considering only these values, it was predicted that these three porphyrin derivatives would not have good interaction to the target. However, these porphyrin derivatives may have affinity to the target because of similar position in the binding site (e.g., Figure 6. The analysis of interactions mode between the protein and ligand (e.g., Figure 7) show that the positive values arose due to some unfavorable bonds between the protein and ligand which appear as a steric effect in the docking simulations performed by applying the principle of the rigid protein's structure and flexible ligand. DBECPDPzP was predicted having the best interaction to the REV-ERBβ with the free binding energy of −29.75 kJ/mol. The interaction (Figure 8) was constructed by nineteen hydrogen bonds (with Val383, Cys384, Phe443, Gly478, Gly480, Leu482, Leu483, Thr410, Thr442, Met447, Phe450, His568, Glu571, and Leu572), four π-π interactions (with Trp402, Phe405, Phe409, and His568), and twelve π-alkyl interactions (with Val383, Cys384, Pro385, Met386, Phe409, Val413, Phe443, Met447, Ala479, Met486, Leu572, and Phe575). The best pose of DBECPDPzP to the REV-ERBβ receptor was selected for running the molecular dynamic simulation.

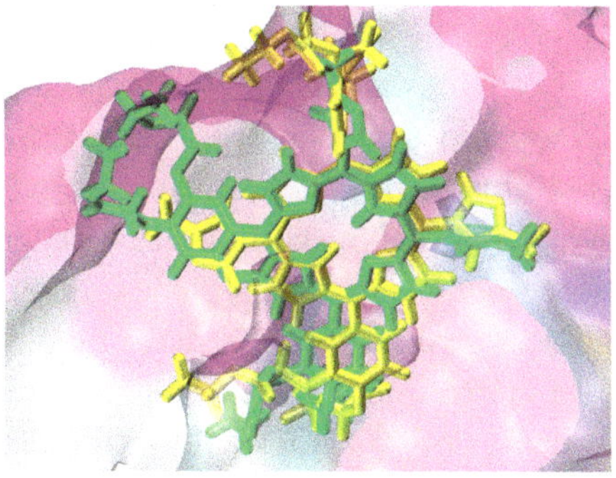

Figure 6. Overlay the docking pose of cDBECPDPzP (green) and DBECPDPzP (yellow) in the binding site of 4N73.

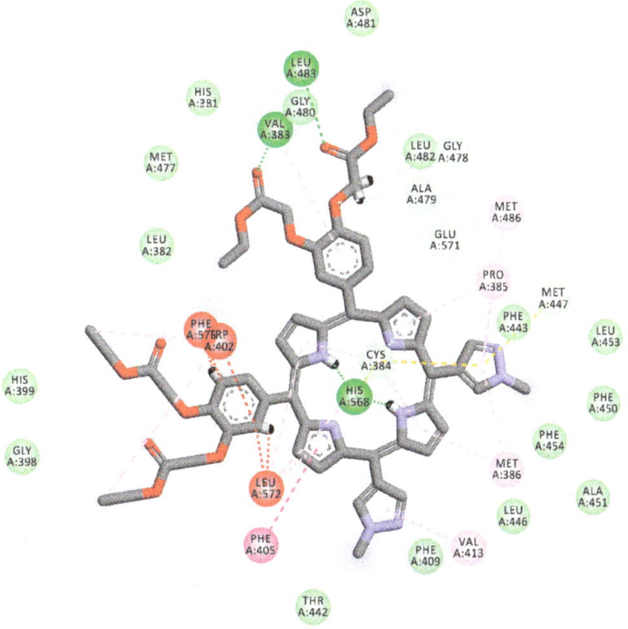

Figure 7. 2D interaction between cDBECPDPzP and REV-ERBβ, which contains an unfavorable bond (red interaction) due to steric effects.

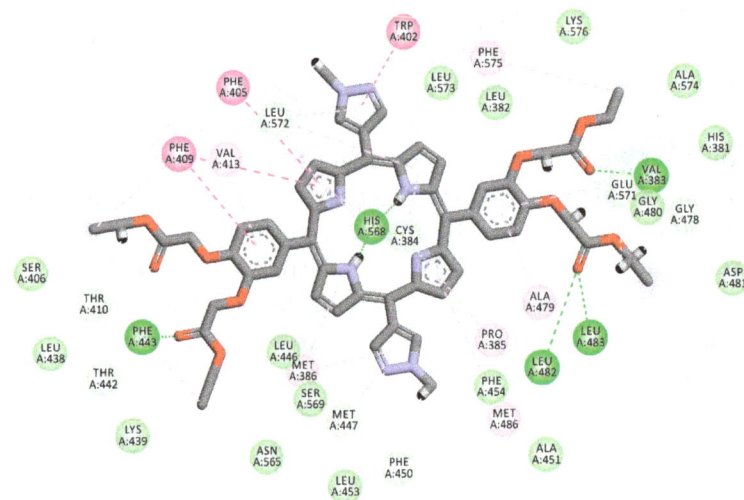

Figure 8. 2D interaction between DBECPDPzP and REV-ERBβ.

Figure 1 shows the RMSD of both complexes, which was used to evaluate their stability. The complexes are stable if the RMSD are constant and do not show large fluctuation. The 5FL6-TrTMNP complex shows better stability compared to 4N73-DBECPDPzP during the simulation. However, both complexes showed a minor movement with the RMSD of less than 3 Å [31].

Figures 2 and 3 show the visualization of the complex during simulation, in which the TrTMNP pose shows significant changes, especially its nitrophenyl moeity. Comparing the pose at 0 ns to that at 50 ns, the pose of TrTMNP rotated nearly 90°. The CAIX structure binding site also encountered some changes to accommodate the proper interaction with TrTMNP. In the case of REV-ERBβ, no significant changes in the binding site were observed, but the DBECPDPzP structure could move inside the binding pocket. Likewise, no significant changes in the pose of DBECPDPzP and only the rotation in the side chain (BECP structure) were observed during the simulation, and the whole structure was translated to achieve a proper interaction.

MM/PBSA calculation was applied to predict more accurate on the binding free energy of protein-ligand complexes, and the results showed that their binding free energies were better than that observed in the docking simulation. Table 2 showed that ΔG_{Bind} of both complexes were dominated by ΔE_{vdw}. The result confirms that the docking simulation gives proper information in which the interaction between porphyrin and the protein target was dominated by van der Waals interaction. The docking results showed some electrostatic interaction between the porphyrin derivatives and the target. However, the MM/PBSA calculation suggested that the ΔE_{ele} gives no significant effect to the ΔG_{Bind}. Both complexes have good stability during molecular dynamic simulation, and 4N73-DBECPDPzP showed stronger binding interaction compared to that of 5FL6-TrTMNP, as expressed by the larger negative ΔG_{Bind}.

3.2. Synthesis of Porphyrin Derivatives

All of porphyrin derivatives used in this study were synthesized by the Adler method (Scheme 1).

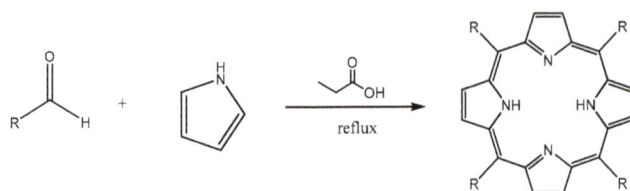

Scheme 1. General Adler method to synthesize porphyrin derivatives.

The synthesis of porphyrin derivatives were carried out by the Adler method because the purification and isolation of the product was relative simple [32], although the yield was relative low (usually below 20%). For the five known porphyrin derivatives, the aldehyde reagents were commercially available, so it can be directly reacted with pyrrole. However, in the case of three novel porphyrins containing *bis*-3,4 ethylcarboxymethylenoxyphenyl (BECP) as one of the meso-subtituents, the related aldehyde was not available commercially. Consequently, the aldehyde should be firstly synthesized. *Bis*-3,4 ethylcarboxymethylenoxy benzaldehyde (BECB) was prepared according to Scheme 2 [33].

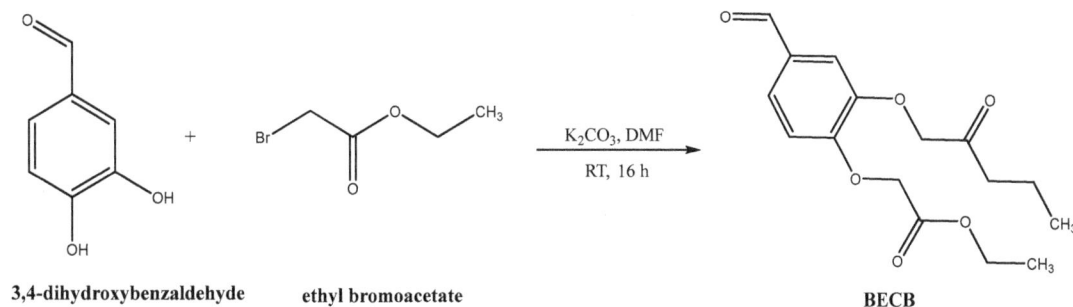

3,4-dihydroxybenzaldehyde   **ethyl bromoacetate**   **BECB**

Scheme 2. Synthetic route of BECB.

The purpose of introducing the BECP as a meso-substituent was to increase the polarity of porphyrin derivatives. Increasing the polarity can contribute to better solubility in water. This is an important issue because most of anticancer drugs will be administered as an injection dosage form. Moreover, porphyrins containing BECP as the meso-substituent showed good affinity to the receptor as described in the in silico study, thus, it was predicted that these compounds be promising candidates for further in vitro cytotoxicity studies.

3.3. Cytotoxicity Test

From the data in Table 3, it can be concluded that all porphyrin derivatives were categorized as marginally-active compounds against tested cell line because they have IC_{50} in the range of 1 to 5000 µM [34], except for TrTMNP against T47D cell line, TrTMNP against the Vero cell line, as well as TTP against the Vero cell line. Comparing the value of IC_{50} against the cancer cell line and normal cell line (Vero cell line) can be used to proof that almost all synthesized porphyrins have higher anti-proliferation activities towards cancer cells compared to those of normal cells. Among the studied porphyrin derivatives, TTP and TrTMNP show better selective cytotoxic effect to the cancer cell compared to that of normal cell. Furthermore, if we refer the assumption that the compounds having IC_{50} less than 100 µM are potential candidates as anti-proliferative agents [35], the three novel porphyrins (cDBECPDPzP, DBECPDPzP, and DBECPDTP) also still have chance to be further investigated. These three novel porphyrins also show selective cytotoxic effects on cancer cells compared to the normal cells. Generally, increasing the polarity of the porphyrin by changing its meso-substituent can increase the cytotoxic effect on cancer cell lines, such as HepG2 and MCF-7. The result also showed that BECP as the meso-substituent of novel porphyrin derivatives increased the polarity of porphyrin derivatives and increase the cytotoxic effect on the cancer cell line.

CAIX was firstly identified as membrane-bonded protein on the surface of HeLa cells [36,37]. CAIX is a hypoxia-induced enzyme that is overexpressed in cancer cells [11]. The function of CAIX is to produce and manage the intracellular pH according to the proper environment for growth and survival of cancer cells. Thus, an inhibitor of CAIX can be a promising anticancer agent. Based on in silico study, all synthesized porphyrins have good binding interaction to CAIX. They also showed good cytotoxic activities against the HeLa cell line with an $IC_{50} < 2$ mM. DBECPDTP shows the highest anti-proliferative effect to the HeLa cell line with an IC_{50} of 201.7 μM. This is slightly lower than that of TrTMNP, which was predicted as the best ligand based on in silico study of the CAIX target.

Previous study showed that REV-ERBβ is dominant (more than 75%) in the MCF-7 cell line and the HepG2 cell line, whereas REV-ERBα is dominant in normal cells [5]. As observed in the in silico study, all porphyrin derivatives have interactions with REV-ERBβ, the in vitro test also confirmed that they have cytotoxicity activity to the MCF-7 and HepG2. DBECPDTP has the strongest cytotoxicity against MCF-7 cells with an IC_{50} of 42.1 μM, while cDBECPDPzP has the strongest cytotoxicity against HepG2 cells with an IC_{50} of 28.6 μM. Based on the above results, porphyrin derivatives which have low IC_{50} values are prospective compounds for further detailed pharmacological evaluation with respect to cellular accumulation, phototoxicity, as well as the mechanism of action.

4. Materials and Methods

4.1. In Silico Study

4.1.1. Macromolecule Preparation

Macromolecules used in this study were carbonic anhydrase IX (CA IX) and nuclear receptor REV-ERBβ. Both receptor's structures were downloaded from the Protein Data Bank with PDB ID 5FL6 and 4N73, respectively. The preparations of macromolecules were conducted by removing the water molecules and natural ligand, adding the polar hydrogen atoms, and calculating the Kollman charges.

4.1.2. Ligand Preparation

Ligands used in the present study were eight porphyrin derivatives, of which five are known porphyrin derivatives and three are novel porphyrin derivatives (Figure 9). The ligand's structures were prepared by GaussView 5.0.8 and optimized by Gaussian09 [38] using Density Functional Theory method with 6–31 basis sets. The optimized structure and the partial charges data were used as input for molecular docking studies.

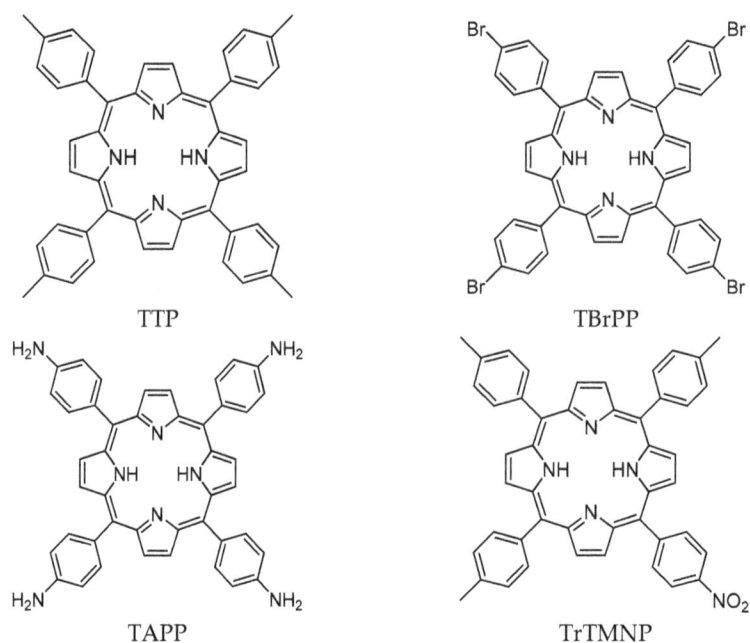

TTP

TBrPP

TAPP

TrTMNP

Figure 9. *Cont.*

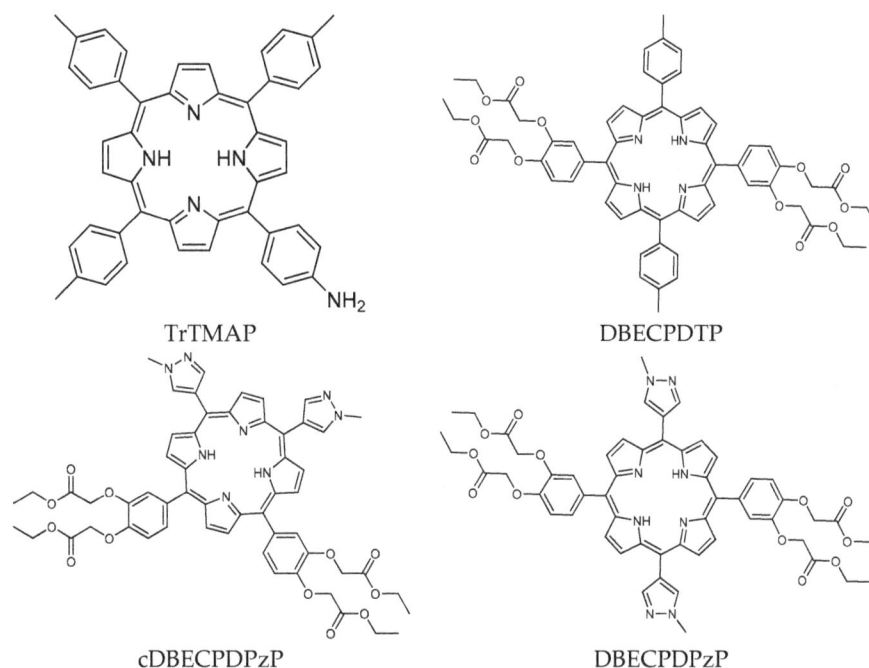

Figure 9. Structure of porphyrin derivatives.

4.1.3. Molecular Docking Simulation

Molecular docking simulations were performed by AutoDock 4.2 with MGLTools 1.5.6 [39,40]. All ligands for this simulation were set as maximum torsion [41]. All simulations were performed using a grid box $64 \times 60 \times 60$ points with 0.375 Å spacing. The Lamarckian Genetic Algorithm [40] was used with 100 conformations. All other docking parameters were set as default. Analysis of the results of the docking simulation was performed with VMD 1.9.2 [42] and Discovery Studio 2016 [43].

4.1.4. Molecular Dynamic Simulation

Molecular dynamic simulations were performed for two complexes having the best value of binding free energy in each receptor. The simulations were performed by Gromacs2016 [44–50] and the analyses were performed with VMD 1.9.2 [42] and Discovery Studio 2016 [43]. AMBER99SB-ILDN force field [51] was used to parameterize the protein, while the ligand was parameterized using ACPYPE [52]. Long-range electrostatic force was determined by the Particle Mesh Ewald method [53,54]. Neutralization of the system was performed by adding Na^+ and Cl^- ions. The cubic of TIP3P water model was used to solvate the system. The step of the simulation was included minimization, heating until 310 K, temperature equilibration (NVT), pressure equilibration (NPT), and production run with a 2 fs timestep for 50 ns. The stability of the system was verified by analysis of the energy, temperature, pressure, and root mean square deviation (RMSD).

4.1.5. MM/PBSA Calculation

MM/PBSA calculation was performed by the g_mmpbsa package [55,56] integrated in Gromacs software. Polar desolvation energy was calculated with the Poisson-Boltzmann equation with a grid size of 0.5 Å. The dielectric constant of the solvent was set to 80 to represent water as the solvent [57,58]. Nonpolar contribution was determined by calculation of the solvent accessible surface area with the radii of the solvent as 1.4 Å. Binding free energy of the complex was determined based on 100 snapshots taken from 49 to 50 ns molecular dynamic simulation trajectories of the complex.

4.2. Synthesis of Porphyrin Derivatives

4.2.1. Materials

Pyrrole (WAKO) and *p*-tolualdehyde (TCI) were distilled under reduce pressure before use. Phosphoryl chloride (WAKO), *p*-nitrobenzaldehyde (WAKO), *p*-bromobenzaldehyde (TCI), 1-methylpyrazole (TCI), 3,4-dihidroxybenzaldehyde (WAKO), ethyl bromoacetate (TCI), and $SnCl_2 \cdot 2H_2O$ (WAKO) were used as received. Other chemicals and solvents were of analytical grade and were purchased from Kanto Chemicals and WAKO. ^{1}H-NMR and ^{13}C-NMR spectra were recorded in the solvents indicated at 300 MHz (on JNM-LA 300 spectrometer) and 125 MHz (on Agilent Varian 500 MHz), respectively, and the chemical shift are reported in parts per million (ppm, δ). Mass spectra were recorded on a Brucker Ultraflex I MALDI-TOF LRMS or a Waters LCT-Premier ESI-LRMS.

4.2.2. Procedure of Synthesis

Synthesis of 5,10,15,20-*tetrakis*(*p*-tolyl)porphyrin (TTP)

TTP was synthesized regarding reported method [32,59] with slightly modification. Distilled *p*-tolualdehyde (9.4 mL, 80 mmol) was added to the 300 mL of refluxing propionic acid. Pyrrole (5.6 mL, 80 mmol) was then added to the mixture and the mixture was refluxed for 2 h. After 2 h, the mixture was cooled to room temperature and filtered. The residue was then washed by hot water and methanol. The residue was dried in vacuum desiccator and purified by silica column chromatography using chloroform as eluent. Evaporation of the solvent resulted purple solid (4.47 g, 33.4% yield). ^{1}H-NMR (CDCl$_3$, 300 MHz): −2.79 ppm (s, 2H), 2.70 ppm (s, 12H), 7.54 ppm (d, *J* = 7.8 Hz, 8H), 8.09 ppm (d, *J* = 7.8 Hz, 8H), 8.84 ppm (s, 8H). ^{13}C-NMR (CDCl$_3$, 125 MHz): 21.5 ppm (CH$_3$-tolyl), 120.1 ppm (C-*meso*), 127.3 ppm (C 3′,5′-tolyl), 127.4 ppm (C β-pyrrole), 134.5 ppm (C 2′,6′-tolyl), 134.5 ppm (C 4′-tolyl), 137.3 ppm (C 1′-tolyl), 139.3 ppm (C α-pyrrole). Melting point > 300 °C. UV/Vis (CH$_2$Cl$_2$): 420 nm (B-band), 516, 551, 591, and 647 nm (Q-band). MALDI-TOF LRMS: m/z = 671.007 [M + H]$^+$ (exact mass = 671.318).

Synthesis of 5,10,15,20-*tetrakis*(*p*-bromophenyl)porphyrin(TBrPP)

TBrPP was synthesized regarding reported method [60] with slightly modification. *p*-bromobenzaldehyde (1.85 g, 10 mmol) was added to the 38 mL of refluxing propionic acid. Pyrrole (0.7 mL, 10 mmol) was then added to the mixture and the mixture was refluxed for 2 h. After 2 h, the mixture was cooled to room temperature and filtered. The residue was then washed by hot water and methanol. The residue was dried in vacuum desiccator and purified by silica column chromatography using chloroform as eluent. Evaporation of the solvent resulted dark purple solid (795.1 mg, 34.2% yield). ^{1}H-NMR (CDCl$_3$, 500 MHz): −2.86 ppm (s, 2H), 7.91 ppm (d, *J* = 8 Hz, 8H), 8.08 ppm (d, *J* = 8 Hz, 8H), 8.86 ppm (s, 8H). ^{13}C-NMR (CDCl$_3$, 125 MHz): 118.6 ppm (C-*meso*), 122.6 ppm (C 4′-bromophenyl), 130.0 ppm (C 2′,3′,5′,6′-bromophenyl), 131.5 ppm (C β-pyrrole), 135.8 ppm (C 1′-bromophenyl), 140.8 ppm (C α-pyrrole). Melting point > 300 °C. UV/Vis (CH$_2$Cl$_2$): 420 nm (B-band), 515, 549, 590, and 646 nm (Q-band). ESI LRMS: m/z = 927.317 [M + 2H]$^{2+}$ (exact mass = 927.905).

Synthesis of 5,10,15,20-*tetrakis*(*p*-aminophenyl)porphyrin (TAPP)

TAPP was synthesized in accordance with the reported method [61] with slight modification. A solution of *p*-nitrobenzaldehyde (7.34 g, 48 mmol) and acetic anhydride (7.8 mL, 82 mmol) in 200 mL propionic acid was refluxed. Then pyrrole (3.4 mL, 48 mmol) was added dropwise as a solution in 6 mL propionic acid. The mixture was stirred for 30 min. The reaction was cooled to room temperature, filtered, and the collected residue was washed with hot water until the washings were colorless. Then the black residue was rinsed with methanol and dried in a vacuum desiccator. The residue was then mixed with 100 mL DMF and stirred for one hour at around 80 °C, cooled to room temperature, and the solution was stored in a refrigerator for 1.5–2 days. The mixture was filtered and the solid was washed with acetone until the washings were colorless. The dark purple product was dried under vacuum at room temperature to give 5,10,15,20-*tetrakis*(p-nitrophenyl)porphyrin (TNPP). The product (504 mg, 5.3% yield) was not soluble in common organic solvents and used for the next step without further purification. UV-VIS (tetrahydrofuran): 422 nm (B-band), 515, 549, 591, and 647 nm (Q-band).

A mixture of TNPP (500 mg, 0.63 mmol) and hydrochloric acid (12 M, 25 mL) was put in three-neck flask. A solution of $SnCl_2 \cdot 2H_2O$ (2.50 g, 11 mmol) in concentrated hydrochloric acid (5.4 mL) was added to the porphyrin mixture and the reaction mixture was heated using a water bath at 75–80 °C for 1.5 h. The hot-water bath was removed and replaced with a cold water bath, and then with an ice-water bath. The reaction was neutralized with sodium hydroxide solution. The mixture was then filtered and the black solid material was collected, washed twice with water. Extract the TAPP by using Soxhlet with acetone (250 mL). Evaporating the acetone afforded a shiny purple solid (322.7 mg, 76% yield). ^{1}H-NMR (CDCl$_3$, 300 MHz): −2.72 ppm (bs, 2H), 4.01 ppm (bs, 8H), 7.05 ppm (d, J = 8.4 Hz, 8H), 7.98 ppm (d, J = 8.4 Hz, 8H), 8.89 ppm (s, 8H). ^{13}C-NMR (CDCl$_3$, 125 MHz): 113.4 ppm (C-*meso*), 120.1 ppm (C 4′-aminophenyl), 130.9 ppm (C β-pyrrole), 132.7 ppm (C 2′,3′,5′,6′-aminophenyl), 135.7 ppm (C 1′-aminophenyl), 145.9 ppm (C α-pyrrole). Melting point > 370 °C. UV/Vis (CH$_2$Cl$_2$): 427 nm (B-band), 522, 563, 596, and 655 nm (Q-band). ESI LRMS: m/z = 675.314 [M + H]$^+$ (exact mass = 675.299).

Synthesis of 5,10,15-*tris*(tolyl)-20-mono(p-nitrophenyl)porphyrin (TrTMNP)

TrTMNP was synthesized regarding reported method [62] with slightly modification. Propionic acid (200 mL) was put into a three-neck flask, then distilled pyrrole (3.4 mL, 48 mmol), p-tolualdehyde (7.2 mL, 72 mmol), and p-nitrobenzaldehyde (1.835 g, 12 mmol) were added. The mixture was stirred and refluxed for 2 h. After 2 h, the mixture was cooled to room temperature. The mixture was filtered using a glass filter and washed with hot water. The desired material was extracted from the glass filter using chloroform. The mixture was purified using column chromatography with silica as the stationary phase. The first column using chloroform as mobile phase to separate the dark material and all porphyrin compounds. A second column using chloroform/n-hexane = 5/1 was used to collect the desired porphyrin. TrTMNP was in the second band. Evaporating the solvent gave a purple solid (453.6 mg, 5.4% yield). ^{1}H-NMR (CDCl$_3$, 300 MHz): −2.77 ppm (s, 2H, broad), 2.72 ppm (s, 9H), 7.56 ppm (d, J = 8.1 Hz, 6H), 8.09 ppm (d, J = 7.8 Hz, 6H), 8.40 ppm (d, J = 8.7 Hz, 2H), 8.64 ppm (d, J = 8.4 Hz, 2H), 8.72 ppm (d, J = 5.4 Hz, 2H), 8.88 ppm (s, 4H), 8.91 ppm (d, J = 4.2 Hz, 2H). ^{13}C-NMR (CDCl$_3$, 125 MHz): 21.6 ppm (C CH$_3$-tolyl), 116.3 ppm (C-15 *meso*), 120.7 ppm (C 10,20-*meso*), 121.2 ppm (C 5-*meso*), 121.8 ppm (C 3′,5′-nitrophenyl), 127.5 ppm (C 3′,5′-tolyl), 127.5 ppm (C β-pyrrole), 132.0 ppm (C β-pyrrole), 134.5 ppm (C 2′,6′-tolyl), 137.5 ppm (C 2′,6′-nitrophenyl), 137.5 ppm (C 4′-tolyl), 139.0 ppm (C 1′-tolyl), 139.0 ppm (C α-pyrrole), 147.6 ppm (C 4′-nitrophenyl), 149.4 ppm (C 1′-nitrophenyl). Melting point > 300 °C. UV/Vis (CH$_2$Cl$_2$): 425 nm (B-band), 517, 552, 591, and 647 nm (Q-band). MALDI-TOF LRMS: m/z = 702.731 [M + H]$^+$ (exact mass = 702.287).

Synthesis of 5,10,15-*tris*(tolyl)-20-mono(p-aminophenyl)porphyrin (TrTMAP)

TrTMAP was synthesized according to the reported method [62] with slightly modification. A mixture of TrTMNP (150 mg, 0.214 mmol) and HCl (12 M, 20 mL) was put in a two-neck flask. A solution of $SnCl_2 \cdot 2H_2O$ (300 mg, 1.33 mmol) in concentrated HCl (5 mL) was added to the porphyrin mixture and the reaction mixture was heated using a water bath at 65–70 °C for two hours. The hot-water bath was removed and replaced with a cold water bath, and then with an ice-water bath. The reaction was neutralized with a sodium hydroxide solution. The mixture was then extracted with chloroform. The crude material was purified using column chromatography with chloroform/n-hexane = 3/1. Evaporating the solvent afforded a purple solid (50.7 mg, 35.3% yield). ^{1}H-NMR (CDCl$_3$, 300 MHz): −2.75 ppm (s, 2H), 2.71 ppm (s, 9H), 4.04 ppm (s, 2H), 7.06 ppm (d, 2H, J = 8.4 Hz), 7.55 ppm (d, 6H, J = 7.8 Hz), 8.00 ppm (d, 2H, J = 8.4 Hz), 8.09 ppm (d, 6H, J = 7.5 Hz), 8.85 ppm (s, 4H), 8.92 ppm (d, 2H, $J = 4.8$ Hz). ^{13}C-NMR (CDCl$_3$, 125 MHz): 21.5 ppm (C CH$_3$-tolyl), 113.4 ppm (C 3′,5′-aminophenyl), 119.8 ppm (C 5-*meso*), 120.0 ppm (C 10,20-*meso*), 120.5 ppm (C 15-*meso*), 127.4 ppm (C 3′,5′-tolyl), 127.4 ppm (C β-pyrrole), 131.1 ppm (C β-pyrrole), 132.6 ppm (C 4′-aminophenyl), 134.5 ppm (C 2′,6′-tolyl), 135.6 ppm (C 2′,6′-aminophenyl), 137.3 ppm (C 4′-tolyl), 139.3 ppm (C 1′-tolyl), 139.4 ppm (C 1′-aminophenyl), 145.8 ppm (C α-pyrrole). Melting point > 300 °C. UV/Vis (CH$_2$Cl$_2$): 421 nm (B-band), 518, 554, 593, and 650 nm (Q-band). MALDI-TOF LRMS: $m/z = 672.421$ [M + H]$^+$ (exact mass = 672.313).

Synthesis of *bis*(3,4-ethylcarboxymethylenoxy) Benzaldehyde (BECB)

BECB was synthesized in accordance with the reported method [33] with slight modification. 3,4-dihydroxybenzaldehyde (1.35 g, 9.78 mmol) and anhydrous potassium carbonate (5.4 g, 39.13 mmol) were added in a two-neck flask, then dissolved in dry DMF (20 mL) and stirred for 30 min until it changed into a yellow solution. The mixture was cooled to 0–5 °C using an ice bath. Ethyl bromo acetate (4.9 g, 29.34 mmol) was then added dropwise. The mixture was stirred at 0–5 °C for 30 min and then stirring continued at room temperature for 16 h. After 16 h, the mixture was extracted with brine and dichloromethane. The water phase was washed by dichloromethane, and the organic phase was then collected. The organic phase was extracted again with brine to remove DMF from the mixture. Sodium sulfate was added to the organic phase, filtered, and then evaporated. Purification of the crude product was performed by column chromatography for three times (using silica as stationary phase and ethyl acetate as mobile phase). The solvent was evaporated and the residue was kept under vacuum to obtain yellow oily product (1.3688 g, yield 45.2%).

^{1}H-NMR (CDCl$_3$, 300 MHz): 9.85 ppm (s, 1H), 7.49 ppm (dd, $J = 1.8/8.4$ Hz, 1H), 7.39 ppm (d, $J = 1.5$ Hz, 1H), 6.94 ppm (d, $J = 8.4$Hz, 1H), 4.81 ppm (s, 2H), 4.77 ppm (s, 2H), 4.28 ppm (q, $J = 7.2$ Hz, 4H), 4.12 ppm (q, $J = 7.2$ Hz, 4H), 1.32 ppm (t, $J = 7.2$ Hz, 3H), 1.28 ppm (t, $J = 7.2$ Hz, 3H).

Synthesis of 1-Methylpyrazole-4-carbaldehyde

1-Methylpyrazole-4-carbaldehyde was synthesized regarding reported method [22,63]. Dry dimethylformamide (34 mL) was cooled in an ice bath at 1–10 °C, then phosphoryl chloride (40 mL) was added dropwise. The reaction mixture was then stirred at room temperature for one hour. It was then heated to 90 °C and 10.2 mL of 1-methylpyrazole was added dropwise. The temperature was then increased to 90–95 °C for 1 h, 105–110 °C for 3 h, and 120–125 °C for 1 h. The still hot mixture was poured into about 500 mL of ice and the mixture was then diluted with 200 mL of water. The reaction mixture was left at room temperature overnight. Sodium bicarbonate was added until pH 5–6 and the solution was then extracted with dichloromethane. The organic phase was washed with brine and dried with sodium sulfate. The solvent was then evaporated and then the vacuum distillation was performed to obtain a yellowish liquid 1-methyl pyrazole-4-carbaldehyde (4.35 g, yield 32.22 %).

^{1}H-NMR (CDCl$_3$, 300 MHz): 9.85 ppm (s, 1H), 7.96 ppm (s, 1H), 7.90 ppm (s, 1H), 3.98 ppm (s, 3H).

Synthesis of 5,15-di-[*bis*(3,4-ethylcarboxymethylenoxy)phenyl]-10,20-di(*p*-tolyl)porphyrin (DBECPDTP)

p-tolualdehyde (0.1 mL, 1 mmol) and BECB (310 mg, 1 mmol) were added to 20 mL refluxing propionic acid. Pyrrole (0.14 mL, 2 mmol) was then added and the mixture was refluxed for 4 h. Propionic acid was removed by distillation under reduced pressure to give a dark residue. This was put into a minimum amount of dichloromethane and subjected to silica column chromatography. The elution with dichloromethane gave a major product on the second band (reddish). Re-column chromatography of this crude on longer silica column chromatography and elution with chloroform gave the major dark red product on the second band. Evaporation of the solvent afforded pure DBECPDTP as a purple solid (14.6 mg, yield 1.39%). ^{1}H-NMR (CDCl$_3$, 300 MHz): −2.84 ppm (bs, 2H),

1.13 ppm (t, J = 7.2 Hz, 6H), 1.40 ppm (t, J = 7.2, 6H), 2.70 ppm (s, 6H), 4.18 ppm (q, J = 7.2 Hz, 4H), 4.39 ppm (q, J = 7.2 Hz, 4H), 4.84 ppm (s, 4H), 5.01 ppm (s, 4H), 7.22 ppm (d, J = 8.7 Hz, 2H), 7.72 ppm (s, 2H), 7.77 ppm (d, J = 8.4 Hz, 2H), 8.84 ppm (s, 8H). ^{13}C-NMR (CDCl$_3$, 125 MHz): 14.1 ppm (C CH$_3$-BECP), 14.3 ppm (C CH$_3$-BECP), 21.5 ppm (C CH$_3$-tolyl), 61.3 ppm (C CH$_2$-BECP), 61.5 ppm (C CH$_2$-BECP), 66.5 ppm (C methylene-BECP), 66.9 ppm (C methylene-BECP), 113.3 ppm (C 2'-BECP), 119.0 ppm (C 5'-BECP), 120.3 ppm (C *meso*), 121.4 ppm (C 6'-BECP), 127.4 ppm (C 3',5'-tolyl), 128.7 ppm (C β-pyrrole), 134.5 ppm (C 1'-BECP), 135.4 ppm (C 2',6'-BECP), 135.7 ppm (C 4'-tolyl), 136.4 ppm (C 1'-tolyl), 137.4 ppm (C α-pyrrole), 139.1 ppm (C 3'-BECP), 146.0 ppm (C 4'-BECP), 147.8 ppm (C α-pyrrole), 168.8 ppm (C carboxyl-BECP), 169.2 ppm (C carboxyl-BECP). UV/Vis (CH$_2$Cl$_2$): 421 nm (B-band), 517, 550, 591, and 651 nm (Q-band). MALDI-TOF LRMS: m/z = 1051.696 [M + H]$^+$ (exact mass = 1051.413).

Synthesis of 5,10-di-[*bis*(3,4-ethylcarboxymethylenoxy)phenyl]-15,20-di-(methylpyrazole-4-yl) porphyrin (cDBECPDPzP)

1-Methylpyrazole-4-carbaldehyde (110 mg, 1 mmol) and BECB (310 mg, 1 mmol) were added to 20 mL refluxing propionic acid. Pyrrole (0.14 mL, 2 mmol) was then added and the mixture was refluxed for 4 h. Propionic acid was removed by distillation under reduced pressure to give a dark residue. This was taken into a minimum amount of dichloromethane and subjected to silica column chromatography. The elution with dichloromethane gave product on the second band (reddish). Re-column chromatography of this crude on longer silica column chromatography and elution with chloroform gave the major dark red product on the fourth band. Evaporation of the solvent afforded pure cDBECPDPzP as a purple solid (28.2 mg, yield 5.47%). ^{1}H-NMR (CDCl$_3$, 300 MHz): −2.78 ppm (bs, 2H), 1.16 ppm (t, J = 7.2 Hz, 6H), 1.41 ppm (t, J = 7.2 Hz, 6H), 4.19 ppm (q, J = 7.2 Hz, 4H), 4.33 ppm (s, 6H), 4.40 ppm (q, J = 7.2 Hz, 4H), 4.86 ppm (s, 4H), 5.02 ppm (s, 4H), 7.73–7.78 ppm (m, 6H), 8.18 ppm (s, 2H), 8.33 ppm (s, 2H), 8.83 ppm (s, 2H), 8.86 ppm (d, J = 4.8 Hz, 2H), 9.10 ppm (d, J = 4.8 Hz, 2H), 9.13 ppm (s, 2H). ^{13}C-NMR (CDCl$_3$, 125 MHz): 14.1 ppm (C CH$_3$-BECP), 14.3 ppm (C CH$_3$-BECP), 39.5 ppm (C CH$_3$-pyrazolyl), 61.4 ppm (C CH$_2$-BECP), 61.5 ppm (C CH$_2$-BECP), 66.5 ppm (C methylene-BECP), 66.9 ppm (C methylene-BECP), 110.5 ppm (C 2'-BECP), 113.3 ppm (C 4'-pyrazolyl), 119.2 ppm (C 5'-BECP), 121.6 ppm (C 15,20-*meso*), 122.7 ppm (C 5,10-*meso*), 128.8 ppm (C 6'-BECP), 128.9 ppm (C 5'-pyrazolyl), 131.0 ppm (C β-pyrrole), 134.0 ppm (C 1'-BECP), 136.4 ppm (C 3'-pyrazolyl), 143.6 ppm (C 3'-BECP), 146.1 ppm (C 4'-BECP), 147.9 ppm (C α-pyrrole), 168.8 ppm (C carboxyl-BECP), 169.1 ppm (C carboxyl-BECP). UV/Vis (CH$_2$Cl$_2$): 422 nm (B-band), 520, 558, 595, and 653 nm (Q-band). MALDI-TOF LRMS: m/z = 1033.925 [M + 3H]$^{3+}$ (exact mass = 1033.410).

Synthesis of 5,15-di-[*bis*(3,4-Ethylcarboxymethylenoxy)phenyl]-10,20-di-(methylpyrazole-4-yl) porphyrin (DBECPDPzP)

1-Methylpyrazole-4-carbaldehyde (110 mg, 1 mmol) and BECB (310 mg, 1 mmol) were added to 20 mL refluxing propionic acid. Pyrrole (0.14 mL, 2 mmol) was then added and the mixture was refluxed for 4 h. Propionic acid was removed by distillation under reduced pressure to give a dark residue. This was taken into a minimum amount of dichloromethane and subjected to silica column chromatography. The elution with dichloromethane gave product on the second band (reddish). Re-column chromatography of this crude on longer silica column chromatography and elution with chloroform gave the major dark red product on the third band. Evaporation of the solvent afforded pure DBECPDPzP as purple solid (12.5 mg, yield 2.42%). ^{1}H-NMR (CDCl$_3$, 300 MHz): −2.77 ppm (bs, 2H), 1.17 ppm (t, J = 7.2 Hz, 6H), 1.42 ppm (t, J = 7.2 Hz, 6H), 4.21 ppm (q, J = 7.2 Hz, 4H), 4.34 ppm (s, 6H), 4.42 ppm (q, J = 7.2 Hz, 4H), 4.88 ppm (s, 4H), 5.03 ppm (s, 4H), 7.50–7.60 ppm (m, 2H), 7.70–7.80 ppm (m, 4H), 8.18 ppm (s, 2H), 8.33 ppm (s, 2H), 8.88 ppm (d, J = 4.8 Hz, 4H), 9.10 ppm (d, J = 4.8 Hz, 4H). ^{13}C-NMR (CDCl$_3$, 125 MHz): 14.1 ppm (C CH$_3$-BECP), 14.3 ppm (C CH$_3$-BECP), 39.5 ppm (C CH$_3$-pyrazolyl), 61.4 ppm (C CH$_2$-BECP), 61.5 ppm (C CH$_2$-BECP), 66.5 ppm (C methylene-BECP), 66.9 ppm (C methylene-BECP), 110.0 ppm (C 2'-BECP), 110.7 ppm

(C 5′-BECP), 113.3 ppm (C 4′-pyrazolyl), 119.1 ppm (C 5,15-*meso*), 121.6 ppm (C 10,20-*meso*), 122.8 ppm (C 6′-BECP), 128.8 ppm (C 5′-pyrazolyl), 131.0 ppm (C β-pyrrole), 134.1 ppm (C 1′-BECP), 136.3 ppm (C 3′-pyrazolyl), 143.7 ppm (C 3′-BECP), 146.1 ppm (C 4′-BECP), 147.9 ppm (C α-pyrrole), 168.8 ppm (C carboxyl-BECP), 169.1 ppm (C carboxyl-BECP). UV/Vis (CH_2Cl_2): 422 nm (B-band), 520, 558, 595, and 653 nm (Q-band). MALDI-TOF LRMS: m/z = 1034.477 $[M + 4H]^{4+}$ (exact mass = 1034.417).

4.3. Cytotoxicity Test

4.3.1. Materials

The human epithelioid cervix carcinoma cell line (HeLa), human ductal breast epithelial tumor cell line (T47D), Michigan Cancer Foundation-7 cell line (MCF-7), human colon carcinoma cell line (WIDR), hepatoblastoma-derived cell line (HepG2), and Vero cell line (derived from kidney of African green monkey) were purchased from ATCC by the Faculty of Medicine Gadjah Mada University. The cell lines were cultured in Dulbecco's Modified Eagle Medium (DMEM, Gibco), except for Vero cell line, which was cultured in Medium-199 (M-199, Gibco). Other chemicals, i.e., potassium dihydrogen phosphate, sodium chloride, potassium chloride, sodium hydrogen phosphate, dimethyl sulfoxide, sodium dodecyl sulphate, HEPES, sodium bicarbonate, and 3-(4,5-dimetiltiazol-2-il)-2,5-difeniltetrazolium bromide (MTT) were purchased from Sigma-Aldrich. Fetal bovine serum, trypsin-EDTA 0.25%, and penicillin-streptomycin were purchased from Gibco, whereas Amphotericin B was purchased from Caisson. Phosphate-buffered saline (PBS) was obtained by mixing 0.2 g of KH_2PO_4, 8 g of NaCl, 0.2 g of KCl, 1.15 g of Na_2HPO_4, and 1 L of distilled water.

4.3.2. Procedure

Confluent cells in the Petri dish was harvested by removing the growth media in Petri dish and adding 1 mL of trypsin-EDTA 0.025%. Then the cells was incubated at incubator 37 °C, 5% CO_2 for about three minutes. The suspension of cells was put in centrifuge tube, 2 mL of growth media was added with 7 mL of PBS. The mixture was centrifuged for 10 min at 1200 rpm. The supernatant was separated and 2–3 mL of growth media was added to the pellet cell for counting cell. The cell suspense was cultured in 96-well plates (10,000 cells/well). After 24 h, the porphyrin derivative compounds with series concentration were added to treat the cell cultures for another 24 h. The cells were treated by MTT solution for four hours at incubator (37 °C, 5% CO_2) and the reaction was stopped by stopper solution (SDS 10% HCl). The plate was incubated at room temperature in dark condition for 24 h. The living cells were counted by reading the absorbance at 595 nm. The corresponding IC_{50} values were calculated using non-linear regression analysis (GraphPad Prism 7.0.3). Each test was run in triplicate.

5. Conclusions

In silico study confirmed that DBECPDPzP has good interaction with the REV-ERβ receptor with a binding free energy of −276.46 kJ/mol, while TrTMNP showed appropriate interaction toward CAIX with a binding free energy of −15.50 kJ/mol. Five known porphyrin derivatives and three novel porphyrin derivatives have been successfully synthesized by the Alder method and their structures were confirmed. Cytotoxicity test against five cancer cell lines (HeLa, WIDR, T47D, MCF-7, HepG2) and the normal cell (Vero cell line) revealed that all studied porphyrins are categorized as marginally-active compounds with IC_{50} lower than 1.5 mM, except for TrTMNP against T47D cell line. It was observed that all of the porphyrins showed a selective anti-proliferation activity to cancer cells than to normal cells, except for cDBECPDPzP and DBECPDPzP to the HeLa cell line. The results obtained proved the necessity for further detailed biological investigation for studied porphyrins that showed low IC_{50}.

Acknowledgments: FK wishes to thank PMDSU and PKPI Scholarship 2016 from the Ministry of Research, Technology, and Higher Education (MRTHE), the Republic of Indonesia. This research was financially supported by Hibah PMDSU 2016 and Riset Unggulan Perguruan Tinggi 2016 and 2017 from MRTHE (D.H.T).

Author Contributions: D.H.T. conceived and designed the experiments, analyzed the data, and corrected manuscript; F.K. performed the experiments, collected the data, and drafted the manuscript; Y.M. supported the synthesis work; R.E.K. and A.M. analyzed the data; and N.Y. analyzed the data and corrected the manuscript.

References

1. Seyfried, T.N.; Flores, R.E.; Poff, A.M.; Agostino, D.P.D. Cancer as a metabolic disease: Implications for novel therapeutics. *Carcinogenesis* **2014**, *35*, 515–527. [CrossRef] [PubMed]

2. Siegel, R.L.; Miller, K.D.; Jemal, A. Cancer Statistics, 2017. *CA Cancer J. Clin.* **2017**, *67*, 7–30. [CrossRef] [PubMed]

3. Wu, L.; Qu, X. Cancer biomarker detection: Recent achievements and challenges. *Chem. Soc. Rev.* **2015**, *44*, 2963–2997. [CrossRef] [PubMed]

4. Richter, M.; Zhang, H. Receptor-Targeted Cancer Therapy. *DNA Cell Biol.* **2005**, *24*, 271–282. [CrossRef] [PubMed]

5. Mei, C.D.; Ercolani, L.; Parodi, C.; Veronesi, M.; Vecchio, C.L.; Bottegoni, G.; Torrente, E.; Scarpelli, R.; Marotta, R.; Ruffili, R.; et al. Dual inhibition of REV-ERBβ and autophagy as a novel pharmacological approach to induce cytotoxicity in cancer cells. *Oncogene* **2015**, *34*, 2597–2608. [CrossRef] [PubMed]

6. Nógrádi, A. The Role of Carbonic Anhydrases in Tumors. *Am. J. Pathol.* **1998**, *153*, 1–4. [CrossRef]

7. Maren, T.H. Carbonic anhydrase: Chemistry, physiology and inhibition. *Physiol. Rev.* **1967**, *47*, 595–743. [CrossRef] [PubMed]

8. Tashian, R.E. The carbonic anhydrases: Widening perspectives on their evolution, expression and function. *BioEssays* **1989**, *10*, 186–192. [CrossRef] [PubMed]

9. Hewett-Emmett, D.; Tashian, R.E. Functional diversity, conservation, and convergence in the evolution of the a-, b-, and g-carbonic anhydrase gene family. *Mol. Phylogenet. Evol.* **1996**, *5*, 50–77. [CrossRef] [PubMed]

10. Sly, W.S.; Hu, P.Y. Human carbonic anhydrases and carbonic anhydrase deficiencies. *Annu. Rev. Biochem.* **1995**, *64*, 375–401. [CrossRef] [PubMed]

11. Závada, J.; Závadová, Z.; Pastoreková, S.; Čiampor, F.; Pastorek, J.; Zelnik, V. Expression of MaTu-MN protein in human tumor cultures and in clinical specimens. *Int. J. Cancer* **1993**, *54*, 268–274. [CrossRef] [PubMed]

12. Stanbridge, E.J.; Der, C.J.; Doersen, C.-J.; Nishimi, R.Y.; Peehl, D.M.; Weissman, B.E.; Wilkinson, J.E. Human cell hybrids: Analysis of transformation and tumorigenicity. *Science* **1982**, *215*, 252–259. [CrossRef] [PubMed]

13. Liao, S.Y.; Brewer, C.; Závada, J.; Pastorek, J.; Pastoreková, S.; Manetta, A.; Berman, M.L.; DiSaia, P.J.; Stanbridge, E.J. Identification of the MN antigen as a diagnostic biomarker of cervical intraepithal squamous and glandular neoplasia and cervical carcinomas. *Am. J. Pathol.* **1994**, *145*, 598–609. [PubMed]

14. Schernhammer, E.S.; Laden, F.; Speizer, F.E.; Willett, W.C.; Hunter, D.J.; Kawachi, I.; Colditz, G.A. Rotating night shifts and risk of breast cancer in women participating in the nurses' health study. *J. Natl. Cancer Inst.* **2001**, *93*, 1563–1568. [CrossRef] [PubMed]

15. Schernhammer, E.S.; Laden, F.; Speizer, F.E.; Willett, W.C.; Hunter, D.J.; Kawachi, I.; Fuchs, C.S.; Colditz, G.A. Night-shift work and risk of colorectal cancer in the Nurses' Health Study. *J. Natl. Cancer Inst.* **2003**, *95*, 825–828. [CrossRef] [PubMed]

16. Megdal, S.P.; Kroenke, C.H.; Laden, F.; Pukkala, E.; Schernhammer, E.S. Night work and breast cancer risk: A systematic review and meta-analysis. *Eur. J. Cancer* **2005**, *41*, 2023–2032. [CrossRef] [PubMed]

17. Hansen, J. Increased breast cancer risk among women who work predominantly at night. *Epidemiology* **2001**, *12*, 74–77. [CrossRef] [PubMed]

18. Wang, Y.; Kojetin, D.; Burris, T.P. Anti-Proliferative Actions of a Synthetic REV-ERBα/β Agonist in Breast Cancer Cell. *Biochem. Pharmacol.* **2015**, *96*, 315–322. [CrossRef] [PubMed]

19. Straif, K.; Baan, R.; Grosse, Y.; Secretan, B.; El Ghissassi, F.; Bouvard, V.; Altieri, A.; Benbrahim-Tallaa, L.; Coglianno, V. Monograpgh WHOIARC, Carcinogenicity of shift-work, painting, and fire-fighting. *Lancet Oncol.* **2007**, *8*, 1065–1066. [CrossRef]

20. Urruticoechea, A.; Alemany, R.; Balart, J.; Villanueva, A.; Vinals, F.; Capella, G. Recent Advances in Cancer Therapy: An Overview. *Curr. Pharm. Des.* **2010**, *16*, 3–10. [CrossRef] [PubMed]

21. Sebastian, R. Nanomedicine-the Future of Cancer Treatment: A review. *J. Cancer Prev. Curr. Res.* **2017**, *8*, 00265. [CrossRef]

22. Tjahjono, D.H.; Akutsu, T.; Yoshioka, N.; Inoue, H. Cationic porphyrins bearing diazolium rings: Synthesis and their interaction with calf thymus DNA. *Biochim. Biophys. Acta* **1999**, *1472*, 333–343. [CrossRef]

23. Tjahjono, D.H.; Yamamoto, T.; Ichimoto, S.; Yoshioka, N.; Inoue, H. Synthesis and DNA-binding properties of bisdiazoliumylporphyrins. *J. Chem. Soc. Perkin Trans.* **2000**, *1*, 3077–3081. [CrossRef]

24. Subbarayan, M.; Shetty, S.J.; Srivastava, T.S.; Noronha, O.P.D.; Samuel, A.M. Evaluation studies of technetium-99m-porphyrin (T3,4BCPP) for tumor imaging. *J. Porphyr. Phthalocyanines* **2001**, *5*, 824–828. [CrossRef]

25. Muttaqin, F.Z. Sintesis, Pelabelan, dan Uji Biodistribusi Meso-5,15-di [3,4-bis (karboksimetilenoksi)fenil] Porfirin dan Meso-5,15-di [3,4-bis (karboksimetilenoksi) fenil], 10,20-Difenil Porfirin Sebagai Ligan Radiofarmaka Teranostik. Ph.D. Thesis, Sekolah Farmasi Institut Teknologi Bandung, Bandung, Indonesia, 2014.

26. Jia, Z.; Deng, H.; Luo, S. Rhenium-labelled meso-tetrakis [3,4-bis (carboxymethyleneoxy)phenyl] porphyrin for Targeted Radiotheraphy : Preliminary Biological Evaluation in Mice. *Eur. J. Nucl. Med. Mol. Imaging* **2008**, *35*, 734–742. [CrossRef] [PubMed]

27. Izbicka, E.; Wheelhouse, R.T.; Raymond, E.; Davidson, K.K.; Lawrence, R.A.; Sun, D.Y.; Windle, B.E.; Hurley, L.H.; von Hoff, D.D. Effect of Cationic Porphyrins as G-quadruplex Interactive Agents in Human Tumor Cells. *Cancer Res.* **1999**, *59*, 639–644. [PubMed]

28. Hurley, L.H.; Wheelhouse, R.T.; Sun, D.; Kerwin, S.M.; Salazar, M.; Fedoroff, O.Y.; Han, F.X.; Izbicka, E.; von Hoff, D.D. G-quadruplex as Targets for Drug Design. *Pharmacol. Ther.* **2000**, *85*, 141–158. [CrossRef]

29. Kuhn, B.; Kollman, P.A. A Binding of diverse set of ligands to avidin and streptavidin: An accurate quantitative prediction of their relative affinities by a combination of molecular mechanics and continuum solvent models. *J. Med. Chem.* **2000**, *43*, 3786–3791. [CrossRef] [PubMed]

30. Ferrari, A.M.; Degliesposti, G.; Sgobba, M.; Rastelli, G. Validation of an automated procedure for the prediction of relative free energies of binding on a set of aldose reductase inhibitors. *Bioorg. Med. Chem.* **2007**, *15*, 7865–7877. [CrossRef] [PubMed]

31. Arba, M.; Tjahjono, D.H. The binding modes of cationic porphyrin-anthraquinone hybrids to DNA duplexes: In silico study. *J. Biomol. Struct. Dyn.* **2015**, *33*, 657–665. [CrossRef] [PubMed]

32. Adler, A.D.; Longo, F.R.; Finarelli, J.D.; Assour, J.; Korsakoff, L. A simplified synthesis for meso-tetraphenylporphine. *J. Org. Chem.* **1967**, *32*, 476. [CrossRef]

33. Ni, J.; Auston, D.A.; Freilich, D.A.; Muralidharan, S.; Sobie, E.A.; Kao, J.P.Y. Photochemical Gating of Intracellular Ca^{2+} Release Channel. *J. Am. Chem. Soc.* **2007**, *129*, 5316–5317. [CrossRef] [PubMed]

34. Mysinger, M.M.; Carchia, M.; Irwin, J.J.; Shoichet, B.K. Directory of Useful Decoys, Enhanced (DUD-E): Better Ligands and Decoys for Better Benchmarking. *J. Med. Chem.* **2012**, *55*, 6582–6594. [CrossRef] [PubMed]

35. Dodoff, N.I.; Iordanov, I.; Tsoneva, I.; Grancharov, K.; Detcheva, R.; Pajpanova, T.; Berger, M.R. Cytotoxic Activity of Platinum(II) and Palladium(II) Complexes of N-3-Pyridinylmethanesulfonamide: The Influence of Electroporation. *Z. Naturforsch. C* **2009**, *64*, 179–185. [CrossRef] [PubMed]

36. Pastorekova, S.; Zavadova, Z.; Kostal, M.; Babusikova, O.; Zavada, J. A novel quasi-viral agent, MaTu, is a two-component system. *Virology* **1992**, *187*, 620–626. [CrossRef]

37. McDonald, P.C.; Winum, J.; Supuran, C.T.; Dedhar, S. Recent Development in Targeting Carbonic Anhydrase IX for Cancer Therapeutics. *Oncotarget* **2012**, *3*, 84–97. [CrossRef] [PubMed]

38. Frisch, M.J.; Trucks, G.W.; Schlegel, H.B.; Scuseria, G.E.; Robb, M.A.; Cheeseman, J.R.; Scalmani, G.; Barone, V.; Mennucci, B.; Petersson, G.A.; et al. *Gaussian 09*, revision C.01; Gaussian, Inc.: Wallingford, CT, USA, 2010.

39. Goodsell, D.S.; Morris, G.M.; Olson, A.J. Automated docking of flexible ligands: Applications of autodock. *J. Mol. Recogn.* **1996**, *9*, 1–5. [CrossRef]

40. Morris, G.M.; Goodsell, D.S.; Halliday, R.S.; Huey, R.; Hart, W.E.; Belew, R.K.; Olson, A.J. Automated docking using a Lamarckian genetic algorithm and an empirical binding free energy function. *J. Comput. Chem.* **1998**, *19*, 1639–1662. [CrossRef]

41. *AutoDockTools*, version 1.5.6; The Scripps Research Institute: La Jolla, CA, USA, 2015.

42. Humphrey, W.; Dalke, A.; Schulten, K. VMD: Visual molecular dynamics. *J. Mol. Graph.* **1996**, *14*, 33–38. [CrossRef]

43. *Dassault Systemes BIOVIA, Discovery Studio Modeling Environment, Release 2017*; Dassault Systemes: San Diego, CA, USA, 2016.

44. Berendsen, H.J.C.; van der Spoel, D.; van Drunen, R. GROMACS: A message-passing parallel molecular dynamics implementation. *Comput. Phys. Commun.* **1995**, *91*, 43–56. [CrossRef]

45. Lindahl, E.; Hess, B.; van der Spoel, D. GROMACS 3.0: A package for molecular simulation and trajectory analysis. *J. Mol. Mod.* **2001**, *7*, 306–317. [CrossRef]

46. van der Spoel, D.; Lindahl, E.; Hess, B.; Groenhof, G.; Mark, A.E.; Berendsen, H.J.C. GROMACS: Fast, Flexible and Free. *J. Comput. Chem.* **2005**, *26*, 1701–1719. [CrossRef] [PubMed]

47. Hess, B.; Kutzner, C.; van der Spoel, D.; Lindahl, E. GROMACS 4: Algorithms for highly efficient, load-balanced, and scalable molecular simulation. *J. Chem. Theory Comput.* **2008**, *4*, 435–447. [CrossRef] [PubMed]

48. Pronk, S.; Páll, S.; Schulz, R.; Larsson, P.; Bjelkmar, P.; Apostolov, R.; Shirts, M.R.; Smith, J.C.; Kasson, P.M.; van der Spoel, D.; et al. GROMACS 4.5: A high-throughput and highly parallel open source molecular simulation toolkit. *Bioinformatics* **2013**, *29*, 845–854. [CrossRef] [PubMed]

49. Abraham, M.J.; Murtola, T.; Schulz, R.; Páll, S.; Smith, J.C.; Hess, B.; Lindahl, E. GROMACS: High performance molecular simulations through multi-level parallelism from laptops to supercomputers. *SoftwareX* **2015**, *1*, 19–25. [CrossRef]

50. Páll, S.; Abraham, M.J.; Kutzner, C.; Hess, B.; Lindahl, E. Tackling Exascale Software Challenges in Molecular Dynamics Simulations with GROMACS. *Solving Softw. Chall. Exascale* **2015**, *8759*, 3–27.

51. Aliev, A.E.; Kulke, M.; Khaneja, H.S.; Chudasama, V.; Sheppard, T.D.; Lanigan, R.M. Motional timescale predictions by molecular dynamics simulations: Case study using proline and hydroxyproline sidechain dynamics. *Proteins* **2014**, *82*, 195–215. [CrossRef] [PubMed]

52. Da Silva, A.W.S.; Vranken, W.F. ACPYPE—AnteChamber Python Parser interface. *BMC Res. Notes* **2012**, *5*, 367. [CrossRef] [PubMed]

53. Darden, T.; York, D.; Pedersen, L. Particle mesh Ewald—An NlogN method for Ewald sums in large systems. *J. Chem. Phys.* **1993**, *98*, 10089–10092. [CrossRef]

54. Essmann, U.; Perera, L.; Berkowitz, M.L.; Darden, T.; Lee, H.; Pedersen, L.G. A smooth particle mesh Ewald method. *J. Chem. Phys.* **1995**, *103*, 8577–8593. [CrossRef]

55. Baker, N.A.; Sept, D.; Joseph, S.; Holst, M.J.; McCammon, J.A. Electrostatics of nanosystems: Application to microtubules and the ribosome. *Proc. Natl. Acad. Sci. USA* **2001**, *98*, 10037–10041. [CrossRef] [PubMed]

56. Kumari, R.; Kumar, R.; Open Source Drug Discovery Consortium; Lynn, A. g_mmpbsa—A GROMACS Tool for High-Throughput MM-PBSA Calculations. *J. Chem. Inf. Model.* **2014**, *54*, 1951–1962. [CrossRef] [PubMed]

57. Hou, J.Q.; Chen, S.B.; Tan, J.H.; Ou, T.M.; Luo, H.B.; Li, D.; Xu, J.; Gu, L.Q.; Huang, Z.S. New Insights into the structures of ligand-quadruplex complexes from molecular dynamics simulations. *J. Phys. Chem. B* **2010**, *114*, 15301–15310. [CrossRef] [PubMed]

58. Špačková, N.; Cheatham, T.E., III; Ryjáček, F.; Lankaš, F.; van Meervelt, L.; Hobza, P.; Šponer, J. Molecular dynamics simulations and thermodynamics analysis of DNA—drug complexes. Minor groove binding between 4′,6-diamidino-2-phenylindole and DNA duplexes in solution. *J. Am. Chem. Soc.* **2003**, *125*, 1759–1769.

59. Sun, Z.; She, Y.; Zhou, Y.; Song, X.; Li, K. Synthesis, Characterization and Spectral Properties of Substituted Tetraphenylporphyrin Iron Chloride Complexes. *Molecules* **2011**, *16*, 2960–2970. [CrossRef] [PubMed]

60. Liu, X.; Xu, Y.; Guo, Z.; Nagai, A.; Jiang, D. Super absorbent conjugated microporous polymers: A synergistic structural effect on the exceptional uptake of amines. *Chem. Commun.* **2013**, *49*, 3233–3235. [CrossRef] [PubMed]

61. Ormond, A.B.; Freemand, H.S. Effects of substituents on the photophysical properties of symmetrical porphyrins. *Dyes Pigments* **2013**, *96*, 440–448. [CrossRef]

62. Sol, V.; Blais, J.C.; Carre, V.; Granet, R.; Guilloton, M.; Spiro, M.; Krausz, P. Synthesis, Spectroscopy, and Photocytotoxicity of Glycosylated Amino Acid Porphyrin Derivatives as Promising Molecules for Cancer Phototherapy. *J. Org. Chem.* **1999**, *64*, 4431–4444. [CrossRef]

63. Finar, I.L.; Lord, G.H. The formylation of the pyrazole nucleus. *J. Chem. Soc.* **1957**, *0*, 3314–3315. [CrossRef]

12

Looking for Novel Capsid Protein Multimerization Inhibitors of Feline Immunodeficiency Virus

Natalia Sierra [1], Christelle Folio [2], Xavier Robert [2] (iD), Mathieu Long [2], Christophe Guillon [2,*] (iD) and Guzmán Álvarez [1,*] (iD)

[1] Laboratorio de Moléculas Bioactivas, CENUR Litoral Norte, Universidad de la República, Ruta 3 (km 363), Paysandú C.P. 60000, Uruguay; nataliasierraben@gmail.com

[2] Equipe Rétrovirus et Biochimie Structurale, Université de Lyon, CNRS, MMSB, UMR 5086 CNRS/Université de Lyon, IBCP, C.P. 69367 Lyon, France; folio.christelle@gmail.com (C.F.); xavier.robert@ibcp.fr (X.R.); mathieu.long@ibcp.fr (M.L.)

* Correspondence: christophe.guillon@ibcp.fr (C.G.); guzmanalvarezlqo@gmail.com (G.Á.)

Abstract: Feline immunodeficiency virus (FIV) is a member of the retroviridae family of viruses. It causes acquired immunodeficiency syndrome (AIDS) in worldwide domestic and non-domestic cats and is a cause of an important veterinary issue. The genome organization of FIV and the clinical characteristics of the disease caused by FIV are similar to human immunodeficiency virus (HIV). Both viruses infect T lymphocytes, monocytes, and macrophages, with a similar replication cycle in infected cells. Thus, the infection of cats with FIV is also a useful tool for the study and development of novel drugs and vaccines against HIV. Anti-retroviral drugs studied extensively with regards to HIV infection have targeted different steps of the virus replication cycle: (1) disruption of the interaction with host cell surface receptors and co-receptors; (2) inhibition of fusion of the virus and cell membranes; (3) blocking of the reverse transcription of viral genomic RNA; (4) interruption of nuclear translocation and integration of viral DNA into host genomes; (5) prevention of viral transcript processing and nuclear export; and (6) inhibition of virion assembly and maturation. Despite the great success of anti-retroviral therapy in slowing HIV progression in humans, a similar therapy has not been thoroughly investigated for FIV infection in cats, mostly because of the little structural information available for FIV proteins. The FIV capsid protein (CA) drives the assembly of the viral particle, which is a critical step in the viral replication cycle. During this step, the CA protein oligomerizes to form a protective coat that surrounds the viral genome. In this work, we perform a large-scale screening of four hundred molecules from our in-house library using an in vitro assembly assay of p24, combined with microscale thermophoresis, to estimate binding affinity. This screening led to the discovery of around four novel hits that inhibited capsid assembly in vitro. These may provide new antiviral drugs against FIV.

Keywords: assembly inhibitors; immunodeficiency virus; microscale thermophoresis

1. Introduction

Since its first isolation in 1986, feline immunodeficiency virus (FIV) has been observed worldwide, and FIV infection remains a major health problem among cats, especially in countries with large populations of free-roaming cats [1]. FIV is a lentivirus which causes an immunodeciency syndrome in cats and all the members of the *Felidae* family [2]. FIV closely resembles the human immunodeficiency virus (HIV) in its genomic, biochemical, and morphologic characteristics, as well as clinical and hematological manifestations [3]. As a result, FIV infection of domestic cats is dubbed "feline AIDS" and is considered to be an excellent small animal model for testing prophylactic and therapeutic strategies against human AIDS [4]. A number of antiretroviral drugs for HIV-1, including the prototype nucleoside analogue 3′-azido-3′-deoxythymidine (AZT), have been tested using the FIV model [5]. Several reports have described the in vitro inhibition of FIV by nucleoside-analogue reverse transcriptase inhibitors, such as AZT and 9-(2-phosphonomethoxyethyl)adenine. Moreover, some 4-amino-3,6-disulphonato-1,8-naphthalimide derivatives, such as dextran sulphate, pradimicin A, heparin, phosphonoformate, 2′3′-dideoxythymidine, 2′3′-dideoxyadenosine, and 2′3′-dideoxyinosine, have also been shown to have in vitro activity against FIV in various assays [6]. However, to date, no efficient drug or vaccine for FIV infection has been brought to the market [7].

Recent progress in the combination therapy of several antiretroviral drugs, such as the highly active antiretroviral therapy, has achieved long-term control of HIV replication in vivo [8] and clinical outcome is improved when plasma viral burden is reduced [9]. In the treatment of humans with AIDS, specific targeting of HIV is important. Single-agent treatments are no longer recommended for the treatment of HIV-infected individuals because it promotes the rapid emergence of mutated HIV strains which become resistant to the antiviral agent. Highly active antiretroviral therapy of HIV-infected patients involves the administration of combinations of antiviral drugs from different drug classes, resulting in a slower occurrence of resistant strains [10]. To our knowledge, combination treatment with drugs from different drug classes has not been assessed in FIV-infected cats. This is mainly due to the fact that, despite similarities between the HIV-1 and FIV proteases, all but one of the currently available HIV-1 protease inhibitors failed to inhibit the protease of FIV [11] because of structural differences around the active site [12].

Virion assembly in lentiviruses is the result of a series of steps driven by the multimerization of the structural polyprotein Gag at the plasma membrane of the infected cell. Indeed, the intrinsic biological property of Gag to self-assemble into spherical virus-like particles both in cell cultures or in vitro systems is well documented [4,13,14]. Within the virion, the viral capsid is the protein shell that contains the viral ribonucleoprotein complex, which consists of genomic RNA, nucleocapsid protein, reverse transcriptase, and integrase. Being a lentivirus, lentiviral capsids are conical in shape and consist of a polymer of a single viral protein, the capsid protein (p24 or CA). As in the case of HIV, FIV is assembled as an immature particle, in which CA is released from the Gag polyprotein during proteolytic cleavage by the viral protease and maturation of the particles. After release, CA self-assembles to form the final closed conical structure [15]. Despite that, the CA of FIV represents an interesting therapeutic target which has not yet been exploited.

The viral capsid plays a crucial role in the first steps of the retroviral infection, including reverse transcription, entry to the nucleus, and integration. In HIV-1, most amino acid substitutions in CA that disrupt the structure and/or stability of the capsid are detrimental to the infection [16,17]. Several host factors interact with CA, and amino-acid substitutions or chemical inhibitors that disrupt these interactions can inhibit HIV infection [18,19]. For example, inhibitors of HIV-1 PF74 and BI-2 (Figure 1D) bind to a pocket between the N-terminal (NTD) and C-terminal (CTD) domains of CA and prevent interactions of the viral capsid with cellular proteins CPSF6 and Nup153 [20–23]. Additionally, compounds or peptides such as CAP-1 or NYAD-1 (Figure 1B,D), which prevent the formation of the mature functional viral capsid, inhibit the replication of the virus [23–25]. An interesting feature of the CA protein as a pharmacological target is its highly conserved sequence in the circulating strains of infected individuals, resulting in a low propensity to develop resistance [26,27]. On the other hand, the inhibitory effect of compound C (Figure 1C) can be reversed with a simple substitution of an amino acid at the N-terminal compound binding site of CA. Thus, the binding site in CA is important because some areas seem more vulnerable to mutations with the concomitant loss of binding to the compound [17]. In another way, inhibition of the capsid assembly acting on DNA control, as done by the drug Bevirimat, produces non-infective viral particles (Figure 1F) [9].

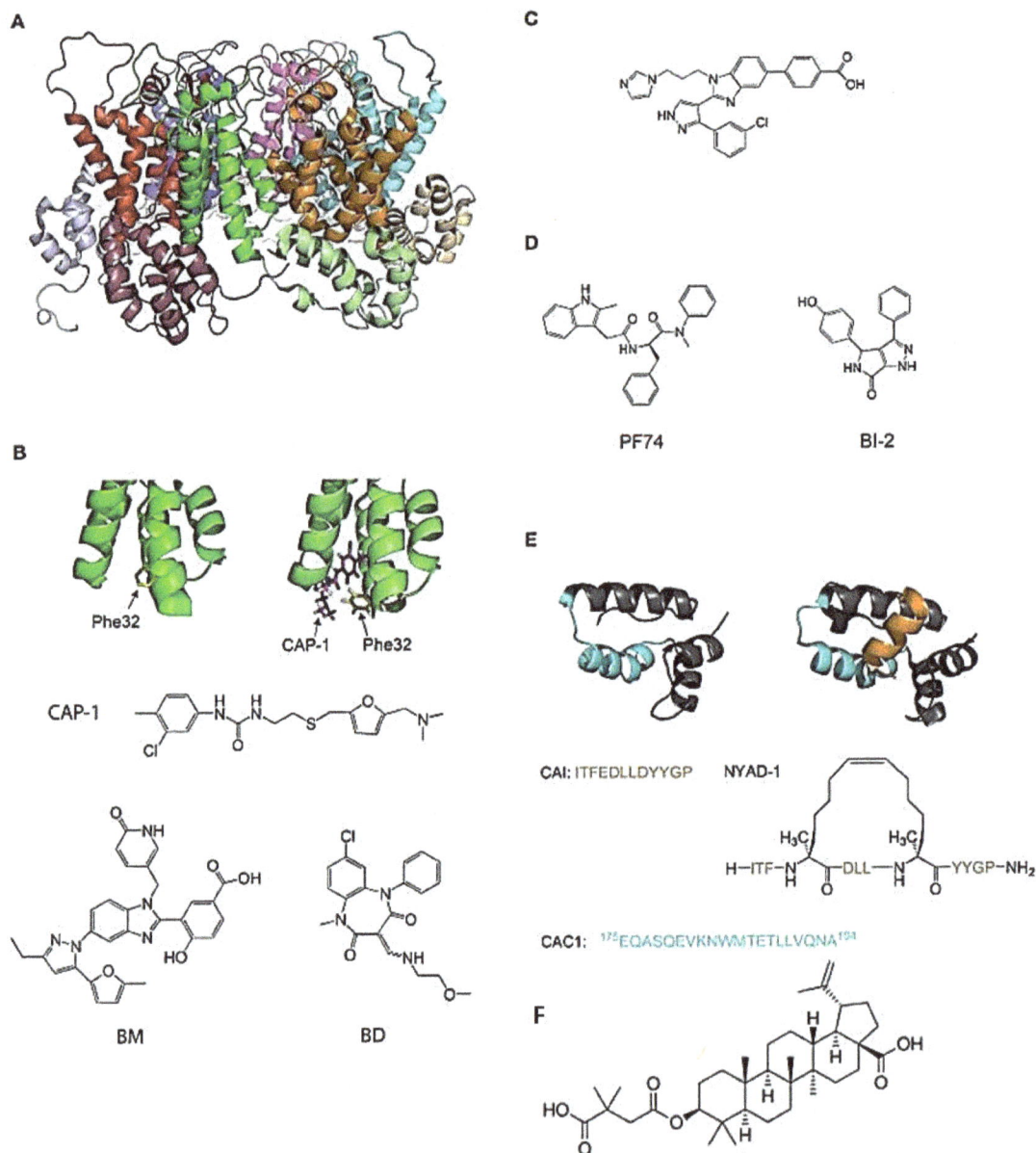

Figure 1. Molecules which inhibit the assembly of HIV-1 viral capsid [16]. (**A**) The structure of the hexamer of the HIV-1 CA protein (PDB ID: 1VUU). The different monomers are green, red, blue, magenta, cyan, and orange. The NTD and the CTD of each monomer are in different shades of the same color; (**B**) The structure of HIV-1 p24 NTD in the absence (**left**) and presence (**right**) of CAP-1. Phe32 is shown in yellow. CAP-1 is shown in magenta (PDB IDs: 1VUU and 2JPR); (**C**) Formula of the CA-binding compound described by Lemke et al. [26]; (**D**) Formula of the CA-binding compounds PF74 and BI-2; (**E**) Structure of the CA protein of HIV-1 CTD in the absence (**left**) and presence (**right**) of the capsid pool inhibitor (CAI, orange). The helix from which the CAC1 peptide was derived is cyan. The sequence of CAI and the structure of the optimized peptide NYAD-1 are given below (PDB IDs: 1AUM and 2BUO); (**F**) The structure of the Bevirimat [9].

In this work we performed a large screening of around four hundred molecules from our in-house library to identify leads of compounds blocking the assembly of FIV CA. We used an in vitro assembly assay of CA, combined with microscale thermophoresis, to estimate binding affinity, and we used docking studies to get a hint into the protein compounds interfaces. This led to the identification of several lead compounds which warrant further investigation for the development process of new anti-FIV drugs.

2. Results and Discussion

2.1. Our In-House Library

Most of the compounds tested in this study were synthetized previously as part of our ongoing program in drug development for the Chagas disease and other human diseases, such as cancer and aging disease. This resulted in a library containing, to date, more than 2000 compounds [28–30]. We selected some compounds which harbored structural similarity with the reported HIV-1 p24 assembly inhibitors, as well as compounds randomly selected to representing all of the chemical families present in our library (Figure 2). A database with all the compounds from our library was generated using the ChemOffice® 12.0 software package (Cambridge, MA, USA). Then, structural similarities with known HIV capsid inhibitors were estimated using the ChemFinder tool from ChemOffice®. For the selection process, we used a structural similarity criteria of 80% with the reported inhibitor of CA as a search filter (Supplementary Figure S1). As an example, this resulted in the identification of 18 molecules from our library which harbor 80% similarity with the CAP-1 HIV-1 inhibitor (Figure 1), from which the compound with the best score was selected [9,22–24,31–33]. The random selection of the other compounds was performed based on several criteria: abundance of the compound, solubility, cost-effective synthetic procedures, and compounds with toxicology data. The structural details of the selected molecules are in Table S1 (Supporting Information), with some examples in Figure 2, and include families like benzofuroxanes, furanes and thiophenes, 4-substituted-1,2,6-thiadiazines and its synthetic precursors, quinoxaline 1,4-dioxides, phenazine 5,9-dioxides, furoxanes, imidazole N-oxide, indazoles, thiazoles, 1,2,4-triazine N-oxides, flavonoids, nitroalkenes, and others.

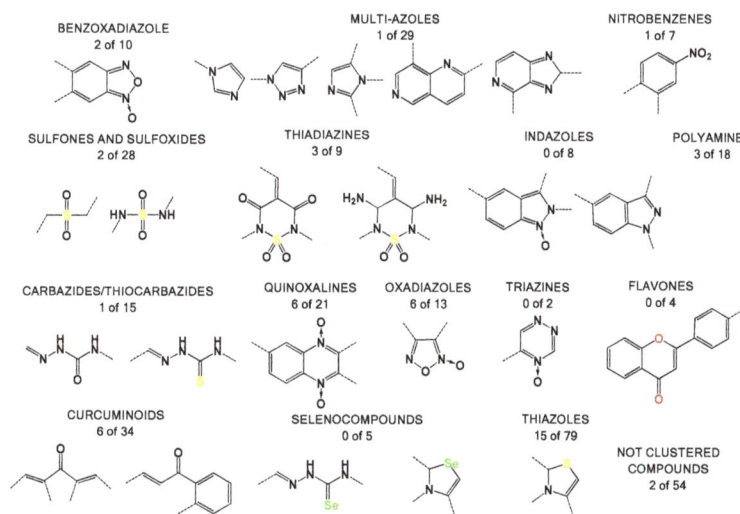

Figure 2. Representation of the compound families used in this work. There are 15 clustered families and 54 compounds with high diversity of structures. The numbers below the families' names are the molecules with inhibitory effects in our assembly assay versus the total molecules of the family that we tested (see below). For example, we identified two molecules of the benzoxadiazole family which inhibit in vitro assembly out of the 10 molecules tested.

2.2. In Vitro Assembly Studies

To find novel chemical structures as a backbone for the design of new antiviral drugs targeting the capsid assembly of the virus, we optimized a CA assembly in vitro assay for screening purposes [34].

Indeed, our initial assay used light scattering and could only monitor the assembly of one sample per experiment on 40 min kinetics [35]. This resulted in using almost 20 mg of protein in a 14 h period to test 10 compounds, in duplicate, using light scattering, which was not adequate for screening methods. The use of the spectrometric technique to follow capsid assembly has been described for

HIV [24] and is based on the detection of capsid assembly via the measurement of the increase of medium turbidity. The use of this technique to monitor FIV p24 assembly allowed us to use 384-well plates, reducing the volume of protein to 15 µL per sample and allowing a testing of 10 compounds, in duplicate, in 40 min. Moreover, in this format, the protein concentration (5 mg/mL) was enough to start the assembly without needing the high concentration of salt used in the HIV in vitro assembly assay. High salt concentration could cause a problem by interfering with the solvation and solubility of some molecules and the loss of their interaction with the target. The only limitation of this method using low volumes was the risk of introducing air bubbles in the reaction, which interfere negatively in the absorbance measurement. However, this issue was solved by a careful manipulation in the filling process of the plates.

The most important limitations in screening our compounds in the assembly assay were the dimethyl sulfoxide (DMSO) concentration. In the case of the CA assembly, the maximal concentration of DMSO was 0.25–0.5% v/v. This makes sense because the assembly process depends on a weak interaction of the protein surface. As DMSO is a surfactant, presence of DMSO might "solubilize" the CA monomers. However, this maximal DMSO concentration is too low for several lipophilic molecules, and many molecules could not be tested for that reason. To get better solubility, we replaced DMSO with glycerol for some compounds which, in some cases, was useful but was not sufficient to solubilize some compounds.

With this spectrometric assembly assay, we were able to discriminate two different behaviors for compounds interfering with the assembly of FIV CA: the enhancement of the assembly or its inhibition. The enhancement of assembly is associated with an increase of the diameter of the assembled objects and could result in a disordered or altered capsid with a loss of function. Inhibition is the classical effect which would impair the formation of the capsid (Figure 3).

The compounds were selected as an active compound when the inhibition of the assembly process was more than 40% at 50 or 25 µM. The oxadiazoles family was the most active, with 50% of its members showing assembly inhibition activity. High nitrogen content heretocycles were not a good source of bioactive molecules. Some compounds with structural similarities with Bevirimat were also active, like some steroid compounds clustered in diverse families. The thiazoles family shows several active compounds, but these are highly diverse and do not show a structural correlation between them. On the other hand, compounds of the thiadiazine family showed active molecules with structures that are closely correlated. We could not find active molecules in four families (i.e., selenium containing compounds, flavones, triazines, and indazoles).

The dose response could not be calculated with this method. To confirm the interaction of our compound with FIV CA and get a dose response, we performed microscale thermophoresis (MST) to confirm the interaction of the active compounds and their affinity for CA.

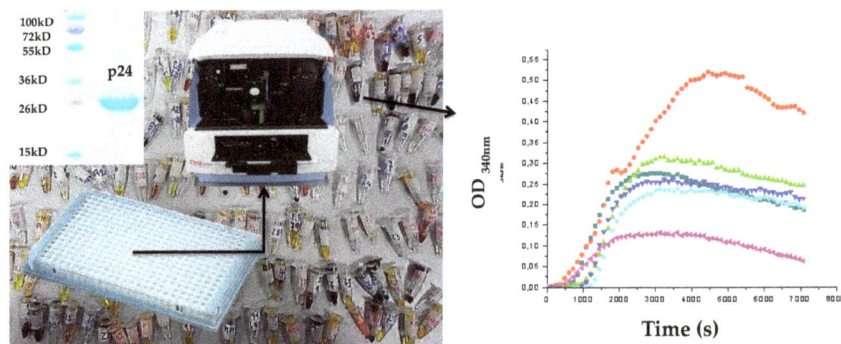

Figure 3. Left panel: general representation of the optimized screening in the assembly assay. Purity of p24 is shown in the inset. Right panel: two discriminable behaviors are visible compared to the control (in dark blue). In red is the enhancement of the process, and in pink is the inhibition of the process. The green and light blue curves are typical for compounds with no effect on the p24 assembly.

2.3. Microscale Thermophoresis Studies

For the active compounds selected from the screening, we checked the binding affinity using MST (Figure 4). Microscale thermophoresis can cope with the presence of 5% of DMSO, resolving the solubility problems that we encountered in the assembly assay for some compounds. Another advantage of MST is that it uses low concentrations of protein (in the nanomolar range), which could be better in analyzing the interaction process because the compound/protein ratios were inverted compared to the assembly assay. The major disadvantage of this method is the interference of the compound with the measurement, either by autofluorescence or quenching. However, from the 48 active compounds which we identified by spectrometric methods, we confirmed using MST that 14 compounds bind to p24 (Figure 5).

We explored the binding affinity at two different times (10 and 60 min) to enhance the poetical interactions. There is a correlation between the time and the binding potency for some of the molecules. The most active compound was thiazole **1136** with an EC_{50} of 83 µM, in comparison with the affinity of one of the first reported assembly inhibitor of HIV-1 compounds, CAP-1 (EC_{50} = 60 µM), which was active in the in vitro infection assay with HIV-1 at 100 µM [24].

A structure motif was repeated in some active molecules, such as carboxylic groups and sulfoxides, granting a further analysis of these families of molecules. These 14 compounds were validated again in our assembly assay by light scattering and spectrophotometry. From these, four molecules were validated with a binding affinity to CA and inhibition of the assembly: compounds **878**, **1136**, **1246**, and **1310** (Figure 5B). Also interestingly, these same molecules were used in the screening of five different enzymes from pathogen parasites but did not display inhibitory effects at 100 µM [36,37], suggesting that our compounds are not unspecific interactors.

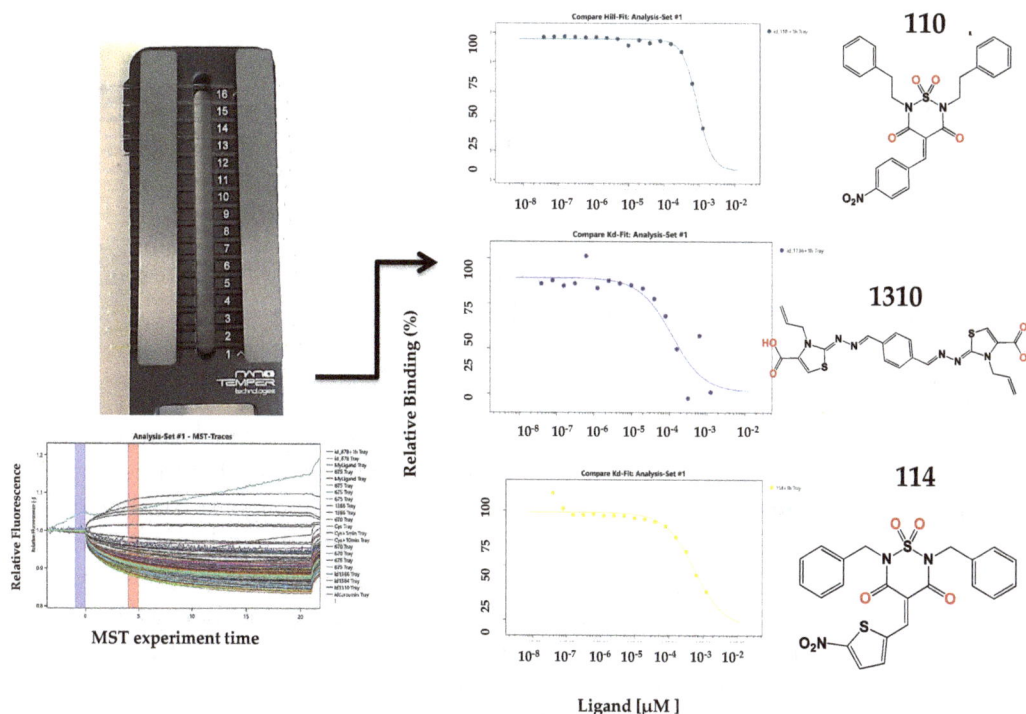

Figure 4. Left panel: schematic representation of the MST assay. It is the cassette with 16 capillary spaces to get 16 points in the doses response assay. On the right are some of the results obtained.

(A)

1136
Binding +
10 min EC$_{50}$ 212μM
1h EC$_{50}$ 83 μM

878
Binding +
10 min EC$_{50}$ 119 μM
1h EC$_{50}$ 166 μM

1246
Binding +
10 min EC$_{50}$ 390 μM
1h EC$_{50}$ 239 μM

1310
Binding +
10 min EC$_{50}$ 655 μM
1h EC$_{50}$ 670 μM

(B)

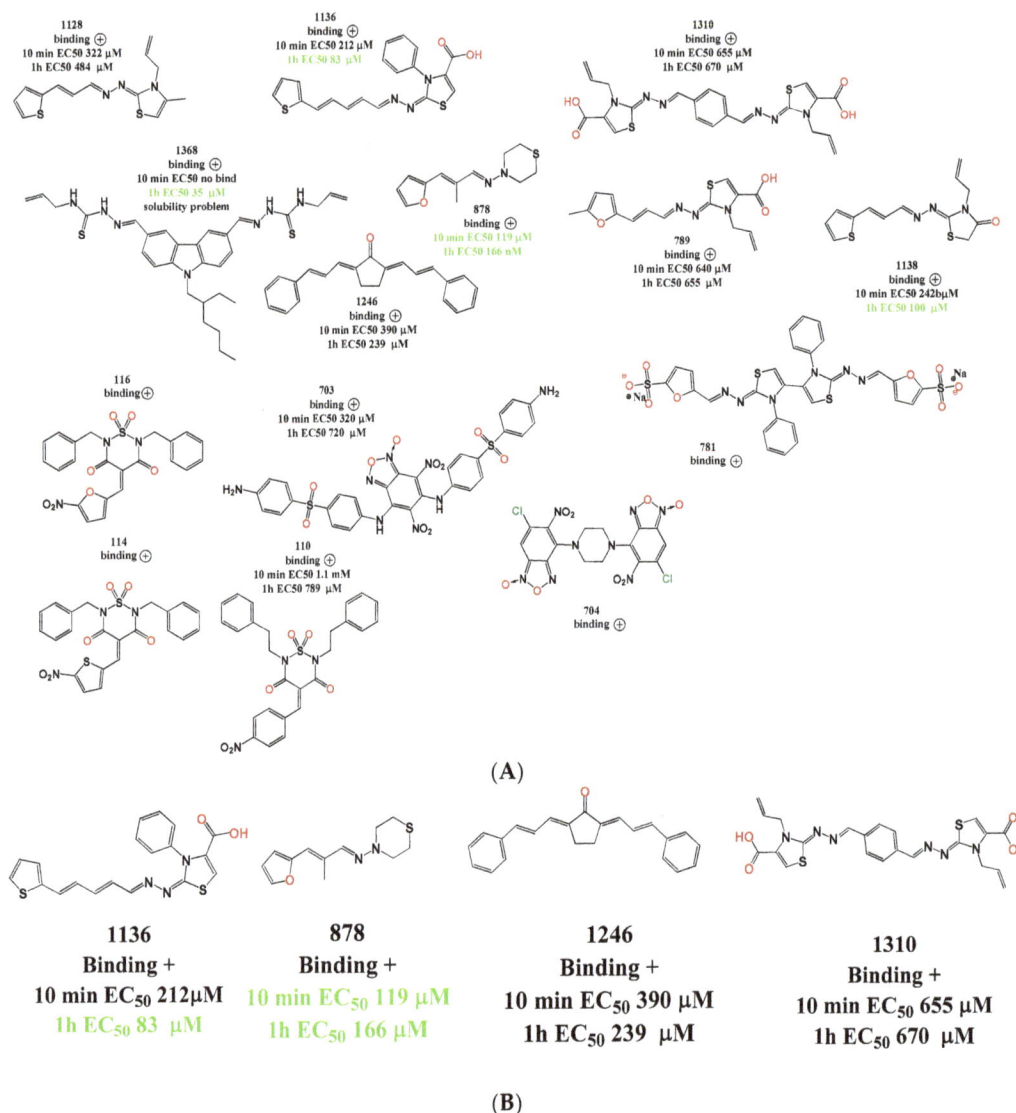

Figure 5. (**A**) Compounds binding to CA identified in the MST screening. With each structure are the binding data and the EC$_{50}$ values; (**B**) Verified hits in the polymerization assay.

2.4. Docking Analysis

To study the different binding modes of these compounds, we performed some computational studies by docking. Surprisingly we found that the compounds bind on the same surface of the protein in the 25-Å-long ridge comprised between helices a4 and a7, although each compound showed a specific binding site. Although this surface is not directly involved in HIV assembly, it is close to the monomer:monomer interface in the published HIV CA hexamer (Figure 6) [38]. Moreover, a recent study identified residues of the FIV capsid, which are important for FIV capsid assembly and are located in helix 4. Although our compounds do not bind directly to these two residues, these compounds could change the conformation of this region upon binding, resulting in the inhibition of p24:p24 interactions during capsid assembly [39].

For each compound, the ten best docking positions were sorted based on their predicted ΔG binding values. Interestingly, predicted K$_D$ values deducted from the dockings are also in the μM range (Table 1). In particular, the K$_D$ value of compound **1136** was predicted to be between 17 and 36 μM, while showing an experimental value of 83 μM when measured by MST (see above).

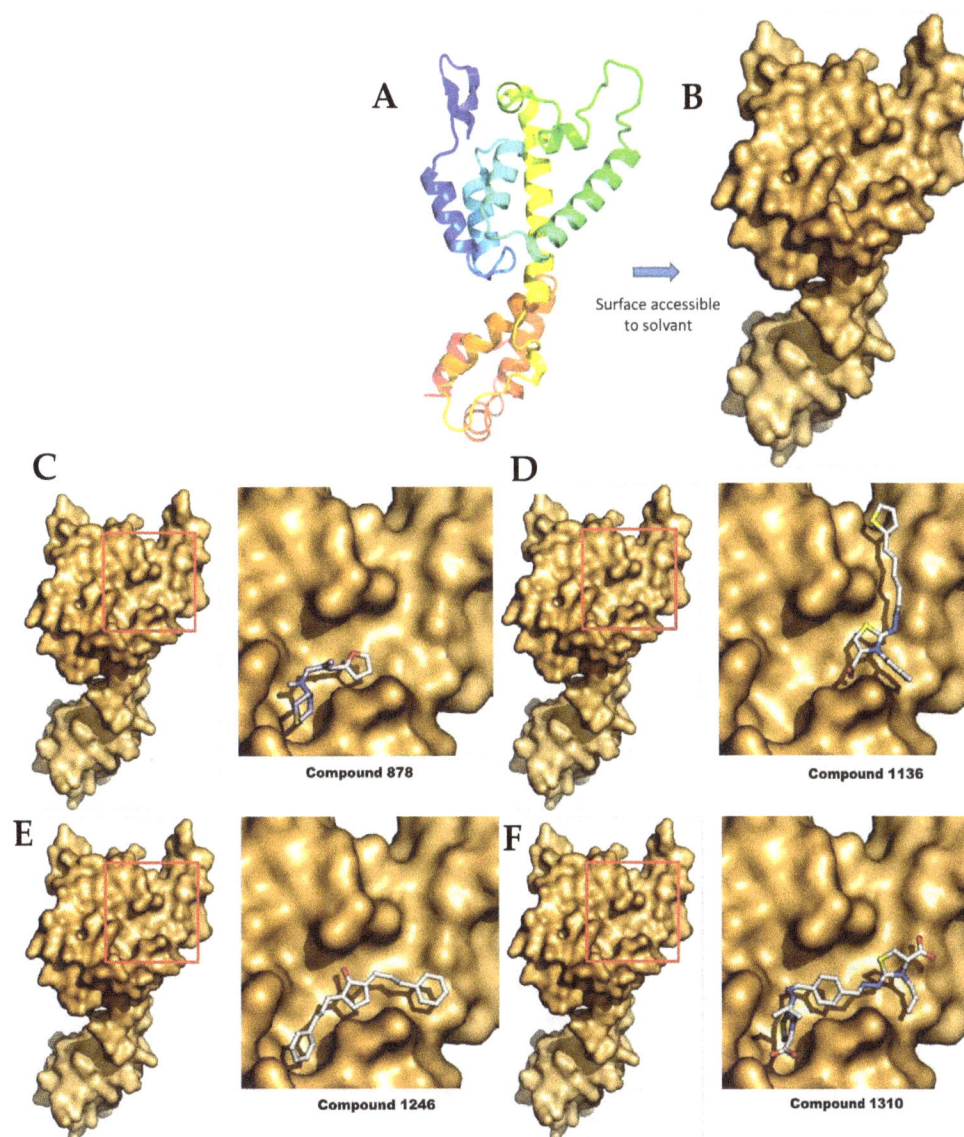

Figure 6. Representation of the CA monomer and the different docking studies from the selected compounds. (**A**) The monomer of CA in cartoons; (**B**) The CA surface accessible to the solvent, computed using PyMol. The best scored positions after docking on CA (**left panel**), with a close-up view (**right panel**) of the binding region (red square) for (**C**) compound **878**; (**D**) compound **1136**; (**E**) compound **1246**; and (**F**) compound **1310**.

Table 1. Data from docking studies with the active compounds identified in the in vitro assay with CA.

Compounds	Predicted Binding ΔG (kcal·mol^{-1}) Range Values	Predicted KD (μM) Range Values
878	−5.2/−4.9	163/269
1136	−6.6/−6.1	17/36
1246	−7.4/−7.0	4/8
1310	−6.3/−6.0	26/43

2.5. Toxicology Data

We explored the toxicology profiles of the active molecules using an online predictor with a database of a hundred thousand molecules. Our selected molecules were considered safe drugs, as deduced from the prediction of the oral toxicity in mice (Figure 7). Cytotoxicity predictions of hepatic toxicity and genotoxicity were also low for these molecules. In the case of **878** and **1246**, cytotoxicity predictions were corroborated by our previous work on these molecules, with a cytotoxicity in murine macrophages of $IC_{50} > 100$ μM [37]. Moreover, the four hits were assayed with two different type of mammalian cell at 100 μM, without cytotoxic effect at this dose (Table S2) [29]. Compound **1246** was used in a murine acute infection model of the Chagas disease and was administrated at 100 mg/kg body with for 15 days, without toxic effect during this period [28].

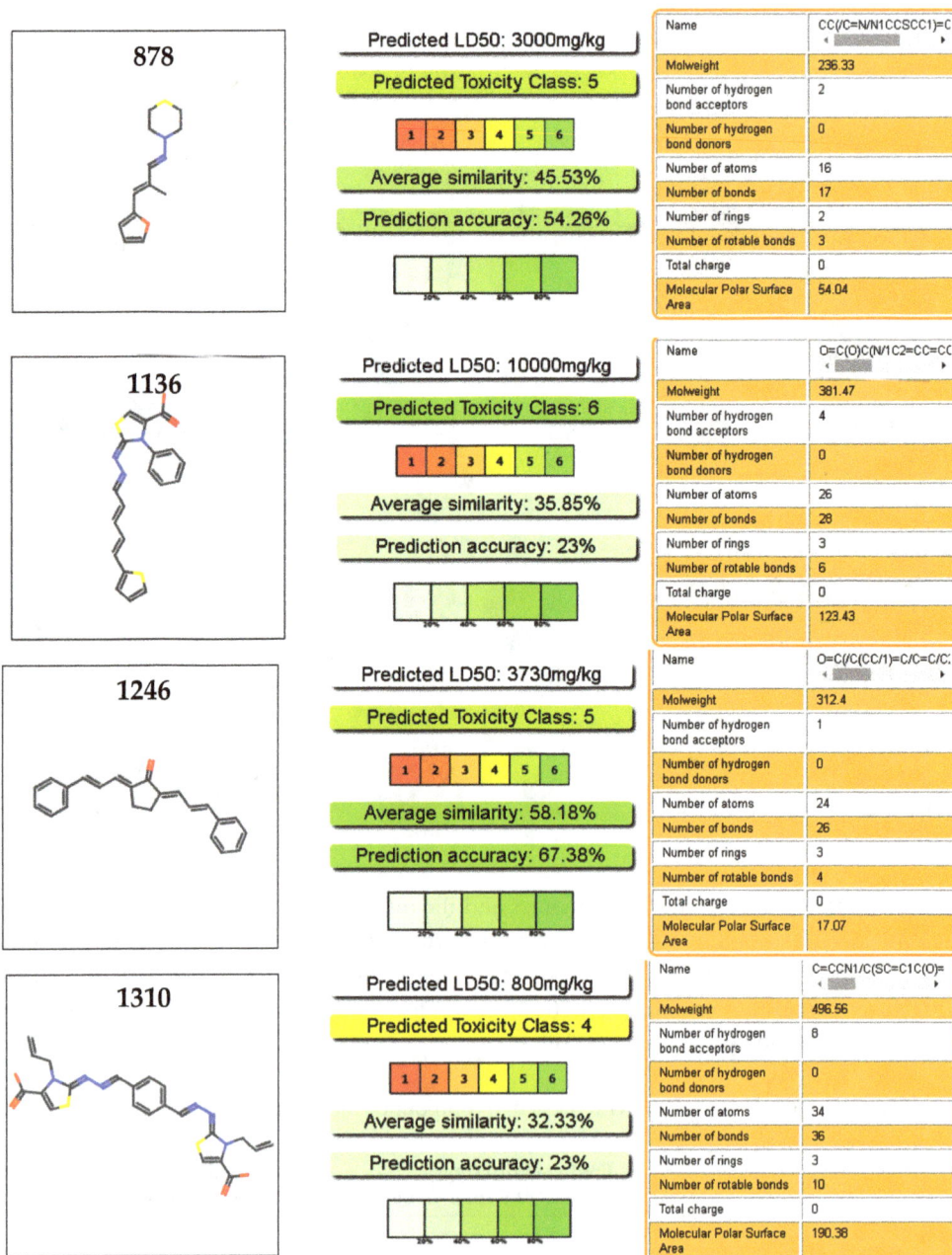

Figure 7. Toxicology profiles of the studied compound calculated from PROTOX (Charite University of Medicine Institute for Physiology Structural Bioinformatics Group Philippstrasse 12, 10115 Berlin, Germany) [40].

3. Experimental Section

3.1. Expression and Purification of CA

The FIV CA protein was expressed and purified mostly as described [35,39]. *Escherichia coli* cells (BL2I (DE3) pLysS, Lucigen, Middleton, WI, USA) transformed with pRSET-p24EDCP-T were grown in Lysogenic broth medium (Sigma-Aldrich, Saint-Quentin-Fallavier, France), supplemented with 50 mg/mL of ampicillin, at 37 °C. When cells reached an OD_{600} value between 0.3 and 0.4, the expression of CA was induced by the addition of 1 mM isopropyl-α-D-1-thiogalactopyranoside (IPTG, Euromedex, Souffelweyersheim, France) for 3 h at 37 °C, then cells were harvested by centrifugation and the pellets were stored overnight at -20 °C. The purification of p24 protein was performed by nickel affinity chromatography, as described [40], using batch incubation with Ni^{2+}-TED resin (Macherey-Nagel, Hoerdt, France)), followed by loading onto a gravity column. The column was washed three times with LEW buffer (50 mM NaH_2PO_4, 300 mM NaCl, pH 8.5), and the elution was performed with LEW buffer containing 50 mM of imidazole. The concentration of CA was quantified by spectrophotometry at 280 nm, using a Nanodrop (Thermo Fisher, Waltham, MA, USA). The purity of the protein at homogeneity was checked using SDS-PAGE analysis before further processing (Figure 3). Buffer exchange, using ultrafiltration devices (10 kD MWCO, Sartorius, Aubagne, France), was performed against a HEPES/NaCl Buffer (50 mM HEPES pH 6.5, 100 mM NaCl).

3.2. Assembly Assay by Spectrophotometry [24]

The CA assembly assay was performed in a final volume of 50 μL in 384-well plates, with a final concentration of 5 mg/mL of purified recombinant FIV p2 in 50 mM NaH_2PO_4 and 1 M NaCl, pH 7.4. Absorbance is measured at 340 nm every 30 s in a multiplate reader Varioskan™ Flash Multimode Reader (Thermo Scientific™, Waltham, MA, USA) at 38 °C for 30 min. The compounds were tested at a fixed initial dose of 25 or 50 μM (at 0.5% DMSO v/v) by adding 1 μL of the concentrated ligand were added to the well before starting the measurement. The controls were CA at 5 mg/mL in only 0.5% DMSO v/v and CA without DMSO. The criteria to select active compounds were the observation of at least 50% of assembly inhibition at these doses, based on the reduction of the OD value at 340 nm at the plateau value compared to the controls.

3.3. Microscale Thermophoresis [41]

MTS experiments were performed according to the NanoTemper technologies protocol in a Monolith NT.115 (green/blue) instrument (NanoTemper Technologies, München, Germany). With this technique, the diffusion behavior of a labeled protein is measured when an infrared light excites the movement of the protein in capillaries. This behavior is the combination of two effects: the fast, local environment dependent responses of the fluorophore to the temperature jump and the slower diffusive thermophoresis fluorescence changes. It will be modified when the protein is complexed with increasing amounts of unlabeled partners, leading to titration curves that can be fit for Kd estimation [41]. In practice, CA was labeled with the Monolith His-Tag Labeling Kit RED-tris-NTA (NanoTemper Technologies, München, Germany), as described by the manufacturer. The experiments were performed using 20% and 40% MST power and between 20–80% LED power at 24 °C. The MST traces were recorded using the standard parameters: 5 s MST power off, 30 s MST power on, and 5 s MST power off. The compounds were used at high concentrations (around 5 mM) in the bindings check assay with DMSO at 5% v/v. If the binding check was positive, then the affinity determination was performed with the same experimental settings, with serial 2× dilutions of the compound of interest.

3.4. Docking

The crystal structure of the full-length FIV CA that we previously solved (PDB entry 5NA2) [40] was used as a target protein in the subsequent docking experiments. In this PDB entry, CA NTD and CA CTD domains are in a compact form, due to an artifactual intermolecular disulfide bond. In order to obtain its open form, we used the hexameric crystal structure of the HIV-1 capsid protein CA as template (PDB entry 5HGN) [38]. CTD and NTD domains from FIV CA were superimposed to those of HIV-1, and the linker region (residues 137–141) was reconstructed manually using COOT [42], respecting the backbone and side-chains conformational restraints.

Compounds were modelled using the smiles code from the Chemoffice software. Then, CA in its open form and compounds were prepared using AutoDockTools v1.5.6 [43]. The polar hydrogen atoms were added, the non-polar hydrogens were merged, and the Gasteiger partial atomic charges were computed. Finally, all the possible rotatable bonds were assigned for each compound molecule.

A "blind docking" was then carried out with the program AutoDock Vina v1.1.2 [44]. Compounds were treated as flexible while the target protein was treated as rigid. The search space was defined in order to encompass the entire surface of the target protein, and a large exhaustiveness value of 1000 was used regarding the wide search space ($76 \times 60 \times 44$ Å^3). A visual examination of the resulting docking poses was carried out using PyMOL 1.5 (Schrödinger, Delano Scientific, LLC, New York, NY, USA).

3.5. Cytotoxicity Assay in Mammalian Cells

Vero cell lines (ATCC, Rockville, MD, USA) were cultivated in Dulbecco's modified Eagles medium (DMEM) with 10% FCS in a humid atmosphere of 5% CO_2 at 37 °C. Vero cells were seeded in 96-well plates at an initial density of 5×10^3 cells per well. J774.1 murine macrophage cells (ATCC, Manassas, VA, USA) were grown in DMEM culture milieu containing 4 mM L-glutamine and supplemented with 10% FCS. The cells were seeded in a 96-well plate (5×10^4 cells in 200 µL culture medium) and incubated at 37 °C in a 5% CO_2 atmosphere for 48 h, to allow cell adhesion prior to drug testing. Both cell lines were exposed for 48 h (at 37 °C and 5% CO_2) to the compounds (100 µM) or the solvent (0.4% DMSO) for the control, and additional controls (cells in medium) were used in each test. The cytotoxicity of the compounds was evaluated by MTT reduction assays. To proceed with the MTT assay, 20 µL of 3-(4,5-dimethylthiazol-2-yl)-2,5-diphenyl-2H-tetrazolium bromide (MTT) 5 mg/mL solution dissolved in $1\times$ PBS was added to the wells and incubated for 4 h at 37 °C in a 5% CO_2 controlled atmosphere. Next, the medium was aspirated and 100 µL of DMSO was added to each well and incubated at room temperature in the dark for 15 min with moderate orbital shaking. Optical density (OD) was read in a plate spectrophotometer (Thermo Scientific Varioskan® Flash Multimode, Waltham, MA, USA) at 570 and 690 nm wavelengths. Each experiment was performed in triplicate. For the statistical analyses, the GraphPad Prism 6 was used. Dunnett's multiple comparison tests and Student's T-test were used when we compared the averages of each condition with the control [45].

4. Conclusions

In this work, we performed a large screening of 400 molecules from a large library of compounds, looking for new hits for antiretroviral drug development against the FIV assembly. For this, we optimized methods towards a cost-effective screening method for FIV assembly inhibitors. Then, we combined the complementary methods using the CA protein (i.e., assembly assay, MST, and docking), allowing the identification of four compounds which represent interesting leads for the design of CA assembly disrupters. Interestingly, these compounds also showed no cytotoxic effects in mammalian cells, thus representing interesting candidate molecules which will now be tested in in vitro infection assays with live viruses.

Author Contributions: N.S. and C.F. performed expression and purification of protein and assembly assays, N.S. and M.L. performed the thermophoresis experiments, X.R. performed the docking analysis, C.G. and G.Á. designed and coordinated the experiments, analyzed the data and wrote the paper.

Funding: ECOS-Sud program (Uruguay—France, action U14S01)

Acknowledgments: PEDECIBA Uruguay, CSIC Universidad de la República. This work was supported by the ECOS-Sud program (Uruguay—France, action U14S01). We thank Pierre Soule (Nanotemper) and Roland Montserret (MMSB) for helpful advices with MST.

References

1. Schwartz, A.M.; McCrackin, M.A.; Schinazi, R.F.; Hill, P.B.; Vahlenkamp, T.W.; Tompkins, M.B.; Hartmann, K. Antiviral efficacy of nine nucleoside reverse transcriptase inhibitors against feline immunodeficiency virus in feline peripheral blood mononuclear cells. *Am. J. Vet. Res.* **2014**, *75*, 273–281. [CrossRef] [PubMed]

2. Mohammadi, H.; Bienzle, D. Pharmacological inhibition of feline immunodeficiency virus (FIV). *Viruses* **2012**, *4*, 708–724. [CrossRef] [PubMed]

3. Yamamoto, J.K.; Sanou, M.P.; Abbott, J.R.; Coleman, J.K. Feline immunodeficiency virus model for designing HIV/AIDS vaccines. *Curr. HIV Res.* **2010**, *8*, 14–25. [CrossRef] [PubMed]

4. Luttge, B.G.; Freed, E.O. FIV Gag: Virus assembly and host-cell interactions. *Vet. Immunol. Immunopathol.* **2010**, *134*, 3–13. [CrossRef] [PubMed]

5. Hart, S.; Nolte, I. Long-Term Treatment of Diseased, FIV-Seropositive Field Cats with Azidothymidine (AZT). *J. Vet. Med. Ser. A* **1995**, *42*, 397–409. [CrossRef]

6. Smyth, N.R.; McCracken, C.; Gaskell, R.M.; Cameron, J.M.; Coates, J.A.; Gaskell, C.J.; Hart, C.A.; Bennett, M. Susceptibility in Cell Culture of Feline Immunodeficiency Virus to Eighteen Antiviral Agents. *J. Antimicrob. Chemother.* **1994**, *34*, 589–594. Available online: http://www.ncbi.nlm.nih.gov/pubmed/7532645 (accessed on 17 May 2018). [CrossRef] [PubMed]

7. Hosie, M.; Techakriengkrai, N.; Bęczkowski, P.; Harris, M.; Logan, N.; Willett, B. The Comparative Value of Feline Virology Research: Can Findings from the Feline Lentiviral Vaccine Be Translated to Humans? *Vet. Sci.* **2017**, *4*, 7. [CrossRef] [PubMed]

8. Kashiwase, H.; Katsube, T.; Iida, K.; Komai, T.; Nishigaki, T. Investigation into the mode of action of R-91650, an arylpiperazinyl fluoroquinolone, on feline immunodeficiency virus replication inhibitory activity. *Arch. Virol.* **2000**, *145*, 859–869. [CrossRef] [PubMed]

9. Timilsina, U.; Ghimire, D.; Timalsina, B.; Nitz, T.J.; Wild, C.T.; Freed, E.O.; Gaur, R. Identification of potent maturation inhibitors against HIV-1 clade C. *Sci. Rep.* **2016**, *6*, 27403. [CrossRef] [PubMed]

10. Grinsztejn, B.; Hosseinipour, M.C.; Ribaudo, H.J.; Swindells, S.; Eron, J.; Chen, Y.Q.; Wang, L.; Ou, S.S.; Anderson, M.; McCauley, M.; et al. Effects of early versus delayed initiation of antiretroviral treatment on clinical outcomes of HIV-1 infection: Results from the phase 3 HPTN 052 randomised controlled trial. *Lancet Infect. Dis.* **2014**, *14*, 281–290. [CrossRef]

11. Hayes, K.A.; Wilkinson, J.G.; Frick, R.; Francke, S.; Mathes, L.E. Early suppression of viremia by ZDV does not alter the spread of feline immunodeficiency virus infection in cats. *J. Acquir. Immune Defic. Syndr. Hum. Retrovirol.* **1995**, *9*, 114–122. [CrossRef] [PubMed]

12. Li, M.; Morris, G.M.; Lee, T.; Laco, G.S.; Wong, C.H.; Olson, A.J.; Elder, J.H.; Wlodawer, A.; Gustchina, A. Structural studies of FIV and HIV-1 proteases complexed with an efficient inhibitor of FIV protease. *Proteins Struct. Funct. Genet.* **2000**, *38*, 29–40. [CrossRef]

13. Nowicka-sans, B.; Protack, T.; Lin, Z.; Li, Z.; Zhang, S.; Sun, Y.; Samanta, H.; Terry, B. Identification and Characterization of BMS-955176, a Second-Generation HIV-1 Maturation Inhibitor with Improved Potency, Antiviral Spectrum, and Gag Polymorphic Coverage. *Antimicrob. Agents Chemother.* **2016**, *60*, 3956–3969. [CrossRef] [PubMed]

14. Tremblay, M.; Bonneau, P.; Bousquet, Y.; DeRoy, P.; Duan, J.; Duplessis, M.; Gagnon, A.; Garneau, M.; Goudreau, N.; Guse, I.; et al. Inhibition of HIV-1 capsid assembly: Optimization of the antiviral potency by site selective modifications at N1, C2 and C16 of a 5-(5-furan-2-yl-pyrazol-1-yl)-1*H*-benzimidazole scaffold. *Bioorg. Med. Chem. Lett.* **2012**, *22*, 7512–7517. [CrossRef] [PubMed]

15. Sundquist, W.I.; Kräusslich, H.G. HIV-1 assembly, budding, and maturation. *Cold Spring Harb. Perspect. Med.* **2012**, *2*, a006924. [CrossRef] [PubMed]

16. Gabizon, R.; Friedler, A.; Jahnke, W. Allosteric modulation of protein oligomerization: An emerging approach to drug design. *Front. Chem.* **2014**, *2*, 9. [CrossRef] [PubMed]

17. Wang, W.; Zhou, J.; Halambage, U.D.; Jurado, K.A.; Jamin, A.V.; Wang, Y.; Engelman, A.N.; Aiken, C. Inhibition of HIV-1 Maturation via Small Molecule Targeting of the Amino-Terminal Domain in the Viral Capsid Protein. *J. Virol.* **2017**, *91*, e02155-16. [CrossRef] [PubMed]

18. Lee, K.; Ambrose, Z.; Martin, T.D.; Oztop, I.; Julias, J.G.; Vandegraaff, N.; Baumann, J.G.; Wang, R.; Takemura, T.; Shelton, K.; et al. Flexible Use of Nuclear Import Pathways by HIV-1. *Cell Host Microbe* **2011**, *7*, 221–233. [CrossRef] [PubMed]

19. Price, A.J.; Fletcher, A.J.; Schaller, T.; Elliott, T.; Lee, K.E.; KewalRamani, V.N.; Chin, J.W.; Towers, G.J.; James, L.C. CPSF6 Defines a Conserved Capsid Interface that Modulates HIV-1 Replication. *PLoS Pathog.* **2012**, *8*, e1002896. [CrossRef] [PubMed]

20. Price, A.J.; Jacques, D.A.; Mcewan, W.A.; Fletcher, A.J.; Essig, S.; Chin, J.W.; Halambage, U.D.; Aiken, C.; James, L.C. Host Cofactors and Pharmacologic Ligands Share an Essential Interface in HIV-1 Capsid That Is Lost upon Disassembly. *PLoS Pathog.* **2014**, *10*, e1004459. [CrossRef] [PubMed]

21. Shi, J.; Zhou, J.; Shah, V.B.; Aiken, C.; Whitby, K. Small-molecule inhibition of human immunodeficiency virus type 1 infection by virus capsid destabilization. *J. Virol.* **2011**, *85*, 542–549. [CrossRef] [PubMed]

22. Thenin-houssier, S.; Valente, S.T.; Sciences, M. HIV-1 capsid inhibitors as antiretroviral agents Suzie. *Curr. HIV Res.* **2017**, *14*, 270–282. [CrossRef]

23. Lamorte, L.; Titolo, S.; Lemke, C.T.; Goudreau, N.; Mercier, J.F.; Wardrop, E.; Shah, V.B.; Von Schwedler, U.K.; Langelier, C.; Banik, S.S.R.; et al. Discovery of novel small-molecule HIV-1 replication inhibitors that stabilize capsid complexes. *Antimicrob. Agents Chemother.* **2013**, *57*, 4622–4631. [CrossRef] [PubMed]

24. Tang, C.; Loeliger, E.; Kinde, I.; Kyere, S.; Mayo, K.; Barklis, E.; Sun, Y.; Huang, M.; Summers, M.F. Antiviral Inhibition of the HIV-1 Capsid Protein. *J. Mol. Biol.* **2003**, *327*, 1013–1020. [CrossRef]

25. Kortagere, S.; Madani, N.; Mankowski, M.K.; Schön, A.; Zentner, I.; Swaminathan, G.; Princiotto, A.; Anthony, K.; Oza, A.; Sierra, L.-J.; et al. Inhibiting Early-Stage Events in HIV-1 Replication by Small-Molecule Targeting of the HIV-1 Capsid. *J. Virol.* **2012**, *86*, 8472–8481. [CrossRef] [PubMed]

26. Lemke, C.T.; Faucher, A.; Mason, S.W.; Bonneau, P. A novel inhibitor-binding site on the HIV-1 capsid N-terminal domain leads to improved crystallization via compound-mediated dimerization research papers. *Acta Crystallogr. Sect. D* **2013**, *69*, 1115–1123. [CrossRef] [PubMed]

27. Rihn, S.J.; Wilson, S.J.; Loman, N.J.; Alim, M.; Bakker, S.E.; Bhella, D.; Gifford, R.J.; Rixon, F.J.; Bieniasz, P.D. Extreme Genetic Fragility of the HIV-1 Capsid. *PLoS Pathog.* **2013**, *9*, e1003461. [CrossRef] [PubMed]

28. Aguilera, E.; Varela, J.; Birriel, E.; Serna, E.; Torres, S.; Yaluff, G.; DeBilbao, N.V.; Aguirre-López, B.; Cabrera, N.; DíazMazariegos, S.; et al. Potent and Selective Inhibitors of *Trypanosoma cruzi* Triosephosphate Isomerase with Concomitant Inhibition of Cruzipain: Inhibition of Parasite Growth through Multitarget Activity. *ChemMedChem* **2016**, *11*, 1328–1338. [CrossRef] [PubMed]

29. Álvarez, G.; Varela, J.; Márquez, P.; Gabay, M.; Arias Rivas, C.E.; Cuchilla, K.; Echeverría, G.A.; Piro, O.E.; Chorilli, M.; Leal, S.M.; et al. Optimization of antitrypanosomatid agents: Identification of nonmutagenic drug candidates with in vivo activity. *J. Med. Chem.* **2014**, *57*, 3984–3999. [CrossRef] [PubMed]

30. Álvarez, G.; Martínez, J.; Varela, J.; Birriel, E.; Cruces, E.; Gabay, M.; Leal, S.M.; Escobar, P.; Aguirre-lópez, B.; De Gómez-puyou, M.T.; et al. Development of bis-thiazoles as inhibitors of triosephosphate isomerase from *Trypanosoma cruzi*. Identification of new non-mutagenic agents that are active in vivo. *Eur. J. Med. Chem.* **2015**, *100*, 246–256. [CrossRef] [PubMed]

31. Fader, L.D.; Landry, S.; Goulet, S.; Morin, S.; Kawai, S.H.; Bousquet, Y.; Dion, I.; Hucke, O.; Goudreau, N.; Lemke, C.T.; et al. Optimization of a 1,5-dihydrobenzo[*b*][1,4]diazepine-2,4-dione series of HIV capsid assembly inhibitors 2: Structure-activity relationships (SAR) of the C3-phenyl moiety. *Bioorg. Med. Chem. Lett.* **2013**, *23*, 3401–3405. [CrossRef] [PubMed]

32. Lemke, C.T.; Titolo, S.; von Schwedler, U.; Goudreau, N.; Mercier, J.-F.; Wardrop, E.; Faucher, A.-M.; Coulombe, R.; Banik, S.S.R.; Fader, L.; et al. Distinct effects of two HIV-1 capsid assembly inhibitor families that bind the same site within the N-terminal domain of the viral CA protein. *J. Virol.* **2012**, *86*, 6643–6655. [CrossRef] [PubMed]

33. Thenin-houssier, S.; De Vera, M.S.; Pedro-Rosa, L.; Brady, A.; Richard, A.; Konnick, B.; Opp, S.; Buffone, C.; Fuhrmann, J.; Kota, S.; et al. Ebselen, a Small-Molecule Capsid Inhibitor of HIV-1 Replication. *Antimicrob. Agents Chemother.* **2016**, *60*, 2195–2208. [CrossRef] [PubMed]

34. Obal, G.; Trajtenberg, F.; Carrion, F.; Tome, L.; Larrieux, N.; Zhang, X.; Pritsch, O.; Buschiazzo, A. Conformational plasticity of a native retroviral capsid revealed by X-ray crystallography. *Science* **2015**, *349*, 95–98. [CrossRef] [PubMed]

35. Serrière, J.; Fenel, D.; Schoehn, G.; Gouet, P.; Guillon, C. Biophysical characterization of the feline immunodeficiency virus p24 capsid protein conformation and in vitro capsid assembly. *PLoS ONE* **2013**, *8*, e56424. [CrossRef] [PubMed]

36. Alvarez, G.; Aguirre-Lopez, B.; Varela, J.; Cabrera, M.; Merlino, A.; Lopez, G.V.; Lavaggi, M.L.; Porcal, W.; Di Maio, R.; Gonzalez, M.; et al. Massive screening yields novel and selective *Trypanosoma cruzi* triosephosphate isomerase dimer-interface-irreversible inhibitors with anti-trypanosomal activity. *Eur. J. Med. Chem.* **2010**, *45*, 5767–5772. [CrossRef] [PubMed]

37. Álvarez, G.; Perdomo, C.; Coronel, C.; Aguilera, E.; Varela, J.; Aparicio, G.; Zolessi, F.R.; Cabrera, N.; Vega, C.; Rolón, M.; et al. Multi-anti-parasitic activity of arylidene ketones and thiazolidene hydrazines against *Trypanosoma cruzi* and *Leishmania* spp. *Molecules* **2017**, *22*, E709. [CrossRef] [PubMed]

38. Jacques, D.A.; McEwan, W.A.; Hilditch, L.; Price, A.J.; Towers, G.J.; James, L.C. HIV-1 uses dynamic capsid pores to import nucleotides and fuel encapsidated DNA synthesis. *Nature* **2016**, *536*, 349–353. [CrossRef] [PubMed]

39. Folio, C.; Sierra, N.; Dujardin, M.; Alvarez, G.; Guillon, C. Crystal structure of the full-length feline immunodeficiency virus capsid protein shows an N-terminal β-hairpin in the absence of N-terminal proline. *Viruses* **2017**, *9*, E335. [CrossRef] [PubMed]

40. Drwal, M.N.; Banerjee, P.; Dunkel, M.; Wettig, M.R.; Preissner, R. ProTox: A web server for the in silico prediction of rodent oral toxicity. *Nucleic Acids Res.* **2014**, *42*, 53–58. [CrossRef] [PubMed]

41. Garcia-Bonete, M.J.; Jensen, M.; Recktenwald, C.V.; Rocha, S.; Stadler, V.; Bokarewa, M.; Katona, G. Bayesian Analysis of MicroScale Thermophoresis Data to Quantify Affinity of Protein:Protein Interactions with Human Survivin. *Sci. Rep.* **2017**, *7*, 16816. [CrossRef] [PubMed]

42. Emsley, P.; Lohkamp, B.; Scott, W.G.; Cowtan, K. Features and development of Coot. *Acta Crystallogr. Sect. D Biol. Crystallogr.* **2010**, *66*, 486–501. [CrossRef] [PubMed]

43. Morris, G.; Huey, R. AutoDock4 and AutoDockTools4: Automated docking with selective receptor flexibility. *J. Comput. Chem.* **2009**, *30*, 2785–2791. [CrossRef] [PubMed]

44. Trott, O.; Olson, A. AutoDock Vina: Improving the speed and accuracy of docking with a new scoring function, efficient optimization and multithreading. *J. Comput. Chem.* **2010**, *31*, 455–461. [CrossRef] [PubMed]

45. Fort, R.S.; Mathó, C.; Geraldo, M.V.; Ottati, M.C.; Yamashita, A.S.; Saito, K.C.; Leite, K.R.M.; Méndez, M.; Maedo, N.; Méndez, L.; et al. Nc886 is epigenetically repressed in prostate cancer and acts as a tumor suppressor through the inhibition of cell growth. *BMC Cancer* **2018**, *18*, 127. [CrossRef] [PubMed]

Permissions

All chapters in this book were first published in PHARMACEUTICALS, by MDPI; hereby published with permission under the Creative Commons Attribution License or equivalent. Every chapter published in this book has been scrutinized by our experts. Their significance has been extensively debated. The topics covered herein carry significant findings which will fuel the growth of the discipline. They may even be implemented as practical applications or may be referred to as a beginning point for another development.

The contributors of this book come from diverse backgrounds, making this book a truly international effort. This book will bring forth new frontiers with its revolutionizing research information and detailed analysis of the nascent developments around the world.

We would like to thank all the contributing authors for lending their expertise to make the book truly unique. They have played a crucial role in the development of this book. Without their invaluable contributions this book wouldn't have been possible. They have made vital efforts to compile up to date information on the varied aspects of this subject to make this book a valuable addition to the collection of many professionals and students.

This book was conceptualized with the vision of imparting up-to-date information and advanced data in this field. To ensure the same, a matchless editorial board was set up. Every individual on the board went through rigorous rounds of assessment to prove their worth. After which they invested a large part of their time researching and compiling the most relevant data for our readers.

The editorial board has been involved in producing this book since its inception. They have spent rigorous hours researching and exploring the diverse topics which have resulted in the successful publishing of this book. They have passed on their knowledge of decades through this book. To expedite this challenging task, the publisher supported the team at every step. A small team of assistant editors was also appointed to further simplify the editing procedure and attain best results for the readers.

Apart from the editorial board, the designing team has also invested a significant amount of their time in understanding the subject and creating the most relevant covers. They scrutinized every image to scout for the most suitable representation of the subject and create an appropriate cover for the book.

The publishing team has been an ardent support to the editorial, designing and production team. Their endless efforts to recruit the best for this project, has resulted in the accomplishment of this book. They are a veteran in the field of academics and their pool of knowledge is as vast as their experience in printing. Their expertise and guidance has proved useful at every step. Their uncompromising quality standards have made this book an exceptional effort. Their encouragement from time to time has been an inspiration for everyone.

The publisher and the editorial board hope that this book will prove to be a valuable piece of knowledge for researchers, students, practitioners and scholars across the globe.

List of Contributors

Paul Chukwudi Ikwegbue, Priscilla Masamba and Abidemi Paul Kappo
Biotechnology and Structural Biochemistry (BSB) Group, Department of Biochemistry and Microbiology, University of Zululand, Kwa Dlangezwa 3886, South Africa

Babatunji Emmanuel Oyinloye
Biotechnology and Structural Biochemistry (BSB) Group, Department of Biochemistry and Microbiology, University of Zululand, KwaDlangezwa 3886, South Africa
Department of Biochemistry, Afe Babalola University, PMB 5454, Ado-Ekiti 360001, Nigeria

Joaquim Aguirre-Plans, Janet Piñero, Ferran Sanz, Laura I. Furlong and Baldo Oliva
Research Programme on Biomedical Informatics, the Hospital del Mar Medical Research Institute and Pompeu Fabra University, Dr. Aiguader 88, 08003 Barcelona, Spain

Emre Guney
Research Programme on Biomedical Informatics, the Hospital del Mar Medical Research Institute and Pompeu Fabra University, Dr. Aiguader 88, 08003 Barcelona, Spain
Department of Pharmacology and Personalised Medicine, CARIM, FHML, Maastricht University, Universiteitssingel 50, 6229 ER Maastricht, The Netherlands

Jörg Menche
CeMM Research Center for Molecular Medicine of the Austrian Academy of Sciences, Lazarettgasse 14, AKH BT 25.3, A-1090 Vienna, Austria

Harald H. H. W. Schmidt
Department of Pharmacology and Personalised Medicine, CARIM, FHML, Maastricht University, Universiteitssingel 50, 6229 ER Maastricht, The Netherlands

Ognjen Perišić
Big Blue Genomics, Vojvode Brane 32, 11000 Belgrade, Serbia
Department of Chemistry, New York University, 1001 Silver, 100Washington Square East, New York, NY 10003, USA

Benedikt Fels, Etmar Bulk, Zoltán Pethő and Albrecht Schwab
Institut für Physiologie II, Robert-Koch-Str. 27b, 48149 Münster, Germany

Dorota Olender, Justyna Żwawiak and Lucjusz Zaprutko
Department of Organic Chemistry, Pharmaceutical Faculty, Poznan University of Medical Sciences, Grunwaldzka 6, 60-780 Poznan, Poland

Constain H. Salamanca, Cristhian J. Yarce, Yony Roman and Andrés F. Davalos
Facultad de Ciencias Naturales, Universidad Icesi, Calle 18 No. 122-135, Cali 760031, Colombia

Gustavo R. Rivera
SIT Biotech GmbH, BMZ 2 Otto-Hahn-Str. 15, 44227 Dortmund, Germany

Barbora Waclawiková and Sahar El Aidy
Department of Molecular Immunology and Microbiology, Groningen Biomolecular Sciences and Biotechnology Institute (GBB), University of Groningen, Nijenborgh 7, 9747 AG Groningen, The Netherlands

Andreas Jordan and Ursula Gresser
Internal Medicine, Medical Faculty, Ludwig Maximilians University of Munich, 80539 Munich, Germany

Alicia Vall-Sagarra and Carmen Wängler
Biomedical Chemistry, Department of Clinical Radiology and Nuclear Medicine, Medical Faculty Mannheim of Heidelberg University, Theodor-Kutzer-Ufer 1-3, 68167 Mannheim, Germany

Shanna Litau
Biomedical Chemistry, Department of Clinical Radiology and Nuclear Medicine, Medical Faculty Mannheim of Heidelberg University, Theodor-Kutzer-Ufer 1-3, 68167 Mannheim, Germany
Molecular Imaging and Radiochemistry, Department of Clinical Radiology and Nuclear Medicine, Medical Faculty Mannheim of Heidelberg University, Theodor-Kutzer-Ufer 1-3, 68167 Mannheim, Germany

Björn Wängler
Molecular Imaging and Radiochemistry, Department of Clinical Radiology and Nuclear Medicine, Medical Faculty Mannheim of Heidelberg University, Theodor-Kutzer-Ufer 1-3, 68167 Mannheim, Germany

Clemens Decristoforo
Department of Nuclear Medicine, University Hospital Innsbruck, Medical University Innsbruck, Anichstrasse 35, 6020 Innsbruck, Austria

Ralf Schirrmacher
Department of Oncology, Division Oncological Imaging, University of Alberta, 11560 University Avenue, Edmonton, AB T6G 1Z2, Canada

Gert Fricker
Institute of Pharmacy and Molecular Biotechnology, University of Heidelberg, Im Neuenheimer Feld 329, 69120 Heidelberg, Germany

Jorge Ramírez, Gianluca Gilardoni and Erika Ramón
Departamento de Química y Ciencias Exactas, Universidad Técnica Particular de Loja (UTPL), Calle M.Champagnat s/n, 1101608 Loja, Ecuador

Solveig Tosi and Anna Maria Picco
Dipartimento di Scienza della Terra e dell'Ambiente, Università degli Studi di Pavia, Via S. Epifanio 14, 27100 Pavia, Italy

Carlo Bicchi
Dipartimento di Scienza e Tecnologia del Farmaco, Università degli Studi di Torino, Via P. Giuria 9, 10125 Torino, Italy

Giovanni Vidari
Dipartimento di Chimica, Università degli Studi di Pavia, Via T. Taramelli 10, 27100 Pavia, Italy

Fransiska Kurniawan, Rahmana Emran Kartasasmita and Daryono Hadi Tjahjono
School of Pharmacy, Bandung Institute of Technology, Jalan Ganesha 10, Bandung 40132, Indonesia

Youhei Miura and Naoki Yoshioka
Department of Applied Chemistry, Faculty of Science and Technology, Keio University, 3-14-1 Hiyoshi, Kohoku-ku, Yokohama 223-8522, Japan

Abdul Mutalib
Center for Radioisotope and Radiopharmaceutical Technology, National Nuclear Energy Agency (BATAN), Serpong, Tangerang 15310, Indonesia

Natalia Sierra and Guzmán Álvarez
Laboratorio de Moléculas Bioactivas, CENUR Litoral Norte, Universidad de la República, Ruta 3 (km 363), Paysandú C.P. 60000, Uruguay

Christelle Folio, Xavier Robert, Mathieu Long and Christophe Guillon
Equipe Rétrovirus et Biochimie Structurale, Université de Lyon, CNRS, MMSB, UMR 5086 CNRS/Université de Lyon, IBCP, C.P. 69367 Lyon, France

Index

www.ingramcontent.com/pod-product-compliance
Lightning Source LLC
Chambersburg PA
CBHW081710240326
41458CB00156B/4230